Electrodiagnostic Medicine

Nestor Galvez-Jimenez
Alexandra Soriano • John A. Morren
Editors

Electrodiagnostic Medicine

A Practical Approach

Springer

Editors
Nestor Galvez-Jimenez
Braathen Neurological Center
Cleveland Clinic Florida
Weston, FL
USA

Cleveland Clinic Lerner College of Medicine of Case Western Reserve University
Cleveland, OH
USA

Alexandra Soriano
Braathen Neurological Center
Cleveland Clinic Florida
Weston, FL
USA

Cleveland Clinic Lerner College of Medicine of Case Western Reserve University
Cleveland, OH
USA

John A. Morren
Neuromuscular Center
Neurological Institute
Cleveland Clinic, and Cleveland Clinic Lerner College of Medicine of Case Western Reserve University
Cleveland, OH
USA

ISBN 978-3-030-74996-5 ISBN 978-3-030-74997-2 (eBook)
https://doi.org/10.1007/978-3-030-74997-2

This Springer imprint is published by the registered company Springer Nature Switzerland AG
The registered company address is: Gewerbestrasse 11, 6330 Cham, Switzerland

Dedication to Dr. Virgilio Salanga

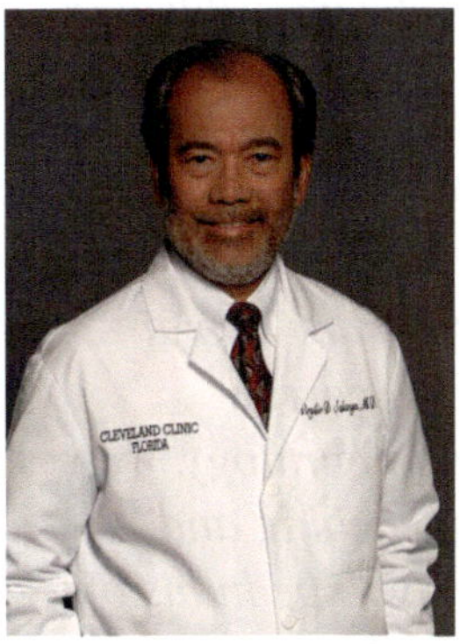

We have been privileged to have worked with some of the best electrodiagnosticians, neurologists, residents, and fellows at Cleveland Clinic. Asa Wilbourn, Maurice Hanson, Kerry Levin, Robert Shields, Richard Lederman, Hiroshi Mitsumoto, and many others come to mind immediately. However, for most of us Dr. Virgilio Salanga, to whom this work is dedicated, had a major influence, and as a consequence made a lasting impact on our interest and understanding in electrodiagnostic medicine. Actually, Virgil taught generations of residents and fellows, both in Ohio and in Florida, many of whom went on to prestigious academic and practice positions in the USA and internationally. Upon his retirement he was the holder of the John and Margaret Krupa distinguished Chair in Neurology at Cleveland Clinic Florida (CCFla) and Chairman of Neurology at CCFla.

Virgil is a Magna Cum Laude graduate with a Doctor of Medicine and Surgery degree from the University of Santo Thomas School of Medicine, in Manila, Philippines. After mixed surgery and internal medicine internships at Michael Reese Hospital and Medical Center in Chicago, Virgil went on to do his residency and neurophysiology training at the Mayo Clinic in Rochester, Minnesota, where he was a student of Edward H. Lambert and Jasper Daube. In Rochester, he confided to us on more than one occasion; he had some of his best formative years, having worked under Arthur Waltz and interacted with Thoralf Sundt both from Mayo, when working on his Master of Science thesis on Regional Cerebral Blood Flow During Stimulation of the Seventh Cranial Nerve. The resultant degree was granted by the University of Minnesota. He had the privilege to study and collaborate with many others who became well-known electrodiagnosticians in their own right, such as Asa Wilbourn, H. Royden Jones Jr., Ludwig Gutmann, Ram Ayyar, and many others. Virgil rose through the ranks at Cleveland Clinic in Cleveland to Vice-chair of Neurology and subsequently moved to Florida in 1988 (with Maurice Hanson and technologist Mary Ronnenberg) to establish the Department of Neurology and the Neurophysiology Laboratory at the Cleveland Clinic in Florida. Upon his retirement, the department had grown to a very busy and academic unit with neurology residents and fellows, in addition to many rotating medical students. Many of us who had the privilege to study and work under him at various times in our academic and professional career, particularly in electrodiagnostic medicine and neurology, were the recipients of an unabated commitment to teaching and excellence. We could not wait to the time of day to be in his office for review of the procedures performed during the day, especially those complex studies in which we wanted to hear his explanation and critical thinking. He was very generous with his time despite the daily clinical responsibility. He was firm, but non-judgmental, and he always expected the best from all of us, never accepting less. In addition, his high-yield lectures were all well attended by residents, fellows, staff, and technologists.

In spirit, this book is the product of the sum of those interactions with our mentors in Cleveland, Ohio, but particularly with Virgilio Salanga to whom this book is dedicated, and to CCFla in which most of the authors and editors have made their academic practice and/or formative years.

Foreword

It is with immense pleasure that I write the foreword to this book that is collaboratively authored by a former colleague, trainees, and laboratory technologists at the Cleveland Clinic—Florida, along with other alumni of the Cleveland Clinic—Ohio. I greatly admire with pride and satisfaction following the careers of my former colleague, Dr. Nestor Galvez-Jimenez, and my former residents and fellows, Drs. Michelle Dompenciel, Raghav Govindarajan, Ramon Lugo, John A. Morren, and Alexandra Soriano. They are all astute clinicians and accomplished electrodiagnosticians.

This book is well written and organized, replete with visually enhancing anatomical and technical illustrations, starting with the underlying principles and practices, optimal techniques of nerve conduction studies, and electromyography. Then specific disorders of the peripheral nervous system are discussed clinically and how properly performed electrodiagnostic studies will complement the clinical neurological assessment. This book will be a valuable resource in the field of electrodiagnostic medicine that trainees and existing practitioners will find very helpful. Beginners and experts and mentors and mentees will find this book a user-friendly guide in correctly performing and reporting clinically meaningful nerve conduction studies and electromyography.

Finally, I am deeply humbled and appreciative that this book is dedicated to me by the editors. It is often said: Teaching is an art that takes time and patience. And that is certainly true of teaching electrodiagnostic studies. I remember how I myself was taught this discipline by my mentors, the late Dr. Jasper Daube and Dr. Edward Lambert, at the Mayo Clinic-Rochester. I am grateful and pleased to have contributed to the training and mentoring of several of the coauthors of this book. I wish them even more success in the future.

Virgilio D. Salanga
Department of Neurology
Cleveland Clinic – Florida
Weston, FL, USA

Preface

Few Antecedent Words of Gratitude from NGJ

When one of us (NGJ) was approached by Springer to work on a book project, the decision to work on a book on electrodiagnostic medicine was easy. The field of electrodiagnostic medicine has grown exponentially with a solid body of evidence based on careful critical thinking, research, mathematical thought, and engineering with the appropriate interfacing of neurophysiological and neuroanatomical concepts. Hence, electrodiagnostic medicine is a field with an interdisciplinary nature to the science, study performance, and approach to patients. Therefore, producing a book of this nature (as has been wisely said many times) is not done in isolation but is the product of a "village." Having asked Drs. John A. Morren and Alexandra Soriano to join me on this project was one of the wisest decisions I made when organizing this project. This is now our work as a team effort. They added editorial expertise, breath of knowledge, a fresh look, and attention to detail so important in projects of this type, particularly as it pertains to electrodiagnostic medicine. My heartfelt thanks go particularly to John A. Morren who added clarity of thought and made what appears complex to explain easy for the reader to understand. This work is as much his work as everyone else's. He read and editorialized each chapter and attended to my many phone calls no matter how basic some of those were to make sure we all understood what was conveyed in each chapter. It was the best decision to have John provide his insight and knowledge and Alex adding her expertise in the performance and understanding on single fiber EMG, an area in which she excels like no one I know, and her ability to write electrodiagnostic reports, which is not as easy as many would make you believe. In addition, I have to give thanks to our technologists from Cleveland Clinic in Ohio and Florida who gave their time and expertise and in many instances were willing to be models for the atlas. My thanks also go to Jessica Galvez, BSc, MEd, PsyD candidate, who, in spite of a busy doctoral study schedule, managed to participate as model for some of the laboratory pictures that needed to be replaced on short notice, saving the day for us. Finally, I will be remiss if I do not acknowledge all the invited authors, all authorities, and accomplished electrodiagnosticians who took time from their very busy schedules to participate in this project.

Using the Book

One of the critical challenges facing trainees and experienced electrodiagnosticians alike is the attention to detail when performing nerve conduction studies (NCS) and needle electrode examination (NEE). This is needed for the coherent interpretation of findings, including when to discard that relatively unimportant finding, recognize an artifact, and ultimately know how to put all the pieces together for a cogent EDX diagnosis. Words matter, and sentences matter in a way that can hardly be more epitomized than with the explanations and conclusions in EDX medicine. Some may argue that an imprecise word or a superfluous comment may lead to confusion and unnecessary assessments by the referring physician, or in the worst-case scenario, even an unnecessary surgical procedure.

The book begins with Chap. 1, which is intended to provide the novice and expert alike with the neurophysiology and neuroanatomical fundamentals on the theory and principles for the practice and understanding of EDX studies. In addition, it provides general concepts on the assessment of common neuromuscular complaints and how to use the EDX techniques to approach and study these patients. More often than not, patients come with symptoms or complaints, and less so with established neuromuscular diagnoses. Hence, the hope is to provide enough knowledge to get a handle on EDX thought process for an appropriate work-up. Chapter 2 describes the most common NCS techniques in great detail using actual individuals in pictures demonstrating the performance of the studies, detailing the pertinent anatomical localization within the segment being evaluated, in addition to helpful tips and common pitfalls. Chapter 3 provides a pictorial survey on the anatomical localization, and appropriate placement of the needle electrode, with similarly helpful tips and common pitfalls for each muscle that may be examined. Further, in Chap. 4, a deeper understanding of the electronics and neurophysiology relating to NEE is facilitated, with explanation of normal and abnormal findings on NEE. This was provided masterfully by Bryan Tsao, MD, who is a leading expert in this area, known for his excellent teaching of the topic, particularly at sessions of the American Association of Neuromuscular and Electrodiagnostic Medicine (AANEM). This is followed by other excellent chapters written by experts in their respective fields and/or academic practices with the hope of providing added insight on the fundamentals of electrodiagnostically assessing patients with neuromuscular conditions. Therefore, these chapters delve into the major conditions often encountered in a busy neuromuscular medicine practice. Chapter 5 expands on the mononeuropathies of the upper and lower extremities with their respective EDX assessments written by Ramon Lugo, MD, and Alexandra Soriano, MD. Chapter 6 written by Megha Dhamne, MD, and John A. Morren, MD, deals with the EDX assessment and nuances of polyneuropathies in a very scholarly fashion. For Chap. 7 on brachial plexopathies, we were extremely lucky to have Mark Ferrante, MD, who is a renowned national and international expert on the topic. He gives his insight and tremendous knowledge on the EDX assessment of patients with brachial plexus lesions. One of us (NGJ) had the privilege to be at the EMG laboratory during residency training when Mark was a fellow at our institution working with Asa

Wilbourn and witnessed how between them, "the book" on the EDX assessment of the brachial plexus and plexopathies was essentially rewritten the way we know it today. Chapter 8 provides another scholarly discussion by Karen Karwa, MD, and John A. Morren, MD, on radiculopathies, the work-up for which is commonly requested in EDX medicine, yet continues to be a source of spurious interpretations and repeat studies, particularly when coming from less experienced laboratories. A major source for neuromuscular consultations and complex EDX assessment is that for patients with disorders of the motor neuron and mimicker conditions. Michelle Dompenciel, MD, provides a discussion of the topic in Chap. 9, and more importantly provides the EDX approach to this complex group of patients. Michelle is an accomplished electrodiagnostician, and we were excited in having her contribute this important chapter.

Chapter 10 by Elanagan Nagarajan, MD, and Raghav Govindarajan, MD, well known in the area of neuromuscular medicine, provides an overview of the pathophysiology and clinical and EDX assessment of patients with neuromuscular junction transmission disorders. Dr. Govindarajan is quite active in the AANEM and one of his main area of interest is that of neuromuscular junction disorders. Their insight and approach to the work-up of these patients, with an emphasis on technical proficiency and interpretation accuracy of this somewhat complex aspect of electrodiagnostic medicine, is of great benefit to the reader. Chapter 11 is contributed by Alexandra Soriano, MD. Alex is an accomplished electrodiagnostician particularly in the assessment, performance, and interpretation of single fiber EMG. She gets referrals from all over the region and country and has been a source of inspiration and along with John A. Morren has provided her expertise and meticulous attention to detail on all matters of EDX medicine. Chapter 12, written by Payam Soltanzadeh, MD, provides an excellent overview, with discourse on core concepts and fundamentals pertaining to the assessment and interpretation of EDX studies in patients with myopathies. The book concludes with Chap. 13 spearheaded by Alex Soriano, MD, and further refined by John A. Morren, MD, providing a succinct overview on how to write an EDX report, particularly in keeping with the recommendations set forth by the AANEM. Just as the practice of EDX medicine is both an art and science, so is the ability to write an EDX report, as this chapter elaborates.

It is the sincere hope of the editors of this work that we have provided a fresh overview on the subject of electrodiagnostic medicine and that this book will serve as a primer to many laboratories, as it will be in ours. We anticipate that it will be very helpful as reference companion, especially to instructors and lifelong learners in the field (not excluding former and future residents and fellows). We also hope that our readers have ever-increasing gratification in the practice of high-quality electrodiagnostic medicine that is not only a meaningful tribute to their mentors in the field but a great service to patients who trust us to do the best for them.

Weston, FL Nestor Galvez-Jimenez
Weston, FL Alexandra Soriano
Cleveland, OH John A. Morren

Contents

1 **Principles of Electrodiagnosis: Introduction** 1
Nestor Galvez-Jimenez, John A. Morren, and Alexandra Soriano

2 **Atlas of Nerve Conduction Studies (NCS)** 25
Nestor Galvez-Jimenez, John A. Morren, Alexandra Soriano, Karin Armstrong, Melissa Goldberg, Lourdes Gonzalez, and Dana Higginbotham

3 **Atlas of Needle Electrode Examination (NEE)**. 43
Nestor Galvez-Jimenez, John A. Morren, and Alexandra Soriano

4 **Introduction to Needle Electromyography** 65
Bryan Tsao

5 **Mononeuropathies** 83
Ramon Lugo and Alexandra Soriano

6 **Polyneuropathies**. 121
Megha Chetan Dhamne and John A. Morren

7 **Brachial Plexopathies** 157
Mark A. Ferrante

8 **Radiculopathies**. 195
Karen A. Karwa and John A. Morren

9 **Motor Neuron Diseases**. 213
Michelle M. Dompenciel

10 **Disorders of the Neuromuscular Junction** 227
Raghav Govindarajan and Elanagan Nagarajan

11 **Single Fiber EMG** 249
Alexandra Soriano

12 **Myopathies**. 255
Payam Soltanzadeh

13 **Recommendations for Writing an Electrodiagnostic Study Report** 265
Alexandra Soriano and John A. Morren

Correction to: Radiculopathies C1

Index. 271

Contributors

Karin Armstrong, C.N.C.T. Neurophysiology Lab, Cleveland Clinic Florida, Weston, FL, USA

Megha Chetan Dhamne, MBBS, MD Department of Neurology, Dr. L H Hiranandani Hospital, Mumbai, Maharashtra, India

Michelle M. Dompenciel, MD Department of Neurology, Cleveland Clinic, Weston, FL, USA

Mark A. Ferrante, MD University of Tennessee Health Science Center, Memphis, TN, USA

Nestor Galvez-Jimenez, MD, MSc, MHA, FACP Braathen Neurological Center, Cleveland Clinic Florida, Weston, FL, USA

Cleveland Clinic Lerner College of Medicine of Case Western Reserve University, Cleveland, OH, USA

Melissa Goldberg, BS, C.N.C.T. Neurophysiology Lab, Cleveland Clinic Florida, Weston, FL, USA

Lourdes Gonzalez, C.N.C.T. Neurophysiology Lab, Cleveland Clinic Florida, Weston, FL, USA

Raghav Govindarajan, MD, FAAN, FANA, FACP Department of Neurology, Neurology Clinics, ALS and MDA Clinic, EMG/Neurophysiology Lab, Clinical Outcomes for Department of Neurology, University of Missouri, Columbia, MO, USA

Department of Neurology, University of Missouri, Columbia, MO, USA

Dana Higginbotham, R.NCS.T. Neurophysiology Lab, Neuromuscular Center, Neurological Institute, Cleveland Clinic, Cleveland, OH, USA

Karen A. Karwa, MD Neurology of the Rockies, Englewood, Colorado, USA

Ramon Lugo, MD Cleveland Clinic Florida, Weston, FL, USA

John A. Morren, MD/MBBS (Hons), FAAN, FAANEM Neuromuscular Center, Neurological Institute, Cleveland Clinic, and Cleveland Clinic Lerner College of Medicine of Case Western Reserve University, Cleveland, OH, USA

Elanagan Nagarajan, MD Department of Neurology, Neurology Clinics, ALS and MDA Clinic, EMG/Neurophysiology Lab, Clinical Outcomes for Department of Neurology, University of Missouri, Columbia, MO, USA

Department of Neurology, University of Missouri, Columbia, MO, USA

Payam Soltanzadeh, MD Neuromuscular Program, Department of Neurology, UCLA, Los Angeles, CA, USA

Alexandra Soriano, MD Braathen Neurological Center, Cleveland Clinic Florida, Weston, FL, USA

Cleveland Clinic Lerner College of Medicine of Case Western Reserve University, Cleveland, OH, USA

Bryan Tsao, MD, MBA, FAAN Department of Neurology, Loma Linda University School of Medicine, Loma Linda, CA, USA

1 Principles of Electrodiagnosis: Introduction

Nestor Galvez-Jimenez, John A. Morren, and Alexandra Soriano

Introduction

Michael Aminoff [1] very eloquently defined the common "misusage" of the term electromyography (EMG) … "*electromyography refers strictly to methods used to record the electrical activity of muscle, …* However … *it has come to have a wider meaning which encompasses also the electrodiagnostic techniques used to study the functional integrity of the peripheral nerves and the neuromuscular junction.*" Therefore, for many physicians and laypersons alike, the EMG is at times shrouded in mystery, often resulting in misguided fears and confusion. Consequently, a frequent and highly frustrating scenario is that of a request for a "screening" study as if the EMG can be equated to an electrocardiogram which may be performed to "see what is found". General statements such as limb pain, or the "rule out" myopathy, neuropathy or radiculopathy all in one *request* or *reason for study* do not provide enough pertinent information and the electrodiagnostician must perform an independent history and examination to better grasp the clinical context in which the study is being utilized. This is considered essential despite ever-escalating pressures a physician has for an increasing number of studies, and other operational and/or insurance and reimbursements pressures to do more with less. Therefore, the "EMG" is best performed when the referring or treating physician has already in mind some tentative conclusions about the patient's symptoms and request the study after having done a careful neurological evaluation. A basic tenet in electrodiagnostic medicine is that the "*EMG is an extension of the neurological examination*", not a replacement for it. Unfortunately, the latter portion of this is often overlooked by referring providers. As Asa Wilbourn admonished us "*…the procedure is ill suited to routine screening for neurologic disease. A total body EMG would require hours to performed, be prohibitively expensive, and cause intolerable patient discomfort*" [2].

N. Galvez-Jimenez (✉) · A. Soriano
Braathen Neurological Center, Cleveland Clinic Florida, Weston, FL, USA

Cleveland Clinic Lerner College of Medicine of Case Western Reserve University, Cleveland, OH, USA
e-mail: galvezn@ccf.org; soriana@ccf.org

J. A. Morren
Neuromuscular Center, Neurological Institute, Cleveland Clinic, and Cleveland Clinic Lerner College of Medicine of Case Western Reserve University, Cleveland, OH, USA
e-mail: morrenj@ccf.org

N. Galvez-Jimenez et al. (eds.), *Electrodiagnostic Medicine*,
https://doi.org/10.1007/978-3-030-74997-2_1

Currently the preferred and accepted term is Electrodiagnostic (EDX) studies, which encompasses two main groups of techniques, namely (a) nerve conduction studies (NCS) which may include F-wave and H-reflex responses, and other special studies such as repetitive nerve stimulation (RNS), and (b) needle electromyography (EMG) recording directly from muscle [alternatively referred to as needle electrode examination (NEE)]. A highly specialized separate technique called single fiber EMG (SFEMG) falls into the latter category. The various components of electrodiagnostic studies may provide information about the peripheral sensory and/or motor nerve fibers (including anterior horn cells), as well as the neuromuscular junction and muscle (see Table 1.1).

EDX studies provide an objective evaluation of a limited portion of the peripheral nervous system, specifically the peripheral portion of some sensory fibers and the motor unit (Fig. 1.1), which includes the anterior horn cell/motor neuron, the neuromuscular junction and all the muscle fibers innervated by the same motor neuron [2].

The study must be tailored to the patient symptoms and neurological findings and be adjusted as the procedure progresses and new findings begin to accrue. For example, a patient who is sent for foot drop may be found to have evidence of abundant active/ongoing axonal loss in many myotomes, and this may require extending the NCS and the EMG to other limbs, paraspinal muscles and/or cranial innervated muscles to exclude a widespread process such as motor neuron disease (MND). The initial reason for the study was foot drop however the initial findings suggested a more widespread and severe disorder and the time spent and studies done may need to be adjusted accordingly. Therefore, it can be inferred from the above that *the purpose of the EDX study is not only to confirm the presence of a peripheral disorder but more importantly to localize where the lesion is (e.g. anterior horn cell, root, plexus, peripheral nerve/nerves, neuromuscular junction, or muscle) and the underlying pathophysiological process, (e.g. demyelinating and/or axonal neuropathy, neuromuscular junction transmission defect, myopathy)*, which in turn will lead to a differential diagnosis that will help cone down the diagnostic possibilities to a few targeted ones, if not one in particular. If the treating physician is uncertain about the diagnosis, the EDX study may help clarify the nature of the patient's symptoms, although when ordered without proper indication—may lead to more confusion and unnecessary further studies (particularly if the EDX studies are not done properly). Therefore, as Campbell [3] emphasized "*... There can be no serious argument that electromyography, in all the ramifications of that term,* ***is the practice of medicine*** *...* ***Extensive background knowledge*** *is required to perform and accurately interpret electrodiagnostic studies. The necessary preparation spans electronics, biomedical engineering, basic neurophysiology, anatomy, neuromuscular pathology, clinical and musculoskeletal disease, the technical aspects of performing nerve conduction studies and needle electromyography, and,* ***most importantly, the correlations between electrodiagnostic findings and clinical disease.***"

Table 1.1 Types of basic electrodiagnostic examinations and peripheral nerve fibers assessed

Motor	Motor NCS, needle electrode examination, F-wave responses, RNS (NMJ study), SFEMG (NMJ study)
Sensory	Sensory NCS
Mixed (Motor and Sensory)	Mixed nerve NCS (e.g. palmar and plantar mixed nerve responses), H-reflexes

NCS nerve conduction studies, *RNS* repetitive nerve stimulation, *SFEMG* single-fiber electromyography, *NMJ* neuromuscular junction

Biases, Advantages and Disadvantages/Limitations (see Tables 1.2, 1.3 and 1.4)

To clearly understand and interpret NCS, we believe understanding the biases, advantages and limitations are important before we delve into the

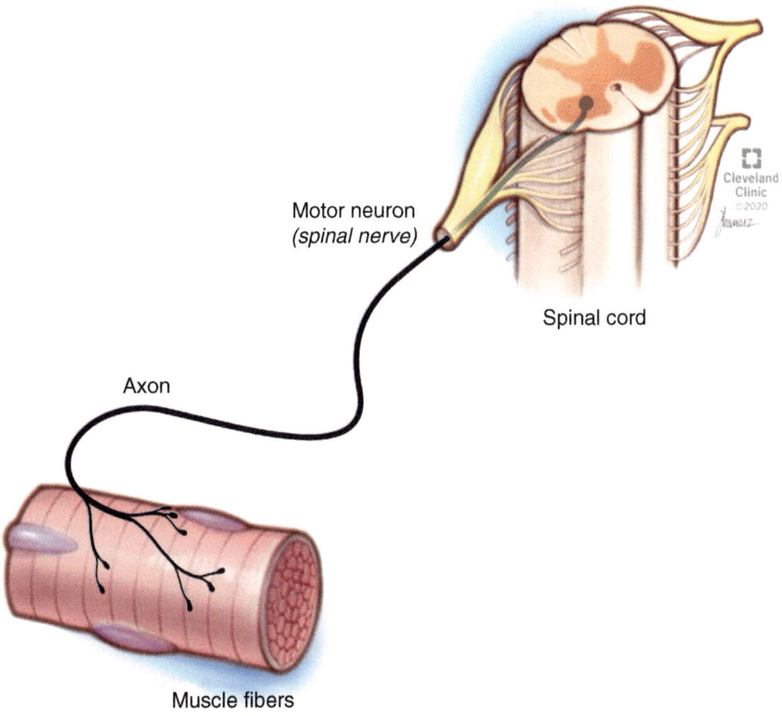

Fig. 1.1 Illustration of the anatomical components of a motor unit: an anterior horn cell/motor neuron and all of the muscle fibers (muscle cells) it innervates

actual NCS. The pathophysiology and physiological basis for clinical EDX practice should be understood. The diagnostic value of EDX studies may be limited, and at times severely so in some patients, particularly those with many co-morbidities such as diabetes mellitus, chronic renal and/or liver failure, prior multiple lumbosacral surgeries, limb edema and many others alone or in combination.

1. When performing and analyzing NCS, the physician must keep in mind that upper and lower extremity NCS are **biased** towards assessing the distal limb nerves and muscles and also towards the C8/T1 and L5/S1 distributions. This is also manifested by the median motor and ulnar motor responses for the routine motor NCS of the upper extremity, and the tibial motor and peroneal (fibular) motor responses for the routine motor NCS of the lower extremities. From a dermatome perspective, often covered is C6 and C8 when routinely performing upper limb sensory NCS: median sensory recording index finger and ulnar sensory recording fifth finger, and S1 when recording sural responses (and/or L5 when recording the superficial peroneal (fibular) sensory response) in the lower extremities. These are mixed nerves (except the sural nerve) and the sensory and motor abnormalities may reflect axonal, demyelinating, neuromuscular and myopathic involvement alone or in combination, therefore the physician must have special knowledge of peripheral neuromuscular anatomy, understanding and recognizing disorders that affect the nerves, muscles and neuromuscular junction, and the observable changes in both the normal and diseased states. Consequently, abnormalities observed in such studies may be reflecting local muscle, NMJ, or distal neuropathic process but also may be reflecting more proximal alterations affecting the root and anterior horn segment. The sensory NCS are extremely useful in localizing the lesion either distal to or proximal to the dorsal root ganglia (DRG)-practically defining the intraspinal localization of the process when the sensory responses are present. Such findings are pivotal when planning the NEE. Abnormalities of sensory

Table 1.2 Biases, advantages and disadvantages of EDX studies

Biases
Routine NCS studies of the upper and lower extremities are biased towards assessing the distal limbs via nerves subserved by the C8/T1 and L5/S1 anterior horn/root segments, and the C6 and C8 and S1 (+/−L5) sensory responses respectively
Advantages
Nerve conduction studies Require only "passive" patient cooperation Usually, particularly when performing routine studies, produces relatively little or minor patient discomfort Permit the evaluation of some sensory fibers Provides information regarding the state of myelination of motor and sensory fibers Very useful in detecting demyelinating block/segmental demyelination and its localization.
Needle electrode examination Allows for a flexible and widespread motor assessment of the peripheral nervous system, and muscle disease Sensitive for detecting motor axonal loss Sensitive for localizing a lesion producing motor axonal loss Sensitive for detecting primary muscle disease (when appropriately performed).
Disadvantages
Nerve conduction studies Evaluates only a limited portion of the peripheral nervous system Does not assess small sensory fibers (those involved in small fiber neuropathy) Are relatively insensitive to axon loss, particularly that affecting motor fibers Relatively insensitive for detecting primary muscle disorders
Concentric/monopolar needle electrode examination Requires active patient cooperation Patients may find it difficult to tolerate and a few may not complete the study Does not evaluate sensory fibers therefore it demonstrates motor axonal loss only May be confusing/difficult to interpret when concomitant myopathy exists Does not sensitively evaluate demyelinating segmental loss along motor fibers. May be affected by temperature changes as well: e.g. features of active/ongoing axonal loss such as fibrillation potentials may disappear if limbs are cold. In monopolar needle studies, the current criteria for MUP analysis are different and must be kept in mind when using such an electrode; must have a ground and reference electrodes connected directly to the patient.

Table 1.3 Limitations of nerve conduction studies due to underlying patient conditions (modified from [4])

Limitations	Results
Unsedated child Confused/Uncooperative patient (e.g.: dementia, encephalopathy)	Poor testing; limited study
Edema (e.g.: lymphedema due to axillary node dissection in the context of breast cancer, Congestive Heart Failure, others)	Low amplitude sensory and motor responses or, if severe, unelicitable responses
Cool/cold extremities	Prolonged distal latencies, slow conduction velocities and high amplitudes
Excessive sweating	Artifact and/or inadequate responses. Poor electrodes adherence to skin with consequent poor contact
Skin lesions (e.g.: rashes, infections, hematomas, skin breakdown)	Inability to test the limb, or to reliably stimulate/record from interest site
Central line, implanted pacemakers or defibrillators, Deep Brain Stimulator (DBS) chest generator	Cannot stimulate near the site, near wires or pacer due to consequent transmission of stimulation to heart (or brain, in case of DBS)
Anterior neck swelling or thickness	Cannot achieve supra-maximal stimulation (e.g.: in brachial plexus, phrenic nerve studies)

latency, amplitude or absence of sensory responses localizes the lesion to a process distal to the DRG.

2. **Age** affects the NCS and EMG. For example: it has been said, however somewhat challenged by some recent data and our own experience, that after age 60 years, sensory responses of the lower extremities (sural and superficial peroneal (fibular)) may be absent as a normal physiological finding, making the assessment for a disorder distal to the dorsal root ganglia such as a neuropathy challenging. Therefore, particularly with lower extremity disease in those above

Table 1.4 Limitations of needle electromyography due to underlying patient conditions

Limitations	Results
Bleeding disorders, Use of anticoagulants, including Novel Oral AntiCoagulants (NOACS)	Concerns about deep-seated bleeding particularly intramuscularly in large muscles, and in deep muscles (e.g.: iliacus, quadriceps), skin and subcutaneous hematomas
Coma or drug induced sedation	Patient unable to participate/ follow commands, with subsequent inability to properly analyze recruitment or MUP morphology
Agitation or inability to relax on command	Unable to reliably assess insertional and/or spontaneous activity. Increased risk of an accidental needle stick to the examiner
ICU conditions such as intubated or restrained patients	Uncooperative, or unable to position patient for, or participate in the study. Unable to easily assess paraspinal and nearby muscles

60 years, what may be normal or abnormal may merge, making the EDX findings less specific [2, 5], and this must be acknowledged by the interpreting physician. Of note, tibial H-reflexes may also be absent as a normal age process after 60 years. However, it may also be the only manifestation of an S1 radiculopathy or a proximal demyelinating block [3, 6, 7].

3. It is of utmost importance to pay attention to detail when performing NCS as any deviation of the norm or external and internal (patient) factors may affect the results. **Temperature, distance measurements, and presence of limb edema may all affect the results**. Cold limbs notoriously lead to widespread distal latency prolongation, conduction velocity slowing and abnormally high amplitudes. Pedal edema may result in abnormally low or absent sensory responses. Flawed measurements, such as an erroneously short measured distance from the below-elbow to wrist site may result in spuriously fast motor conduction velocities. Similar errors may be incurred in ulnar studies when performed with the arm extended at the elbow rather than with elbow flexion at 90 degrees, particularly when assessing velocity slowing or conduction block between the above-elbow and below-elbow sites (elbow segment).
4. Other factors that affect the reliability of the data obtained and must be keep in mind when performing NCS, include **submaximal stimulation or excessive stimulation** with consequent volume conduction, spread to contiguous or nearby nerves, and **electrical interference** (which we experience more commonly in the intensive care unit, or near radiological suites when the electrical cables/ wall outlets have not been properly isolated/ conditioned). This "electrical noise" is quite a problem in many areas particularly in the inpatient hospital setting, making the recording of responses quite challenging at times. This is often most problematic when performing sensory nerve conduction studies and concentric needle electromyography in the ICU. Other important factors include the **correct placement of the stimulator, as well as the recording and reference electrodes**. This may result in abnormal morphology of responses obtained, and/or abnormal latencies and/or conduction velocities.

Physiopathological Basis for the Interpretation of NCS

Details will be provided in the respective chapters (vide infra), however, some introductory remarks are important to have a basic foundation when interpreting these studies.

Firstly, the peripheral nerves are composed of many individual nerve fibers or axons varying in size from 0.5 to 22 microns, surrounded by connective tissue, which is a major component of the peripherals nerves, providing the support or "skeleton" for the axons and Schwann cells. Another important function of the connective tissue is to provide protection and nutrition for the enclosed nerves. It is important to recognize that, comparatively speaking, the area occupied by fascicles, epineurium and perineurium varies from nerve to nerve. This is important as some nerves or fascicles are prone to damage selectively depending on the location of the lesion (as may be seen with pressure-susceptible superficial areas). For example, in some cases of ulnar neuropathy at the elbow, the fibers to the abductor digiti minimi may be spared while those for the first dorsal interossei may be preferentially affected. Kline [8] has reported what was supported by earlier data from Sydney Sunderland [9] that 85% of the cross sectional area of the sciatic nerve at the level of the hip is connective tissue, for example.

The **epineurium** is the outer layer covering the nerve composed of collagen and elastic fibers with abundant epineural vessels longitudinally oriented with small penetrators forming a mesh or network communicating with the perineurium and endoneurium. The perineurium is that connective tissue encircling the nerve fascicles. The **perineurium** is the peripheral nerve equivalent of the blood-brain barrier (blood-nerve barrier) due to the presence of tight junctions with same function as those noted in the central nervous system. Damage to the perineurium may result in axonal loss and demyelination within the fascicle. Finally the **endoneurium** encircles *each* myelinated axon and groups of unmyelinated and thinly/poorly myelinated axons. The endoneurium serves as the last blood-nerve barrier, is composed of micro vessels, tight junctions and collagen fibers.

Schwann cells, similar to the oligodendrocytes in the CNS, forms myelin coverings around axons with the plasma membrane of each Schwann cell wrapping around and fusing with itself forming a thick myelin sheath [7–10].

The peripheral nervous system has a limited repertoire to injury [7, 10]. Common forms of injury include compression, stretching, ischemia, and exposure to toxins including medications (e.g. colchicine), particularly chemotherapeutic agents and antibiotics (e.g.: metronidazole). Despite these varied causes the major responses to injury are axonal loss, demyelination, or a combination of both [5, 7]. Axon loss may result in conduction failure distally from the site of the injury, whereas demyelination—usually a segment or a region of focal demyelination, may result in conduction slowing or (when severe enough) conduction block, as seen with **neurapraxia**. An example of this will be carpal tunnel syndrome, with the main underlying pathophysiological process being focal demyelination resulting in prolonged distal latencies (sensory followed by alteration in the motor latencies); similar also seen in other compressive neuropathies such as ulnar neuropathy at the elbow and/or wrist, also acute or chronic demyelinating polyneuropathies. In other conditions, particularly chronic exposure to toxic/metabolic processes such as diabetes mellitus, there may be both axonal and segmental demyelination. In **axonotmesis**, there is loss of the continuity of the axon with preservation of the connective tissue including endoneurium surrounding the axons. With axonal loss, there is a "dying back" or Wallerian degeneration, which, on average takes about 3 weeks to manifest typical changes during the needle electrode examination, consisting of fibrillation and positive sharp wave potentials. These may be preceded by few days with an increase in insertional activity—however, this is a nonspecific finding. In the chronic phase of significant axon loss nerve injury, there will be muscle atrophy, in addition to muscle weakness. In these cases, there is typically loss of both motor and sensory function, unless the nerve is a pure sensory one (e.g. lateral femoral cutaneous nerve). It is important to recognize that axonotmesis prognosis is distance—dependent as there may be good recovery from axonal re-growth if the target muscle distance to the lesion is less than approximately 20 inches [7, 11]. **Neurotmesis** is the most severe form of injury when the whole structure/continuity of the nerve is lost, either because of severe nerve transection, or crushing injuries. In many instances, there may be proximal axonal growth but once advancing nerve fibers reach the stump, they fail to find their way along the original nerve course, with no recovery of function. Consequently, there will be permanent muscle weakness and atrophy, unless there is successful surgical re-anastomosis [2, 5, 9, 12].

Nerve Conduction Studies

During the performance of nerve conduction studies we are measuring electrical responses elicited by stimulating a peripheral nerve, recording from surface electrodes, or rarely needle electrodes recording from a muscle or sensory fibers. Those recorded from the muscle constitute motor nerve conduction studies, and those from the sensory fibers are the sensory nerve conduction studies. The motor responses are the summation of the electrical potentials generated by a large number of muscle fibers resulting in the compound muscle action potential (CMAP) and are measure in millivolts, whereas sensory fibers responses represent the summation of the direct response from the sensory fibers, which are quite small and are measured in microvolts, and are called sensory nerve action potentials (SNAPs). Because of its size, the sensory fiber responses are smaller and therefore, are more difficult to obtain, are usually affected first in a generalized peripheral neuropathic process, are prone for artifactual effects and technical difficulties related to patient characteristics such as limb edema. In this latter scenario for example, the distance from surface electrode to nerve is increased by the interstitial fluid, with increased electrical resistance and high frequency filtering effects due to accentuation of connective tissue making the recording or eliciting of a reliable sensory response quite challenging. These challenges often converge in the ICU patient who may have limb edema and/or trophic skin changes for a variety of reasons, with the sensory (more than motor) nerve conduction responses further affected by electrical "noise" in the critical care environment.

When performing motor NCS, one must keep in mind that the responses reflect the time it takes for the stimulus to travel to the recording electrode, which is placed on the belly of the muscle where the motor point is located. Hence, motor latency: the time it takes for the stimulation to travel from the stimulus artifact to the onset of the motor response (CMAP), is measured in milliseconds. This parameter reflects the time taken to travel along the fast-conducting large myelinated fibers (abundant myelin sheath and axons), the neuromuscular junction and that needed for the activation of the muscle fibers and resultant muscle contraction. These must be kept in mind when interpreting the motor NCS responses elicited within the specific clinical context of each case. Without a good neuromuscular history and examination, the data may be more difficult to interpret. The sensory NCS latency reflects the time it takes the stimulus to travel via fast-conducting sensory fibers to the sensory response recording point. The sensory latency is measured from the onset of the stimulus artifact to the negative peak and is reported in milliseconds as well. Specific parameters constituting a typical motor and sensory nerve conduction response are shown in Figs. 1.2 and 1.3 respectively.

Amplitude and duration of the compound muscle action potential (CMAP) represent the number of axons and connected muscle fibers in the motor response, along with the degree of synchronization/desynchronization of the different fibers conduction times. This latter point is better assessed by the area under the curve (AUC), and looking at the configuration of the CMAP, particularly when there is low amplitude and dispersion of the motor response (discordant increase in CMAP duration). The AUC is routinely calculated by the computerized software in most NCS/EMG equipment. Amplitude of the CMAP is additionally affected by disorders of the neuromuscular junction as exemplified by the low motor responses observed in patients with Lambert-Eaton myasthenic syndrome.

In our EMG laboratory, we routinely test median motor nerve responses recording from the abductor pollicis brevis (APB) muscle, ulnar motor nerve responses recording from the abductor digiti minimi (ADM) muscle, tibial nerve

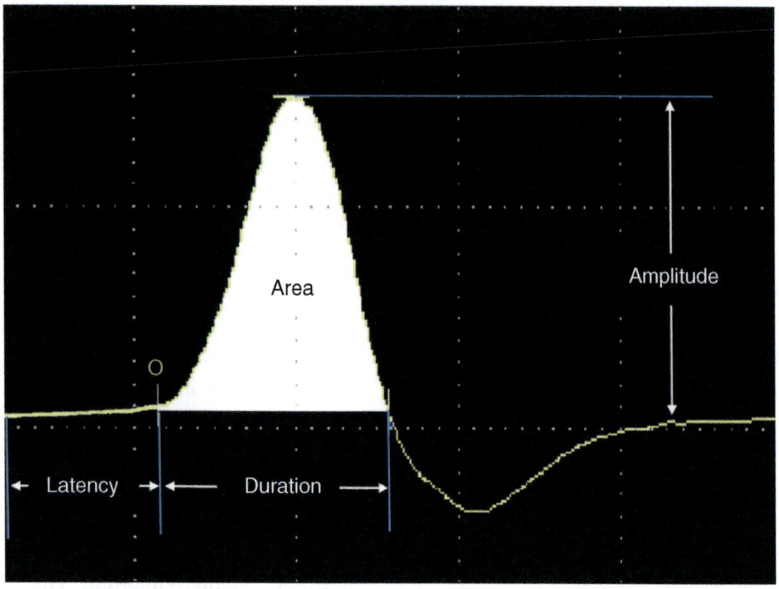

Fig. 1.2 Outline of a typical motor nerve conduction response showing component parameters

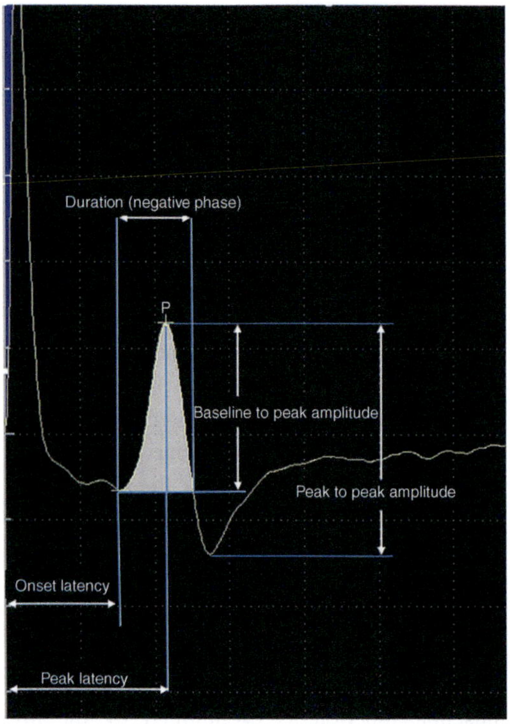

Fig. 1.3 Outline of a typical sensory nerve conduction response showing component parameters

motor responses recording from the abductor hallucis (AH) muscle, and peroneal (fibular) motor nerve response recording from the extensor digitorum brevis (EDB) muscle. Routine sensory responses include median sensory recording index finger, ulnar sensory recording fifth finger, radial sensory recording from the base of the thumb, sural responses recording lateral leg/lateral malleolus and superficial peroneal (fibular) recording lateral leg/dorsal aspect of the ankle. Depending on the clinical situation, other less commonly performed studies are added as needed including medial and lateral antebrachial cutaneous, median sensory recording thumb and middle finger, dorsal ulnar recording dorsum of hand), saphenous recording lower inner leg, axillary nerve recording the deltoid muscle, musculocutaneous nerve recording from the biceps brachii muscle, radial motor nerve recording from the extensor digitorum communis (EDC) muscle, and in the lower extremities femoral nerve recording from the rectus femoris (or vastus lateralis) muscle, peroneal (fibular) motor nerve recording from the tibialis anterior (TA) muscle (this is particularly important in patients with foot drop), ulnar motor nerve recording from the first dorsal interosseous (FDI) muscle (particularly important in patients suspected of an ulnar neuropathy at the elbow due to preferential fascicular involvement in some cases sparing the ADM, however involving the FDI fibers).

Other studies include palmar and plantar mixed nerve responses. The former are per-

Table 1.5 Nerve conduction studies

Motor Nerve Conduction studies
Routine or standard motor NCS in our EMG laboratory
1. Median motor: recording abductor pollicis brevis (APB)
2. Ulnar motor: recording abductor digiti minimi (ADM)
3. Tibial motor: recording abductor hallucis (AH)
4. Peroneal (fibular) motor: recording extensor digitorum brevis (EDB)
Frequently performed motor NCS in our EMG laboratory
1. Ulnar motor: recording first dorsal interosseous (usually performed when an ulnar neuropathy at the elbow is suspected, in addition to the ulnar motor response recording ADM).
2. Radial motor: recording extensor indicis or extensor digitorum (usually performed when a radial neuropathy at the spiral groove is suspected).
3. Musculocutaneous motor: recording biceps brachii (done in cases involving proximal upper extremity weakness/brachial plexus lesion).
4. Axillary motor: recording deltoid: (done in cases involving proximal upper extremity weakness/brachial Plexus lesion).
5. Peroneal (fibular) motor: recording tibialis anterior (TA) (usually performed when a peroneal (fibular) neuropathy at the fibular head is suspected, for example in patients with foot drop).
6. Femoral motor: recording rectus femoris or vastus lateralis (done in cases involving quadriceps weakness when a femoral neuropathy or lumbar plexus lesion is suspected).

Table 1.5 (continued)

Sensory Nerve Conduction studies
Routine or standard sensory NCS in our EMG laboratory
1. Median: recording index finger
2. Ulnar: recording fifth finger
3. Radial: recording thumb base
4. Sural: recording lateral ankle
Other sensory NCS frequently performed
1. Median/ulnar palmar mixed nerve responses (performed almost exclusively for the diagnosis of carpal tunnel syndrome or ulnar neuropathy at the wrist/Guyon's canal).
2. Lateral and Medial antebrachial cutaneous responses (usually performed when a brachial plexus lesions is suspected).
3. Superficial peroneal (fibular) sensory responses (usually performed in cases of suspected common peroneal (fibular) neuropathy, as may occur from compression at the fibular head)
4. Medial plantar mixed nerve responses (usually performed when distal/early generalized large fiber sensorimotor neuropathy or tarsal tunnel syndrome is suspected).
Sensory NCS difficult to elicit and less commonly performed in our laboratory
1. Saphenous responses (may consider in lumbar plexopathy work-ups)
2. Lateral femoral cutaneous (when meralgia paresthetica or lateral femoral cutaneous neuropathy is suspected. However, this response is very difficult to obtain, particularly in patients with increased abdominal girth).
3. Posterior cutaneous nerve of the thigh.

formed almost exclusively when looking for carpal tunnel syndrome, and the latter—particularly the medial plantar response is done when looking for a very early generalized large fiber sensorimotor neuropathy or tarsal tunnel syndrome. These mixed responses evoke both motor and sensory fibers resulting in larger amplitude responses when compared to the pure sensory nerve responses (Table 1.5).

Needle Electrode Examination

When performing needle electromyography the area "visualized" by the electrode is of about 120–300 microns, usually assessing 5–15 muscle fibers at a time. In the case of the concentric needle electromyography, the area examined has a tear drop appearance [13, 14]. When the electrical potential is generated distally to the location of the needle electrode, the potential may have a triphasic configuration. If the origin of the electrical potentials is right at the needle placement area, the configuration may be that of a positive wave or biphasic wave as the needle electrode "do not see" the incoming potential [13]. However, it must be kept in mind that according to Kimura [15], the spatial relationship between the recording needle electrode and individual muscle fibers play the most important role in determining the waveform configuration. Other factors affecting the Motor Unit Action Potential (MUAP) configuration during EMG are temperature (cool limbs increases the duration of the MUP with decreased in amplitude). Motor unit potentials may become polyphasic in cooler limbs. According to Kimura [15] and supported by Dumitru [13], the changes in such MUAP features are due to the effect of temperature resulting in accentuated differential slowing and desynchronization of muscle fiber activation.

When performing the NEE, the examiner first notices the insertional activity and the resistance to needle insertion. In cases of fibrotic muscles, such as some longstanding, there may be a gritty or sand-like sensation when inserting the electrode. In cases of steroid myopathies the insertion may feel as if inserting the needle in butter with minimal resistance. Once the needle is inserted there will be a very short insertional activity that may be increased in cases of muscle membrane instability/irritability such as active/ongoing motor axon loss or myopathic states. After insertional activity, with the needle remaining motionless in the relaxed normal muscle, there should only be electrical silence constituting the normal baseline muscle response. With denervation and/or muscle fiber destruction, fibrillation potentials with the configuration of positive sharp waves or biphasic spikes responses may be observed on average about 3 weeks after the initial insult/injury, with these denervation potentials lasting typically up to 8–10 months (or may persist considerably longer). The presence of positive sharp wave or fibrillation potentials defines the subacute stage of axonal loss. Fibrillation potentials have an almost constant discharge frequency, simulating the tick-tock of a clock (sometimes described as "metronomic"). The amplitude of such responses may be between 100 and 400 microvolts but may also be somewhat larger or smaller. The fibrillation potentials can be conceptualized as representing the pacemaker activity intrinsic to each muscle fiber, which, when devoid of the inhibitory tonic influence of the motor axons, begin to fire independently. Hence, each fiber begin to fire on its own, resulting in the busy screen that may be observed in such situations. Other types of abnormal insertional activity include myotonic potentials, complex repetitive discharges (CRDs), and myokymia (among other grouped repetitive discharges), which will be discussed in subsequent chapters.

Once analysis of the insertional activity has been performed, the next step is to evaluate the motor unit action potential configuration and firing pattern. Usually the MAUP has a triphasic configuration mimicking that observed in the EKG QRS complex, having an amplitude between 120 microvolts to 2 to 3 millivolts and a maximal duration of approximately 15 milliseconds in duration with a rise time, (measure from the first positive peak to the subsequent negative peak), of less than 100 to 200 microseconds. This results in a crisp, sharp sound providing the best indicator to the proximity of the recording needle tip to the muscle fiber. Of course, the duration and amplitude depends on the muscle studied. Larger muscles tend to have larger MUAP, and small muscles such as the orbicularis oculi tend to have a small MUAP. A motor unit is considered polyphasic once more than three crossings over the baseline are present, a phase being the portion of the waveform between the departure from and return to the baseline. Polyphasic MUAP are markers of chronicity and usually represent the desynchronization of muscle fiber activation due to sprouting when a muscle has been denervated or there is destruction/drop-off of muscle fibers. Such polyphasic MUAP are observed in about 10–15% of MUAP in many muscles, particularly proximal larger muscles such as the iliacus, gluteus muscle groups, brachioradialis, supraspinatus, and deltoid. If the turns do not cross the baseline they are serrated MUAP with the same EDX significance. That is, axonal sprouting with reinnervation consistent with chronic changes. Acute/subacute and chronic electromyographic changes commonly co-exist in the same muscle when studied.

Recruitment of motor units is another important aspect during the performance of the NEE. Once a MUAP has been identified at the beginning of activation, the firing frequency is noted, together with the recruitment ratio which is usually observed once the MUAP achieves a 10–15 Hz and a second MUAP is recruited and begin to fire (recruitment ratio = firing frequency of the fastest firing MUAP/the number of different MUAPs on the screen). This is considered normal recruitment. If the muscle increases its force of contraction, a third MUAP is recruited when the first MUAP achieves ~15 Hz and the second MUP achieves ~10 Hz, and so forth. This is known as the 5:1 recruitment ratio or the "rule of 5's" [6, 13].

Late Responses

Routine NCS are biased towards the assessment of the most distal portions of the peripheral nerves. In the upper extremities, when recording from the hand and distal forearm, the sensory and motor responses obtained are those from the distal portions of the median, ulnar and radial nerve territories. In the lower extremities, the NCS often assess the responses from the distal components of the sciatic nerve below the knee namely the peroneal (fibular) and tibial nerves. They do not assess the more proximal segments of these nerve with the stimulation and recording sites employed.

However, there are other responses which may be obtained to assess the more proximal segment of peripheral nerves. With the appropriate technique, three different types of responses may be observed following the CMAP or M responses recorded from the muscle during NCS. Hence, they are collectively known as "late" responses. These are the F-wave, and H-reflex, and the A-wave. The M response in the context of these late responses is essentially the routinely recorded compound muscle action potential during NCS.

F-Wave (Fig. 1.4)

The F wave is a pure motor response. To generate an F-wave response, a supramaximal stimulation is delivered to the nerve, and such a response will be observed after the direct M response/recorded CMAP during NCS. These responses are useful as a measure of the proximal conduction time and motor axon responses, which are elicited antidromically, while recording orthodromically most often from the median, ulnar and tibial innervated muscles. In other words, the afferent/efferent pathway is within the motor fibers of the anterior horn cell. The motor impulse travels up centripetally (antidromically) along the motor neurons, reaching the cell bodies and backfiring

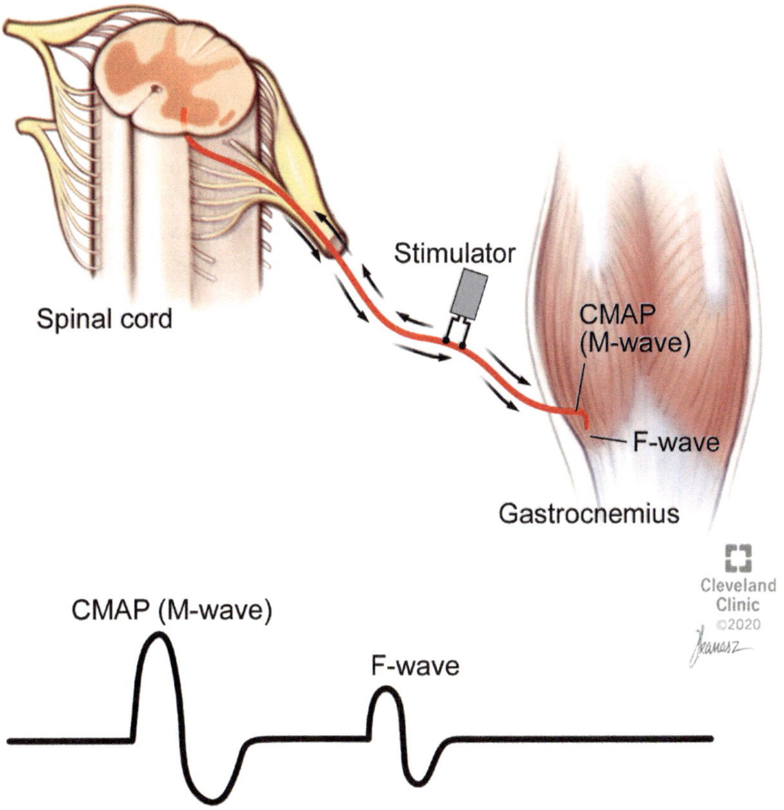

Fig. 1.4 Illustration of the anatomical components and electrical pathway of the tibial F-wave response

via the orthodromic efferent motor axon pathway. There is no synapse involved, but this transmission incurs an estimated minimal lag time of 1.0 ms at the spinal cord motor neuron pool. Therefore, the F-wave provides an assessment of the most proximal portion of the motor axons comprising the peripheral nerve under study. The fibers assessed are the same fast conducting fibers stimulated during routine NCS. According to Kimura, [15] this provides the rationale for the minimal F-wave latency serving as a measure of the fastest conducting motor nerve fibers proximally. There is no sensory component therefore, the F-wave response is not affected by the findings of the sensory NCS. When first described, they were recorded from foot muscles, hence the name "F"-waves.

The F-wave is generated by the random antidromic activation of approximately 1% to 5% of the anterior horn cells (motor neuron) pool. Because of this, there is a need to obtain several responses. In our EDX laboratory we obtain a train of 10 responses, using the one which has the shortest latency as the best response (i.e. "minimal" F-wave latency). There should be a greater than 50% F-wave occurrence rate to be considered normal and, on average, 70% to 80% F-wave occurrence rate is what we usually observe in our laboratory among normal subjects. Because the amplitude of the F-wave is typically 1% to 5% that of the CMAP, if the CMAP is reduced, the F-wave will not be observed. Amplitude, latency and dispersion are variables that may provide useful information when assessed in the appropriate clinical context. Apart from its low amplitude, a key feature that differentiates the F-wave from the M response is its variable inter-response latency. Characteristically, the F-wave latency varies from stimulation to stimulation. Chronodispersion (the difference between the shortest and longest F-wave latencies) is on average, about 4 ms in the upper extremities, and is about 6 ms in the lower extremities. This parameter provides an indication of proximal nerve temporal dispersion. Prolongation of the F-wave latencies indicates proximal nerve segment conduction delay and it may be the only abnormal finding in an otherwise normal NCS in a patient in which an acute inflammatory demyelinating polyradiculoneuropathy (AIDP, or Guillain-Barre syndrome) is suspected. This may be the case in a patient presenting with weakness and areflexia, and yet normal motor and sensory routine NCS (noting as well that often a "sural-sparing" pattern is seen).

It is useful to calculate the F-wave estimate, taking into account the patient's height, which will influence the measured value of the F-wave response (particularly, latency). Because the F-wave assesses the whole length of the nerve, it is generally a very good measure of nerve pathology. If the F-wave latencies are normal and within the range of the F-wave estimate, it is a good indication that the nerve fibers are conducting at the expected velocity, and this excludes a significant pathological (especially demyelinating) process within the length of the nerve. However, if the measured minimal F-wave response is prolonged when compared to the F-wave estimate, this implies a conduction delay in the more proximal nerve segment, likely out of proportion to what would be expected based on the distal motor latency and other findings on routine motor nerve conduction studies. We estimate the F-wave latency by measuring the length of the arm from the stimulation site to the sternoclavicular joint for the upper extremity, and from the site of stimulation to the xiphoid process for the lower extremity. The F-wave latency estimate can be calculated as follows:

$$F[\text{est}] = [(2 \times \text{distance}) / \text{CV}] + \text{DL}.$$

In this formula, the distance is the measured distance from the cathode to the sternoclavicular joint and xyphoid process for the upper and lower extremity, respectively. CV is the calculated conduction velocity, and DL is the motor distal latency for the particular nerve under study. Most current NCS/EMG equipment will calculate this value automatically if the measured distance is entered. Furthermore, most current equipment will provide the FWCV. FWCV is the CV to and from the spinal cord. The FWCV is another measure of the proximal segment conductivity, and accordingly, it is usually affected in disorders in which there is proximal conduction slowing. Of note, there is a variable degree of agreement among many EDX laboratories as to the ultimate usefulness of the F-waves. Utility of F-wave responses is less controversial in certain cases of nerve injury with early or predominant proximal nerve trunk and/or root-level pathology, as in early AIDP. In these cases, the F-wave may be significantly abnormal as an isolated but sensitive finding.

H-reflex (Fig. 1.5)

The tibial H-reflex assesses the proximal portion of tibial nerve by orthodromically activating the afferent Ia sensory fibers (bipolar cell—distal and proximal to the dorsal root ganglion) at the popliteal fossa, stimulating the motor neurons in the anterior horn cells, with the efferent impulse traveling orthodromically via the motor fibers to the muscle, thereby eliciting a CMAP response at the gastrocnemius-soleus muscle complex. The benefits from such a study are the evaluation of the proximal segment of the tibial/S1 nerve/nerve root. This response may be normally absent after age 60 years, and pathologically reduced or absent with proximal processes such as demyelinating polyradiculoneuropathies (e.g. AIDP), and prior laminectomies involving the low lumbar/lumbosacral/S1 region.

The A-wave or Axon Reflex

On occasion, an axon reflex or A-wave is recorded when performing an F wave study. The A-wave is a muscle response just like the CMAP but of lower amplitude and stable configuration and latency as opposed to the F wave which is quite variable in latency and configuration. The A-wave, when present, is always abnormal and is usually observed in patients with radiculopathies or other proximal nerve/nerve root disorders

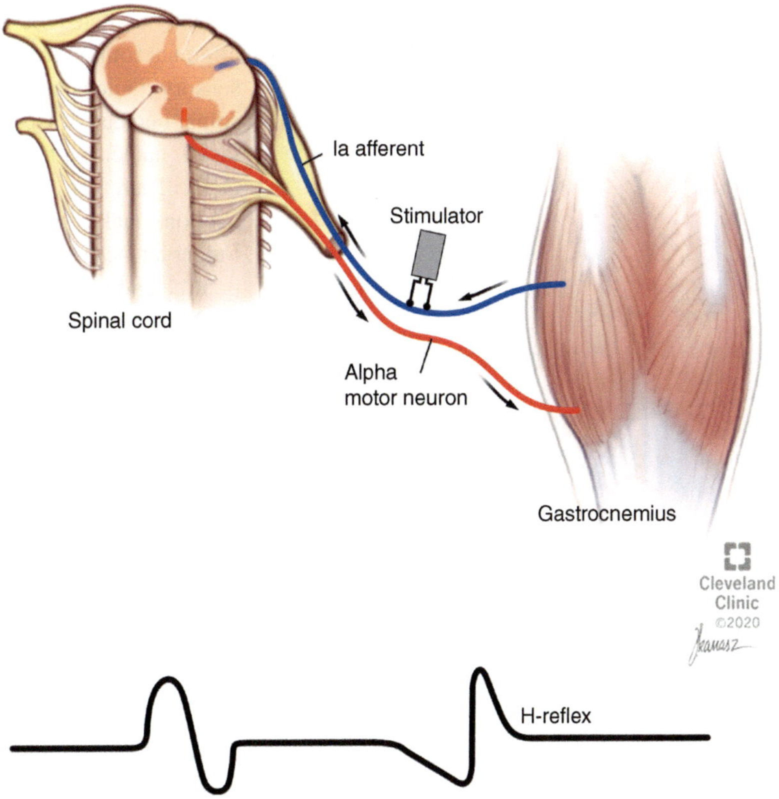

Fig. 1.5 Illustration of the anatomical components and electrical pathway of the tibial H-reflex response

resulting in chronic axon loss. The origins of the A-wave are not certain. However, they may represent either "cross–talk" or ephaptic communication between injured axons proximally, or be the result of collateralization during axon sprouting. The A-wave is usually recorded in between the M response and the F-wave. However, in some cases it may be recorded after the F-wave. This later response has been attributed to the ephaptic transmission mentioned above due to demyelination-related conduction slowing through the collaterals.

Blink Reflexes

The neurophysiological correlate of the corneal reflex is the blink reflex. The underlying polysynaptic reflex arc is the basis of the blink reflex that is measured in the EDX laboratory. Afferents travel via the first (ophthalmic) division of the trigeminal nerve (V_1) to the main sensory nucleus of the trigeminal nerve in the mid-pons, as well as the spinal nucleus of this nerve (i.e. cranial nerve V) in the medulla, connecting via interneurons to the pontine facial nuclei, with facial nerve (cranial nerve VII) efferents ultimately supplying the orbicularis oculi to produce blinking (Fig. 1.6).

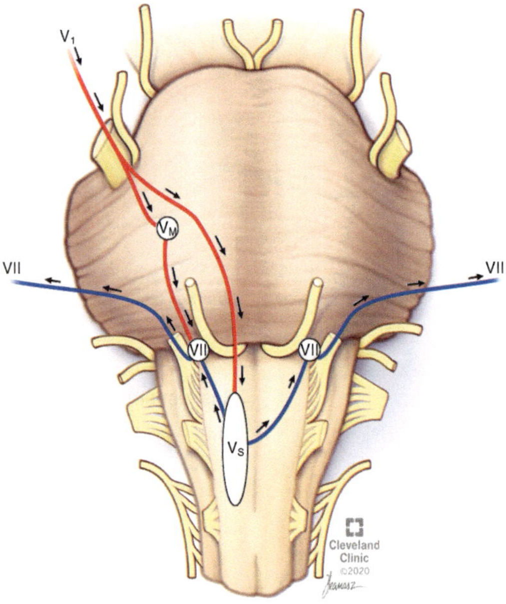

Fig. 1.6 Illustration of the anatomical components and electrical pathway of the blink reflex response

The normal response results in two clearly defined components, ipsilateral orbicularis oculus M response labeled R1 and R2 (mediated primarily by CrN V main sensory nucleus and spinal tract nucleus, respectively), and a contralateral R2 (R2C) response, mediated primarily by the CrN V spinal tract nucleus (Fig. 1.7).

These responses can be measured electrophysiologically by stimulating the supraorbital nerve [typical stimulus intensity of 8.0 mA, stimulus duration 0.2 ms] resulting in an early R1 ipsilateral response with an average latency of 10 ms [maximum 13 ms (8–13 ms)] and subsequent bilateral R2 responses of approximately 30 ms [maximum ipsilateral 33 ms (29–41 ms), and maximum contralateral 34 ms (29–44 ms)]. The most reliable response is R1, which is a pontine reflex mediated by a disynaptic reflex arc formed by the V1 trigeminal afferent to the main sensory nucleus of CrN V, and the pontine nucleus of CrN VII and corresponding facial efferents. R2 responses, which are polysynaptic reflexes mediated via the reflex arc formed by the afferents coming from CrN V, bypassing the main sensory nucleus and synapsing directly with the spinal nucleus of CN V, then to bilateral pontine facial nuclei with efferents to the orbicularis oculi. Therefore, these latter polysynaptic connections make for a longer response onset (i.e. longer latency), considering that R2 is a complex pontine and lateral medullary reflex.

A side-to-side R1 latency difference exceeding 1.2 ms is usually considered abnormal. The side-to-side difference between the ipsilateral R2 latencies and the contralateral R2 latencies should be less than 5 ms and 7 ms, respectively. The R2 responses may vary according to the state of hyper-excitability of the inter-neurons, and can habituate upon repetitive stimulation. However, R2 responses are very important for localization. R1 abnormalities may be produced by disruption in any of the components of the pontine arc: namely the trigeminal afferents, facial efferents or the corresponding pontine nuclei. Whereas with an abnormal or delayed R2, further localization may be made, as an abnormality will help determine

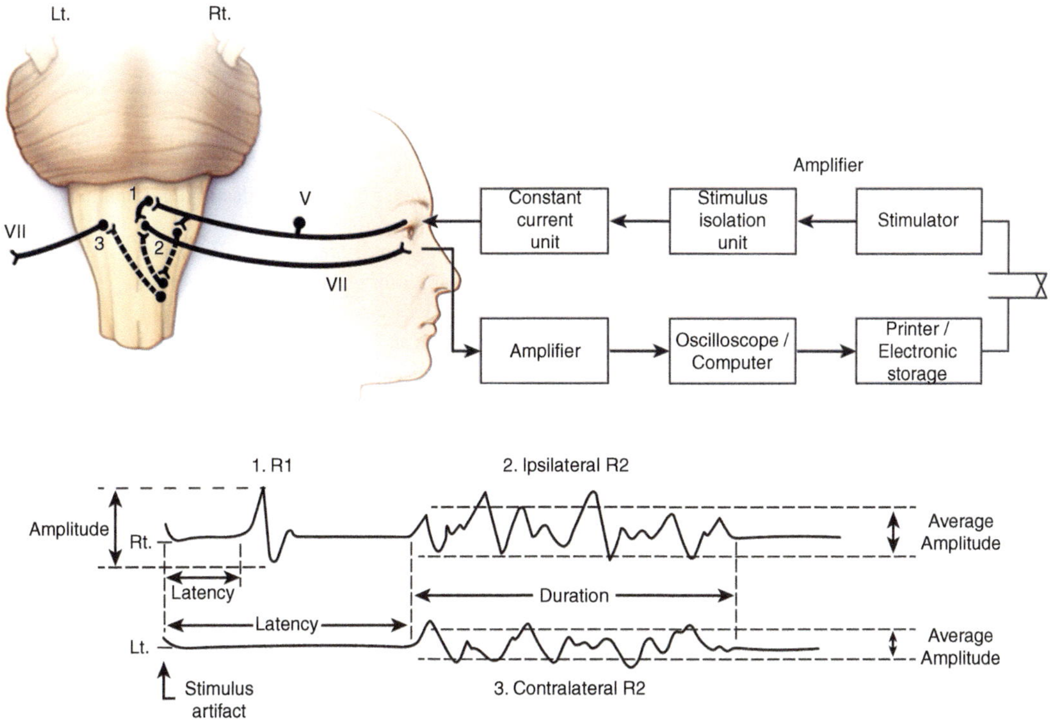

Fig. 1.7 Blink reflex-normal responses and measurements

whether an abnormal R1 is due to an afferent CrN V or efferent CrN VII process. An ipsilateral and contralateral R2 delay, when the affected side is stimulated, indicates a trigeminal nerve lesion. This pattern is known as the "afferent delay". With a lesion of the facial nerve, R2 is delayed on the affected side regardless of the stimulation side/laterality. This is known as "efferent delay" pattern. There are other potentially abnormal patterns, as shown in the figure below (Fig. 1.8). However, using the principles outlined above, a discrete lesion localization can usually be made from the analysis of the R1, R2 and R2C responses.

Facial Nerve Motor Studies

While the blink reflex assesses mostly brainstem components of CrN V afferents and CrN VII efferents, the more distal fibers of CrN VII (that is, distal to the stylomastoid foramen), can be assessed by stimulating the facial nerve as it exits the cranium to innervate facial muscles. The facial nerve has five distinct branches including the temporal, zygomatic, buccal, marginal mandibular, and cervical branches. Stimulating the facial nerve anterior to the mastoid process, slightly above the angle of the jaw over the stylomastoid foramina, recording from the nasalis muscle provides an objective recording of the state of the distal motor fibers. Comparisons are made primarily in amplitude, with a greater than 50% difference in amplitude of the CMAP between sides being abnormal. Just as in routine NCS of the limbs, amplitude provides a measure of the number of functional/intact motor axons, and the motor latency provides a measure of the fastest conducting fibers. In clinical practice, we rely heavily on the side-to-side comparison for these responses. The latencies may be quite variable between individuals and subject to false negatives even in cases of severe facial neuropathies, particularly Bell's palsy. Nonetheless, the reference range for the facial nerve motor latency is generally considered to be between 2.6 and 4.2 ms. Facial nerve studies provide useful information about prognosis, particularly if repeated along the clinical

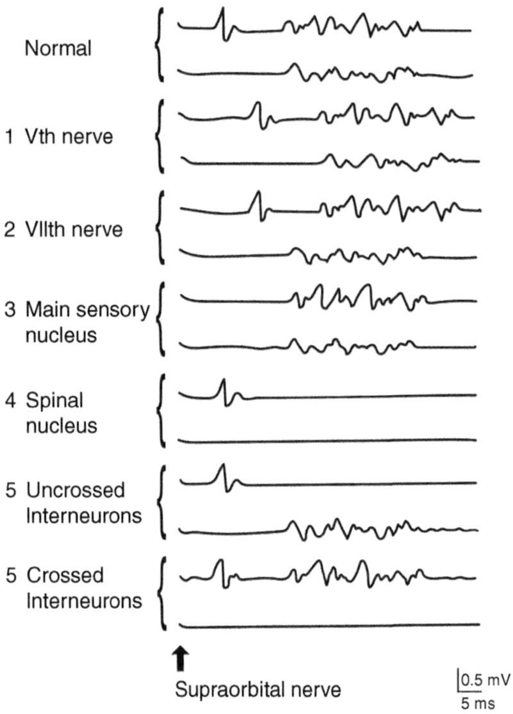

Fig. 1.8 Most common abnormal response patterns observed during analysis of the blink reflex responses

course. A normal facial nerve CMAP response within the first week of injury may indicate a good prognosis for recovery, whereas an abnormal CMAP response lasting beyond 3 weeks, particularly if accompanied by signs of denervation on needle electromyography of facial muscles, portends a worse prognosis. A CMAP difference of 90% between affected and unaffected sides suggests a poorer prognosis. Additionally, a more favorable prognosis may be predicted if the CMAP of the affected side is greater than 25% compared to the unaffected side. Surgical decisions may be based on the results of the facial EDX studies, in the context of the timeline of injury.

Standard Assessments of the Upper and Lower Extremities

Although it should be emphasized that each EDX study should be tailored to the specific case, informed by the history and exam findings and the resulting differential diagnosis, Table 1.6

Table 1.6 Suggested standard assessment of the upper and lower extremities

Upper extremity
Nerve conduction studies
1. Median motor recording Abductor pollicis brevis (APB)
2. Ulnar motor recording Abductor digiti minimi (ADM)
3. Median sensory recording index finger
4. Ulnar sensory recording fifth finger
5. Radial sensory recording forearm
6. Median and ulnar nerve F-wave responses
Needle electrode examination (NEE)
1. Abductor pollicis brevis (APB) [C8/**T1** roots, median nerve, lower trunk/medial cord of brachial plexus]
2. First dorsal interosseous (FDI) [**C8**/T1 roots, ulnar nerve, lower trunk/medial cord of brachial plexus]
3. Extensor indicis (EI) [C7, **C8** roots, radial nerve, middle and lower trunks/posterior cord of brachial plexus]
4. Pronator teres (PT) [C6/C7 roots, median nerve, upper and middle trunk/lateral cord of brachial plexus]
5. Biceps brachii [C5/C6 roots, musculocutaneous nerve, upper trunk/lateral cord of brachial plexus]
6. Triceps [C6, **C7**, C8 roots, radial nerve, upper, middle and lower trunks/posterior cord of brachial plexus]
7. Deltoid [**C5**, C6 roots, axillary nerve, upper trunk/posterior cord of brachial plexus]
8. Cervical paraspinal muscles (if NEE of the upper extremity is normal otherwise, may not perform NEE of the cervical paraspinal muscles at this stage)
Lower extremity
Nerve conduction studies
1. Tibial motor recording Abductor hallucis (AH)
2. Peroneal (fibular) motor recording Extensor digitorum brevis (EDB)
3. Sural responses [peroneal (fibular), tibial, sciatic, lumbosacral plexus, and S1 root work-ups]
4. Tibial H-reflex response
5. Tibial F-wave response
Concentric needle electromyography
1. Extensor digitorum brevis (EDB) [L5/S1 roots, deep peroneal (fibular) nerve, common peroneal (fibular) nerve, sciatic nerve, lumbosacral plexus]
2. Abductor hallucis (AH) [S1 root, tibial nerve, sciatic nerve, lumbosacral plexus]
3. Tibialis anterior (TA) [L4/L5 roots, deep peroneal (fibular) nerve, common peroneal (fibular) nerve, sciatic nerve, lumbosacral plexus]
4. Gastrocnemius medial head (S1/S2 roots, tibial nerve, sciatic nerve, lumbosacral plexus)
5. Tibialis posterior OR flexor digitorum longus (either one is acceptable) [L5 root, tibial nerve, sciatic nerve, lumbosacral plexus]

Table 1.6 (continued)

6. Vastus lateralis [L(2)3/4 roots, femoral nerve, lumbar plexus]
7. Gluteus medius OR tensor fascia lata (either one is acceptable) [**L5**/S1 roots, superior gluteal nerve, sacral plexus)
8. Gluteus maximus [**S1**(S2) > L5 roots, inferior gluteal nerve, sacral plexus]
9. Lumbar/sacral paraspinal muscles (if NEE of the lower extremity is normal otherwise, may not perform NEE of the lumbar/sacral paraspinal muscles at this stage).

discloses the specific NCS and NEE studies that are typically included in "standard" assessments of the upper and lower extremities.

Some Common Scenarios in Which an Electrodiagnostic Study Is Requested

Hand Pain/Numbness/Sensory Disturbance

A common reason for an EDX evaluation in our laboratory is that of hand pain and/or numbness/sensory disturbance with or without associated radicular symptoms. Carpal tunnel syndrome, ulnar neuropathy at the elbow or wrist, or radicular symptoms with involvement of the C6 segment (thumb), C7 (middle finger) and C8 (little finger) dermatomes may all present with numbness/sensory disturbance and/or pain in the hands with or without referred pain to the forearm. Brachial plexopathies may also present with hand numbness/sensory disturbance/pain and weakness (further discussed in the chapter on Brachial Plexopathies). For an in-depth discussion of mononeuropathies and radiculopathies, we also refer the reader to the respective chapters later in this book.

In carpal tunnel syndrome (CTS), patients often complain of hand numbness with or without weakness affecting the thenar muscles (which may undergo atrophy in severe cases). Sensory disturbance may be distributed variably in the thumb, index of middle finger. In some, the whole hand may be involved, and some patients report numbness/sensory disturbance or pain that spreads up to the forearm, sometimes even more proximally. On exam, the sensory perception at the thenar eminence must be spared as the sensory innervation comes from the median palmar sensory branch which originates before (proximal to) the carpal tunnel and it does not travel within this structure.

Our suggested assessment of patients with hand numbness/sensory disturbance/pain includes the standard studies of median motor recording APB, ulnar motor recording abductor digiti minimi, median sensory recording index finger, ulnar sensory recording fifth finger. If these studies are unremarkable, performing palmar mixed nerve median and ulnar orthodromic studies may help increase the sensitivity as it pertains to the detection of a median mononeuropathy at or distal to the wrist. In some laboratories, comparison studies using ulnar sensory responses recording from the fourth finger, stimulating the ulnar nerve at the wrist may add some increased sensitivity when carpal tunnel (or ulnar neuropathy at Guyon's canal) is suspected. One may add a radial sensory study recording at the forearm as it helps to exclude the presence of a polyneuropathy presenting as numbness/sensory disturbance in the hands particularly when the ulnar and median nerves studies demonstrate abnormalities. When a brachial plexus lesion is suspected we add sensory median studies recording thumb and middle finger in addition to the index finger, and add medial and lateral antebrachial cutaneous sensory studies, as well as axillary-deltoid and musculocutaneous-biceps responses when indicated. In CTS, the sensory latencies are first affected due to involvement of the fast-conducting sensory fibers. Depending on the degree of severity, prolongation of the sensory latency may be the only abnormality, followed by reduction in the SNAP amplitude and prolongation of the median motor distal latency recording

APB. When severe, there may be marked decrease or even absence of the median-APB response. When only CTS in present, the ulnar nerve studies are normal. On needle electromyography, we routinely study the APB (median-T1 > C8-lower trunk/medial cord, first dorsal interossei (FDI) [ulnar-C8/T1-lower trunk/medial cord], extensor indices (EI) [radial-C8 > 7-lower and middle trunk/posterior cord], pronator teres [median-C6–C7-upper and middle trunk/lateral cord], biceps brachii (musculocutaneous-C5–C6-upper trunk/lateral cord), triceps (radial-C7(>C6,C8)-middle trunk/posterior cord), deltoid (axillary-C5–C6-upper trunk/posterior cord), and corresponding cervical paraspinal muscles (posterior primary rami).

An ulnar neuropathy must be part of the differential diagnosis of patients with hand numbness/sensory disturbance/pain and/or weakness. The symptoms are often limited to the fourth and fifth fingers with possible radiation of symptoms to the forearm. When assessing an ulnar neuropathy as the cause of such hand symptoms, an ulnar neuropathy at the elbow must be a foremost consideration. With this localization, sensory responses at the hypothenar eminence and dorsal hand are typically reduced (dorsal sensory branch originates in the distal 1/3 of the forearm before entering Guyon's canal). There may be atrophy of the hypothenar muscles and the hand interossei resulting in a claw-appearing hand in many cases, with marked bony prominence of the metacarpal bones and phalanges. Motor axon loss changes in the abductor digiti minimi, first dorsal interosseous, flexor digitorum profundus (to digits 4&5), as well as flexor carpi ulnaris may be evident, depending on severity and/or the presence of fascicular sparing.

As previously mentioned, radiculopathies of the C7 and/or C8 involve the middle and/or the 4th/5th fingers and may present with numbness/sensory disturbance/pain in the respective territories.

In patients with suspected ulnar neuropathy at the elbow, in addition to standard electrodiagnostic studies of the upper extremities, we add recording from the FDI stimulating ulnar, and also the dorsal ulnar sensory response. In many cases of ulnar neuropathy, fibers destined to the FDI may be preferentially affected at the elbow, sparing those destined to the abductor digiti minimi. In patients with an ulnar neuropathy at the elbow, the dorsal ulnar sensory response is usually affected along with the ulnar motor responses recording ADM and/or FDI. On needle electromyography, we add to the standard EMG assessment of the upper extremity, the flexor carpi ulnaris, FDP-4th and 5th, in addition to the ADM and FDI. Of course, in the absence of an intraspinal canal process, the corresponding cervical paraspinal muscles are normal in median and/or ulnar mononeuropathies.

Foot Pain/Numbness/Sensory Disturbance

Another frequent diagnostic challenge is that of patients complaining of foot pain/sensory disturbance/numbness. The pain character may be that of burning, sharp stabbing, or electrical shocks when walking, particularly when applying pressure when walking to the ball of the foot. In most instances, the patient clinical history supports that of a distal neuropathy particularly in the context of diabetes mellitus, glucose intolerance, exposure to chemotherapeutic agents, or other medications (among other possible causes). If burning pain is present a small fiber neuropathy must be considered and in pure small fiber cases the EDX studies are usually normal. However, when a large fiber neuropathy is present, other sensory modalities such as joint position sense and vibratory perception may be diminished with reduced/absent ankle reflexes (and possibly others, depending on severity). Atrophy of the EDB and other distal foot muscles may be present. In these patients, the plantar mixed nerve responses may be absent as the first/earliest manifestation of a distal polyneuropathy. Caution should be applied when interpreting these studies as the sensory responses are of low amplitude and may be affected by many technical factors and patients characteristics such as age, thickness of the skin of the sole of the feet/calluses, and leg/foot edema.

Pain/sensory disturbance/numbness in the foot may be a result of any lesion along the L5/S1 root or segment, lumbosacral plexus, or sciatic, peroneal (fibular) or tibial nerve pathway. Therefore, it is important to remember that all muscles below the knee are innervated via this pathway, with the sciatic nerve dividing at the upper angle of the popliteal fossa in its two main components: the common peroneal (fibular) nerve, and the tibial nerve. The sural nerve, a pure sensory nerve, is composed of fibers coming from the common peroneal (fibular) and tibial nerves via the lateral sural cutaneous nerve (LSCN) and the medial sural cutaneous nerve (MSCN), respectively.

The two main PNS condition causing foot pain/sensory disturbance/numbness in addition to the polyneuropathies are the tarsal tunnel syndrome, and a main trunk tibial neuropathy. It must be kept in mind however, that more common causes of foot pain are musculoskeletal including tendinitis, plantar fasciitis, calcaneus bone degenerative disease (also digital nerve neuromas), and the different causes of foot pain are usually predictable based on the particular area affected, including the anterior, middle and posterior foot regions.

In tarsal tunnel syndrome, the EDX findings are those of abnormal medial/lateral plantar mixed nerve responses (particularly prolongation of distal latency), with low CMAP in the distal tibial-supplied muscles of the lower extremities including the abductor hallucis (AH) and abductor digiti quinti pedis (ADQP). NEE usually demonstrates findings of axon loss in the AH and ADQP. One has to be careful with the electrodiagnosis of this condition given common confounding factors: many patients will have either reduced or absent medial/lateral plantar mixed nerve responses due to local technical or patient-related factors as aforementioned, and often there are "wear and tear" effects in the foot resulting in (mostly chronic) motor axon loss changes in the intrinsic foot muscles. Therefore, in our experience, despite many cases seen in our laboratory for assessment of such a diagnosis, most commonly, a distal polyneuropathy or an S1 radiculopathy is found when there is abnormality. In these cases, the EDX findings include normal sural sensory responses (given the lesion is distal to the tibial contribution to the sural nerve) and usually normal tibial-H reflexes (the H-reflex will be absent if an S1 root involvement is present). As Wilbourn stated, the NCS have the appearance of a severe axon loss lesion involving the S1/S2 root segments [16]. However, if the tibial lesion is proximal to the contribution to the sural nerve the sural nerve response may be normal (or just slightly low in amplitude) due to the possibility of a relatively larger peroneal (fibular) contribution. On NEE, all muscles supplied by the tibial nerve are affected including the tibialis posterior, flexor digitorum longus, AH and ADQP. The more proximal muscles innervated by the tibial nerve are spared including the gastrocnemius, biceps femoris-long head, and other S1-innervated muscles are also spared, namely gluteus maximus and biceps femoris-short head (peroneal (fibular)/S1 above the knee).

Radiculopathies

A common reason for electrodiagnostic consultation in our laboratory is neck or low back pain with radicular symptoms (defined as pain following its dermatomal distribution). However, many patients have pseudo-radicular symptoms due to degenerative disease of the facet joints, discs and other changes seen in spinal osteoarthritis, as well as narrowing of the lateral recesses and foramina, which can present a challenge to the treating physician. Some patients may develop a radiculitis as a reaction to an infectious process such as herpes zoster, borreliosis, sarcoidosis or Behcet's disease. In those cases, an electrodiagnostic study is pivotal in the assessment of patients with suspected radiculopathies. It may not only confirm the presence of a radiculopathy, but the site or level(s) of the lesion/process, the extent/degree of nerve damage, and the nature/pathophysiology of the lesion, i.e.: axon loss vs demyelinating, or a combination of both. Furthermore, it may help exclude a radiculopathy as the cause of the patient's symptoms and may help direct the treating physician to other possibilities or causes.

It is important to recognize a basic tenet of lesion location when assessing radiculopathies with nerve conduction studies. **The sensory nerve conduction responses are typically intact in radiculopathies**. The lesion or process is intraspinal or at the intervertebral foramen, therefore the lesion is proximal to the dorsal root ganglia where the bipolar sensory neuron body resides, resulting in normal sensory nerve conduction responses. However, the patient may complain of numbness, paresthesia or radicular pain, since the afferent pathway is still disrupted. A process distal to the dorsal root ganglia will result in axon loss sequela with reduced or absent sensory responses.

The motor nerve conduction studies may be normal in radiculopathies. However in advanced disease the motor NCS may demonstrate decreased amplitude of the compound muscle action potential recording muscles within the affected myotome.

The motor conduction velocities may be normal or demonstrate mild slowing in keeping with axonal loss. NCS (sensory and motor) are further useful to exclude mimickers of radiculopathies such as peripheral polyneuropathies and mononeuropathies.

The spinal roots divide into the anterior and posterior primary rami once leaving the intervertebral foramen. The posterior primary rami innervate the paraspinal muscles and other midline/truncal muscles and skin areas, and are very helpful in demonstrating the presence of an intraspinal lesion/process (e.g., when paraspinal muscles disclose active/ongoing axon loss changes). The anterior primary rami are the contributors to the plexi, and peripheral nerves of the extremities.

The needle electromyography is the single most important technique to demonstrate, when recording directly from muscle, the involvement of the motor fiber coming from the anterior horn cell. However, it is necessary when performing the NEE to assess multiple muscles belonging to the same myotome (common nerve root innervation), but of different peripheral nerve territories. Therefore, at a minimum and in its most simplistic form, a radiculopathy may be considered when abnormalities are found in two and preferably more muscles innervated by the same nerve root but different peripheral nerves, and normal findings are obtained in muscles supplied by normal adjacent roots. Commonly, an abnormality limited to one muscle is insufficient for diagnosis.

Again, it is important to keep in mind that intrinsic foot muscles, particularly in those older than age 50 years, may disclose normal "wear and tear" and traumatic "physiologic injuries". Accordingly, it is not infrequent to find a low/absent response recording the AH or EDB when stimulating the tibial or peroneal (fibular) nerves respectively, particularly in the elderly. Therefore, recording from the tibialis anterior muscle is recommended. It must be mentioned as well, recording from the tibialis anterior muscle while stimulating the peroneal (fibular) nerve is a must in patient presenting with foot drop (vide infra). Similarly, abnormalities during the NEE of such muscles, namely EDB and AH must be interpreted with caution. In fact, in some laboratories the AH and EDB are no longer examined in patients older than 65 years of age.

Although NEE abnormalities of the paraspinal muscles suggest a radiculopathy, it is a rather non-specific finding in certain circumstances. Paraspinal muscle NEE abnormalities may also be seen compressive myelopathies, anterior horn cell disease, syringomyelia, polio/post-polio, acute flaccid myelitis/myelopathy, spinal muscular atrophy, arachnoiditis and other spinal subarachnoid infiltrative disorders such as meningeal carcinomatosis, diabetes mellitus, porphyria, adult onset acid maltase deficiency, inflammatory myopathies, and as a sequela to laminectomy. Specific NEE findings may include fibrillation potentials, positive sharp waves, myotonic discharges, complex repetitive discharges and fasciculation potentials. On the other hand, the lack of abnormal NEE findings in the paraspinal muscles does not exclude the presence of a motor radiculopathy. Absent or abnormal sensory nerve conduction studies are expected when investigating plexus lesions (should disclose normal NEE findings of the paraspinal muscles). In many patients other comorbidities may be present making the coexistence of root involvement and processes distal to the dorsal root ganglia not an infrequent scenario.

It can be concluded that NEE is pivotal in confirming the presence of a (motor) radiculopathy, but goes further to disclose the underlying pathophysiologic process (such axon loss) and its severity, may help date the process as acute/subacute [especially presence of abundant fibrillation and/or positive sharp wave potentials (including in proximal muscles), commencing about 3 week after injury and remaining until ~8 months to a year after injury (with successful re-innervation); vs more chronic as demonstrated by the presence of long duration, high amplitude (+/−polyphasic) motor unit potentials—indicating collateral sprouting and re-innervation. NEE findings also help exclude muscle disorders—another cause of weakness that may appear on nerve conduction studies as reduced motor responses, with sparing of sensory responses.

Proximal Lower Limb/Anterior Thigh Weakness

Proximal lower limb/anterior thigh weakness may be another common reason for consultation. Frequently, the request is to exclude a proximal myopathy, however other conditions must be excluded such as anterior horn disease (MND), Diabetic lumbosacral radiculoplexus neuropathy (DLRPN) (also called diabetic amyotrophy), other lumbar plexus lesion, obturator and a femoral neuropathies [14, 16]. The process of bipedal motion is quite complex requiring stabilization of the hip, alternating anterior hip rotation, knee locking, anterior heel placement and foot propulsion. Among these, proximal leg weakness may manifest itself as inability/difficulty with getting out of a chair or a low car seat, or rising from a squatting position, as well knee-buckling. When present, this latter phenomenon usually indicates quadriceps muscle weakness (muscle innervated by the femoral nerve-L2, L3, L4 roots/segments—posterior division lumbar plexus). The obturator nerve—(L2–L3–L4 roots/segments—anterior division lumbar plexus) supply the thigh adductor muscles, and the femoral (plus more direct/proximal) motor branches also innervate the iliacus and psoas muscles—[(L1)L2–L3—(via lumbar plexus) for thigh flexion]. The sciatic nerve-[(L4)–L5–S1—lumbosacral trunk-plexus—tibial/peroneal (fibular) nerves]—innervate many muscles in the posterior thigh including the semitendinous, semimembranous, biceps femoris long and short heads, and all muscles below the knee.

When there is anterior thigh weakness or proximal lower limb weakness, it is difficult on clinical grounds alone to determine if the weakness is due to a plexus lesion, L2–L4 radiculopathy, or a femoral neuropathy. Furthermore, a myopathic process often cannot be completely excluded, especially if sensory symptoms are not apparent. Some features may indicate the lesion is proximal to the femoral nerve, including weakness of hip flexion (iliopsoas involvement); obturator nerve involvement via thigh adductor weakness. Involvement of muscles distal to the knee such as the tibialis anterior would suggest a more widespread process involving two or more nerves, or alternatively and more likely, involvement of the lumbar/lumbosacral plexus or even more proximally at the nerve roots. An important clinical observation would be the presence of lateral thigh sensory loss, which is usually indicative of involvement of the lateral femoral cutaneous nerve of the thigh (L2/L3—posterior plexus division).

A suggested EDX assessment of anterior thigh or proximal muscle weakness includes in addition to the standard lower extremity assessment (vide supra) the performance of femoral motor recording quadriceps (rectus femoris or vastus lateralis), and saphenous sensory studies bilaterally (though these responses are technically difficult to obtain in most cases). The NEE must include, in addition to the standard muscles aforementioned, study of the rectus femoris (or vastus lateralis), iliacus, and adductor longus (often useful to also study contralateral muscles).

Femoral mononeuropathies, regardless of etiology often have a similar appearance on EDX studies, i.e. low amplitude CMAP recording quadriceps, and decreased recruitment on NEE, with fibrillation and positive sharp wave potentials if there is active/ongoing denervation. It is important to be mindful of the context in which the suspected process presents to make the appropriate EDX correlation (for e.g. potential focal demyelination/conduction block in a patient with prolonged lithotomy position). It is also important to sufficiently study several adjacent non-femoral innervated muscles, for e.g. the tibialis anterior and adductor muscles and these should be normal to convincingly conclude on a femoral neuropathy. If these muscles are involved, then one has to make the appropriate conclusions of a plexus lesion, multifocal mononeuropathies or root involvement. An example for these latter findings or combinations of them will be diabetic amyotrophy (lumbosacral radiculoplexus neuropathy).

Foot Drop/Weakness

An important muscle to assess when a patient presents with foot drop is the tibialis anterior muscle (the major foot/ankle dorsiflexor). In most cases, the cause of foot drop is a L4/5 radiculopathy or common peroneal (fibular) neuropathy at the fibular head. However, this clinical deficit may also be seen in an anterior horn cell disorder such as a monomelic presentation of MND, a plexopathy, a sciatic mononeuropathy, an isolated deep peroneal (fibular) mononeuropathy, a distal polyneuropathy, neuromuscular junction transmission defect, or muscle disease [particularly distal myopathy or isolated TA myopathic involvement (rare)]. Non PNS causes of foot drop include a focal cortical cerebral infarction, and musculoskeletal disorders/deformities.

A suggested EDX assessment for foot drop in addition to the standard lower extremity assessment includes peroneal (fibular) motor responses recording tibialis anterior, and the superficial peroneal (fibular) sensory responses (bilaterally obtained, if necessary). On NEE, we add to the standard complement—the extensor halluces longus, tibialis posterior, peroneous longus, biceps femoris short head, and semitendinous (with corresponding contralateral lower extremity muscles typically examined when abnormalities are found).

Patients with common peroneal (fibular) neuropathy at the fibular head which commonly results in foot drop may have, according to Katirji and Wilbourn [17] four EDX presentations (see figure):

1. Partial or complete demyelinating block across the fibular head (seen in 30% of the cases)
2. Pure axonal loss, partial (with fascicular sparing) or complete (either seen in 50% of the cases)
3. Mixed demyelinating and axonal loss features (seen in 15–20% of cases)
4. A rare pure deep peroneal (fibular) neuropathy sparing the superficial peroneal (fibular) in less than 5% of the cases.

In those with a focal demyelinating process at the fibular head, they have normal peroneal (fibular) motor responses (recording TA and EDB) when stimulating below the fibular head, but significant drop in or absent amplitude when stimulating above the fibular head, and normal superficial peroneal (fibular) SNAP. In those with a pure axon loss lesion, there is decreased and/or absent motor responses along the peroneal (fibular) nerve path when stimulating above or below the fibular head, in addition to absent superficial peroneal (fibular) SNAP. Those with a mixed lesion will demonstrate low amplitudes of the CMAP recording EDB and TA, partial or total block when stimulating above the fibular head and low/absent superficial peroneal (fibular) SNAP. When the rare pure deep peroneal (fibular) neuropathy is present, there is a low amplitude of the CMAP recording EDB and TA, with normal superficial peroneal (fibular) SNAP.

In patients with an L5 radiculopathy, the most common process is axon loss, usually manifesting itself as a predominantly foot drop with involvement of the tibialis anterior muscle. EDX findings will include a low to unelicitable (when very severe) CMAP responses recording TA and EDB with normal response of the superficial peroneal (fibular) sensory nerve. On NEE, given that the lesion is at the L5 nerve root/segment, all muscles within this myotome will be affected, including those below the knee (common peroneal (fibular) and L5-tibial innervated muscles) and proximal L5 innervated muscles such as the gluteus medius and/or tensor fascia lata.

When a high sciatic neuropathy is suspected as the cause for foot drop, the peroneal (fibular) motor and sensory responses are usually more affected than the derivatives of the tibial nerve. Most lesions are of the axon loss type, with demyelinating lesions rarely being reported in this context. The NCS usually demonstrate decreased to unelicitable responses recording EDB and TA when stimulating the peroneal (fibular) nerve and low to absent SNAP of the superficial peroneal (fibular) sensory. The tibial nerve response recording AH may be normal or decreased in amplitude. It is important to remember that the sural nerve receives fibers from both the common peroneal (fibular) and tibial nerves, therefore the sural response may be low to normal as the sural nerve may be predominantly receiving tibial relatively unaffected sensory fibers. On NEE, the peroneal (fibular)-innervated muscles will typically be more prominently involved—including those supplied by the superficial peroneal (fibular) and deep peroneal (fibular) branches.

Generalized Weakness

Patients with motor neuron disease, neuromuscular junction transmission defects and myopathies are commonly referred to the EMG laboratory when generalized weakness is the main symptom. The clinical history and examination will usually guide the electrodiagnostician to the proper studies.

For those patients with suspected motor neuron disease, we recommend performing a "root search" protocol of the upper and lower extremity (including NEE of muscles which may be a part of a "split-hand" pattern), as well as NEE of the thoracic paraspinal muscles (usually mid and low levels). One may also perform post exercise testing recording APB or FDI to help exclude a neuromuscular junction transmission disorder. If the history suggests a neuromuscular junction transmission defect, we typically perform select motor/sensory studies in the upper and lower extremities such as sural, median motor and sensory, ulnar motor and sensory, and peroneal (fibular) motor. All these motor nerve responses will include a pre- and post-10 s of isometric exercise (particularly, if amplitudes are decreased at baseline). In addition, slow repetitive nerve stimulation of the peroneal (fibular) nerve recording TA, median nerve recording APB, spinal accessory nerve recording trapezius and facial nerve recording nasalis (when indicated, as with cranio-bulbar involvement) is usually performed. In patients suspected to have a myopathic disorder, the NCS usually comprise one motor and sensory response stimulating the median nerve, one motor response in the lower extremity (typically peroneal (fibular) motor recording EDB or TA if EDB abnormal) and a sural sensory response. F-waves of the tibial and median are also usually performed. Additional studies must be informed by the initial findings on these responses. For example, if the initial studies suggest the presence of a polyneuropathy, then additional NCS to complete a polyneuropathy protocol is usually pursued. The reader is referred to the Myopathy/Muscle Disorders chapter for further detailed discussion on this topic.

References

1. Aminoff MJ. Electromyography in clinical practice. 3rd ed. Baltimore: Williams and Wilkins; 1998.
2. Wilbourn AJ. How can electromyography help you? Postgrad Med. 1983;73(6):187–95.
3. Campbell WW. Essentials of electrodiagnostic medicine. Baltimore: Williams & Wilkins; 1999.
4. Neal PJ, Katirji B. Nerve conduction studies: practical guide and diagnostic protocols. AANEM; 2015. www.aanem.org
5. Wilbourn AJ. Nerve conduction studies. Types, components, abnormalities, and value in localization. Neurol Clin N Am. 2002;20:305–38.
6. Rubin DI. Needle electromyography. In: Rubin D, Daube J, editors. Clinical neurophysiology. 4th ed. Oxford: Oxford University Press; 2016.
7. Ferrante MA. EMG what we measure and what we do. AANEM 2012. www.aanem.org
8. Kim DH, Midha R, Murovic JA, Spiner RH. Kline and Hudson's nerve injuries. 2nd ed. Philadelphia: Saunders Elsevier; 2008.
9. Sunderland, Sydney. Nerves and nerve injuries. 2nd ed. New York: Churchill Livingstone; 1978.
10. Kline DG, Hudson AR. Nerve injuries. Operative results for major nerve injuries, entrapments and tumors. Philadelphia: W.B. Saunders; 1995.
11. Ferrante MA. Comprehensive electromyography with clinical correlations. Cambridge: Cambridge University Press; 2018.

12. Isley MR, Krauss GL, Levin KH, Litt B, Shieilds RW, Wibourn AJ. Electromyography/electroencephalography. SpaceLabs Medical. 1993.
13. Dumitru D, Amato AA, Zwarts MJ. Electrodiagnostic medicine. 2nd ed. Philadelphia: Hanley & Belfus, Inc; 2002.
14. Preston DC, Barbara E. Shapiro. electromyography and neuromuscular disorders. Clinical-electrophysiologic correlations. 3th ed. Philadelphia: Elsevier Saunders; 2013.
15. Kimura J. Electrodiagnosis in diseases of nerve and muscle. Principles and practice. 4th ed. Oxford: Oxford University Press; 2013.
16. Wilbourn AJ. Focal weakness, numbness or pain in the lower extremities. American Academy of Neurology. 49th Annual Meeting, April 12–17, 1997.
17. Katirji MB, Wilbourn AJ. Common peroneal mononeuropathy: a clinical and electrophysiological study of 116 lesions. Neurology. 1988;38:1723–8.

Atlas of Nerve Conduction Studies (NCS)

2

Nestor Galvez-Jimenez, John A. Morren, Alexandra Soriano, Karin Armstrong, Melissa Goldberg, Lourdes Gonzalez, and Dana Higginbotham

Introduction

There may be some acceptable variability in certain aspects of NCS, depending on the laboratory performing the testing. What is described in this chapter follows the methodology utilized in our laboratory, which conforms to what is generally considered standard practice in the field of electrodiagnostic medicine.

N. Galvez-Jimenez (✉) · A. Soriano
Braathen Neurological Center, Cleveland Clinic Florida, Weston, FL, USA

Cleveland Clinic Lerner College of Medicine of Case Western Reserve University, Cleveland, OH, USA
e-mail: galvezn@ccf.org; soriana@ccf.org

J. A. Morren
Neuromuscular Center, Neurological Institute, Cleveland Clinic, and Cleveland Clinic Lerner College of Medicine of Case Western Reserve University, Cleveland, OH, USA
e-mail: morrenj@ccf.org

K. Armstrong · M. Goldberg · L. Gonzalez
Neurophysiology Lab, Cleveland Clinic Florida, Weston, FL, USA
e-mail: armstrk@ccf.org; goldbem2@ccf.org; gonzall5@ccf.org

D. Higginbotham
Neurophysiology Lab, Neuromuscular Center, Neurological Institute, Cleveland Clinic, Cleveland, OH, USA
e-mail: higgind2@ccf.org

General Concepts

The performance of NCS is deceptively simple but the importance of standardization in key aspects across laboratories cannot be overemphasized. Accordingly, being consistent and attentive to ensure that the studies are always performed in the same fashion is crucial for reliable NCS results.

Most errors during NCS are caused by incorrect or inconsistent technical components. Otherwise, an anatomical variation may produce apparently spurious NCS results as well, so knowledge of these is also essential. Additionally, it is imperative to maintain the tested limb/region at the recommended temperature (above 32 °C for the upper extremities and above 30 °C for the lower extremities, measured at the dorsum of the hands and feet).

Filter settings are also important, though typically preset in modern machines (e.g. 1 Hz–5 kHz for compound muscle action potentials, 10 Hz–5 kHz for sensory nerve action potentials, 2 Hz–10 kHz for needle EMG, and 500 Hz–10 kHz for single fiber EMG).

E1: recording/active electrode. For motor NCS, this is on the motor point of the muscle (the end plate region). Note: E1 used to be referred to

N. Galvez-Jimenez et al. (eds.), *Electrodiagnostic Medicine*,
https://doi.org/10.1007/978-3-030-74997-2_2

as G1, but use of this term is now discouraged. The "G" designation referred to "grid" derived from the classic electroencephalography literature, but now obsolete.

E2: reference/inactive electrode. For motor NCS, this is usually on the tendon of the muscle.

Note: Similarly, E2 used to be referred to as G2, but this term is now discouraged.

Recorded responses are those obtained from E1 while E2 is silent. However, in some instances, E2 may be active due to inadvertent volume conduction.

The ground electrode should always be between the stimulation site and recording sites.

As previously discussed in Chap. 1, the expected response is that of a negative (upward) potential. For motor NCS, if there is a positive (downward) deflection preceding the negative deflection, is often because the E1 electrode is not adequately over the motor point/end plate region and its position must be adjusted until a negative first potential response is obtained.

Upper Extremities

Sensory NCS

Median Sensory Recording at Index Finger (See Fig. 2.1)

Anatomy: brachial plexus (lateral cord ← upper and middle trunk) ← (mostly) C6–7 dorsal root ganglia (DRG).

Position: Patient is supine with the forearm and hand supinated, resting completely on the bed.

Recording electrode location:

E1: Second metacarpo-phalangeal joint.
E2: Second Distal interphalangeal joint, 3–4 cm distally to E1.

Ground: Between stimulation and recording sites, at the dorsum of the hand.

Stimulation: At the wrist between the tendons of the flexor carpi radialis (FCR) and palmaris longus (PL), 13 cm proximal from E1.

Caveats/Notes: make measurements with fingers extended and abducted.

Median Sensory Recording at the Thumb (See Fig. 2.2)

Anatomy: brachial plexus (lateral cord ← upper trunk) ← (mostly) C6 dorsal root ganglion (DRG).

Position: Patient is supine with the forearm and hand supinated resting completely on the bed.

Recording electrode location:

E1: first metacarpo-phalangeal joint.
E2: first interphalangeal joint.

Ground: Between stimulation and recording sites, at the dorsum of the hand.

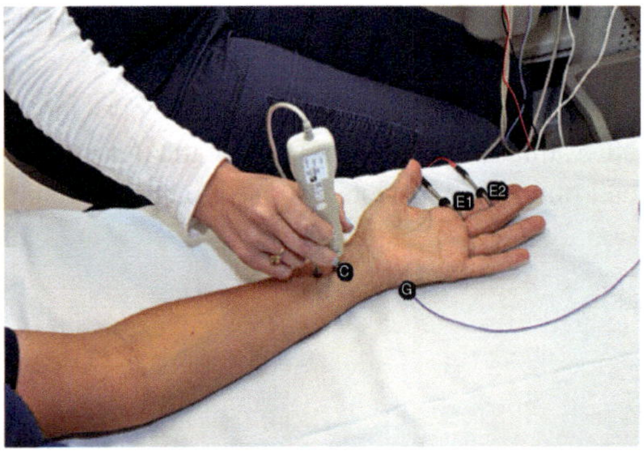

Fig. 2.1 Median sensory response—stimulating at wrist, recording index. C = Cathode; G = Ground

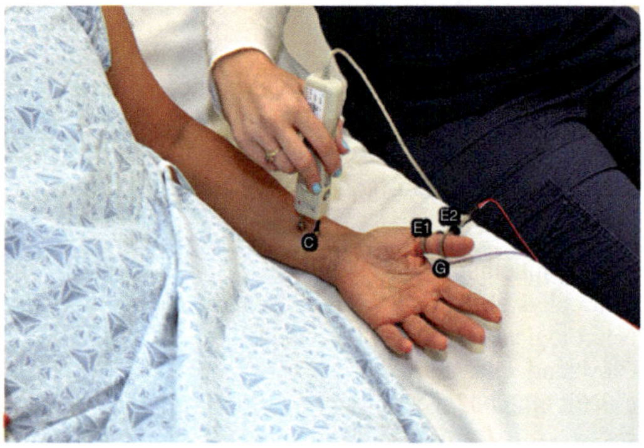

Fig. 2.2 Median sensory response—stimulating at wrist, recording thumb. C = Cathode; G = Ground

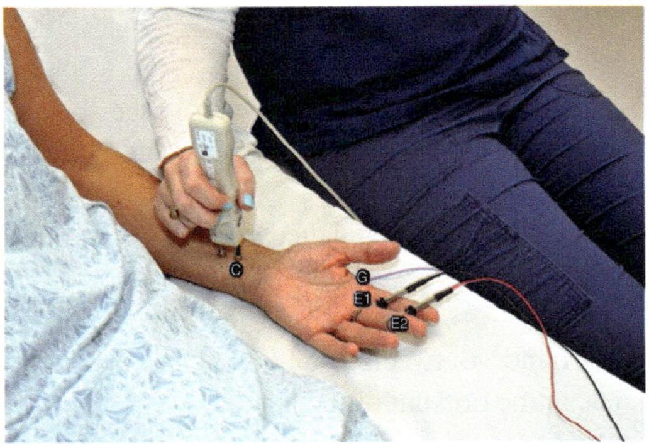

Fig. 2.3 Median sensory response—stimulating at wrist, recording middle finger. C = Cathode; G = Ground

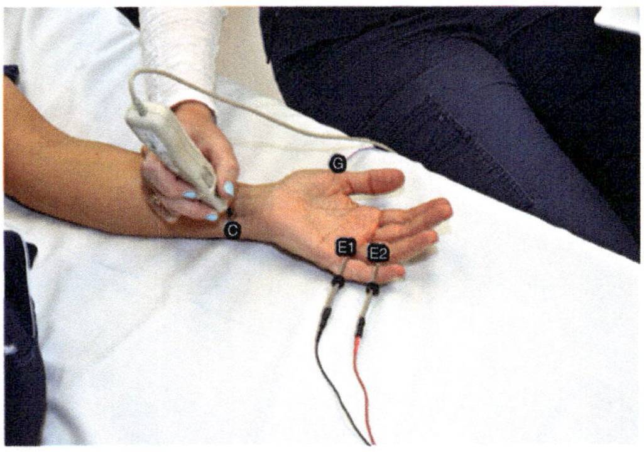

Fig. 2.4 Ulnar sensory response—stimulating at wrist, recording little finger (D5). C = Cathode; G = Ground

Stimulation: At the wrist between the tendons of the flexor carpi radialis (FCR) and palmaris longus (PL), 13 cm proximal from E1.

Caveats/Notes: make measurements with fingers extended and abducted.

Median Sensory Recording at Middle Finger (See Fig. 2.3)

Anatomy: brachial plexus (lateral cord ← middle trunk) ← (mostly) C7 dorsal root ganglion (DRG).

Position: Patient is supine with the forearm and hand supinated resting completely on the bed.

Recording electrode location:

E1: Third metacarpo-phalangeal joint.
E2: Third Distal interphalangeal joint, 3–4 cm distally to E1.

Ground: Between stimulation and recording sites, at the dorsum of the hand.

Stimulation: At the wrist between the tendons of the flexor carpi radialis (FCR) and palmaris longus (PL), 13 cm proximal from E1.

Caveats/Notes: make measurements with fingers extended and abducted.

Ulnar Sensory Recording at Fifth Finger (See Fig. 2.4)

Anatomy: brachial plexus (medial cord ← lower trunk) ← (mostly) C8 dorsal root ganglion (DRG).

Position: Patient is supine with the forearm and hand supinated resting completely on the bed.

Recording electrode location:

E1: Fifth metacarpo-phalangeal joint.
E2: Fifth Distal interphalangeal joint, 3–4 cm distally to E1.

Ground: Between stimulation and recording sites, at the dorsum of the hand.

Stimulation: At the medial wrist between tendons of the flexor carpi ulnaris (FCU) and flexor digitorum profundus (FDP), 11 cm proximal to E1.

Caveats/Notes: make measurements with fingers extended and abducted.

Dorsal Ulnar Cutaneous Sensory Recording at Dorsum of the Hand (See Fig. 2.5)

Anatomy: brachial plexus (medial cord ← lower trunk) ← (mostly) C8 dorsal root ganglion (DRG).

Position: Patient is supine with the forearm and hand pronated, resting completely on the bed.

Recording electrode location.

E1: dorsum of hand between the fourth and fifth finger web space.
E2: 3–4 cm distal to E1, at the base of the fifth finger.

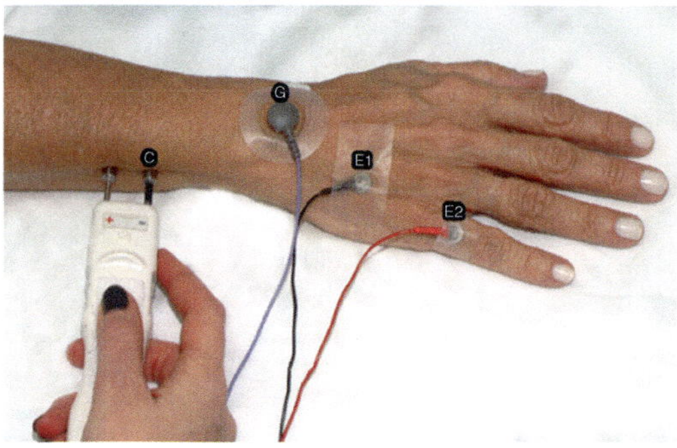

Fig. 2.5 Ulnar sensory response—stimulating at wrist, recording dorsum of hand (dorsal ulnar cutaneous sensory response). C = Cathode; G = Ground

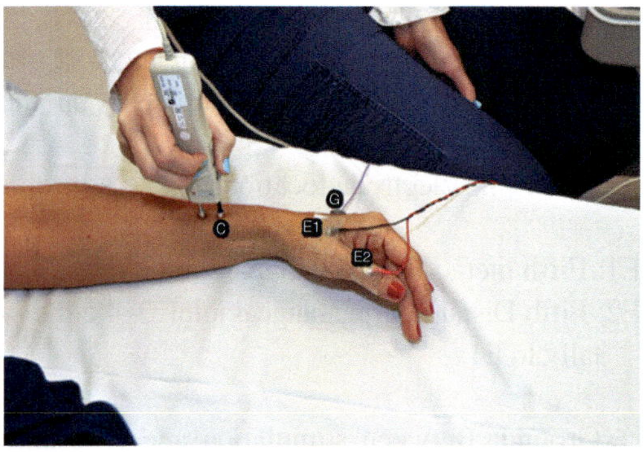

Fig. 2.6 Radial sensory response—stimulating at distal forearm, recording at first web space. C = Cathode; G = Ground

Ground: Between stimulation and recording sites, at the dorsum of the hand.

Stimulation: At the wrist, 10 cm proximal from E1 recording electrode, stimulating between the ulna and flexor carpi ulnaris (FCU) tendon, proximal to the ulna styloid.

Caveats/Notes: Helpful in determining ulnar neuropathy at the elbow, or most other lesions proximal to the wrist, as it is typically spared in an ulnar lesion at the wrist (Guyon's canal).

Radial Sensory Recording at Base of the Thumb (See Fig. 2.6)

Anatomy: brachial plexus (posterior cord ← upper and middle trunk) ← (mostly) C6–7 dorsal root ganglia (DRG).

Position: Patient supine with forearm midway between pronation and supination and resting completely on the bed.

Recording electrode location:

- E1: At the anatomic "V" or web space formed between the index finger and thumb metacarpals.
- E2: First digit interphalangeal joint, 3–4 cm distal to E1.

Ground: Between stimulation and recording sites, at the dorsum of the hand.

Stimulation: over the radius 10 cm proximal to E1.

Median Palmar Mixed Nerve (See Fig. 2.7)

Anatomy: brachial plexus (lateral cord ← upper and middle trunk) ← (mostly) C6–7 dorsal root ganglia (DRG).

Patient position: Patient supine with arm resting comfortably completely on the bed. Palm facing up and fingers abducted.

Important: This is an orthodromic nerve stimulation study.

Recording electrode location:

- E1: at the wrist crease between the flexor carpi radialis and flexor pollicis longus.
- E2: 3 cm proximal to E1, in a straight line.

Ground: dorsum of the hand.

Stimulation: in the palm, 8 cm distal to the E1 in the space between the second and third digits (second metacarpal interspace).

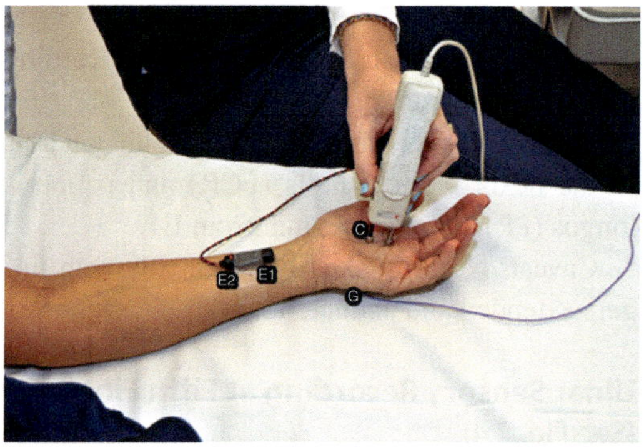

Fig. 2.7 Median palmar mixed nerve study—stimulating the median nerve at the palm, recording at the wrist. C = Cathode; G = Ground

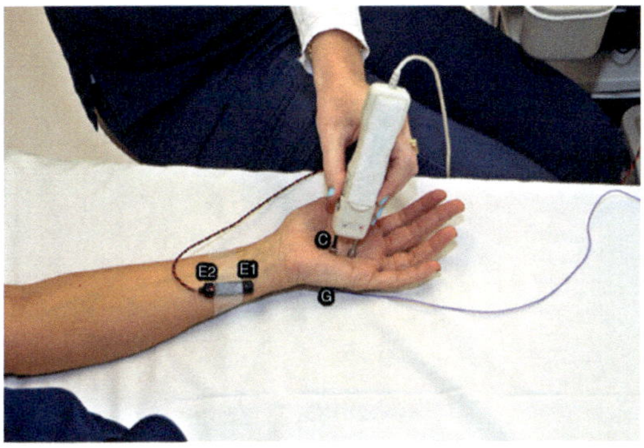

Fig. 2.8 Ulnar palmar mixed nerve study—stimulating the ulnar nerve at the palm, recording at the wrist. C = Cathode; G = Ground

Caveats/Notes: some laboratories use a standardized bar electrode (shown in picture).

Ulnar Palmar Mixed Nerve (See Fig. 2.8)

Anatomy: brachial plexus (medial cord ← lower trunk) ← (mostly) C8 dorsal root ganglion (DRG).

Patient position: Patient supine with arm resting comfortably completely on the bed. Palm facing up and fingers abducted.

Important: This is an orthodromic nerve stimulation study.

Recording electrode location:

E1: at the wrist crease between the flexor carpi ulnaris and flexor digitorum profundus.
E2: 3 cm proximal to E1, in a straight line.

Ground: dorsum of the hand.

Stimulation: at the palm, 8 cm distal to the E1 in the space between the fourth and fifth digits (fourth metacarpal interspace).

Caveats/Notes: some laboratories use a standardized bar electrode (shown in picture).

Medial Antebrachial Cutaneous Sensory Recording Medial Forearm (See Fig. 2.9)

Anatomy: brachial plexus (medial cord ← lower trunk) ← (mostly) T1 dorsal root ganglion (DRG).

Patient position: Patient supine with arm resting comfortably completely on the bed. Palm facing up/forearm supinated and mildly flexed at the elbow.

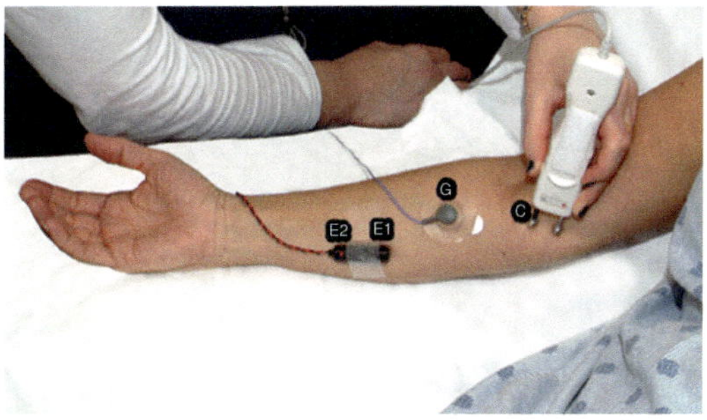

Fig. 2.9 Medial Antebrachial Cutaneous sensory response—stimulating anteromedial elbow, recording medial forearm. C = Cathode; G = Ground

Recording electrode location:

E1: anteromedial forearm 12 cm distal to the stimulation site/cathode (that is, point between the biceps tendon and the medial epicondyle).
E2: 3 cm distal to E1, in a straight line.

Ground: between the stimulation and recording sites.

Stimulation: find the midpoint between the biceps tendon and medial epicondyle, 12 cm proximal to E1.

Caveats/Notes: some laboratories use a standardized recording bar electrode (shown in picture).

Lateral Antebrachial Cutaneous Sensory Recording Lateral Forearm (See Fig. 2.10)

Anatomy: musculocutaneous nerve ← brachial plexus (lateral cord ← upper trunk) ← (mostly) C6 dorsal root ganglion (DRG).

Patient position: Patient supine with arm resting comfortably completely on the bed. Palm facing up/forearm supinated and mildly flexed at the elbow.

Recording electrode location:

E1: anterolateral forearm 12 cm distal to the stimulation site, which is a point lateral to the biceps tendon at the antecubital fossa.
E2: 3 cm distal to E1, in a straight line.

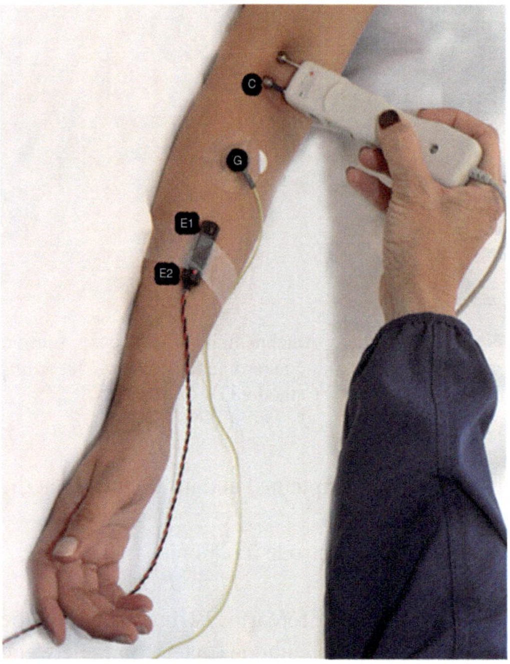

Fig. 2.10 Lateral Antebrachial Cutaneous sensory response—stimulating anterolateral elbow, recording lateral forearm. C = Cathode; G = Ground

Ground: between the stimulation and recording sites.

Stimulation: lateral to the biceps tendon at the antecubital fossa, 12 cm proximal to E1.

Caveats/Notes: some laboratories use a standardized recording bar electrode (shown in picture).

Motor NCS

Median Motor Recording at Abductor Pollicis Brevis (APB)

Anatomy/Innervation: Median nerve ← medial cord ← lower trunk ← C8-T1 spinal nerve roots.

Position: Patient supine with forearm supinated, extended at the elbow and resting completely on the bed.

Recording electrode location:

E1: Motor point, belly of the ABP.
E2: first metacarpophalangeal joint.

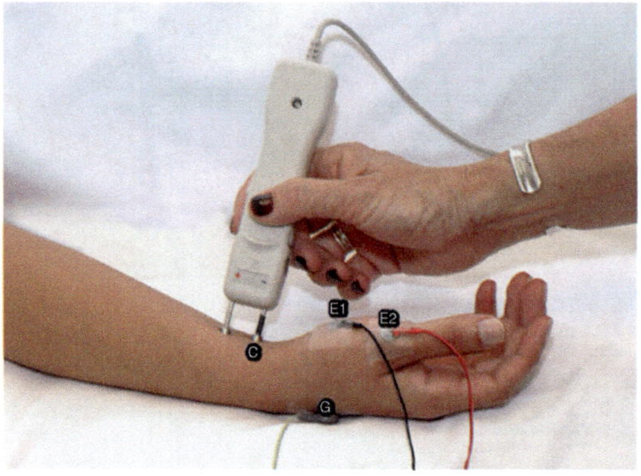

Fig. 2.11 Median motor response recording the abductor pollicis brevis, distal stimulation at the wrist. C = Cathode; G = Ground

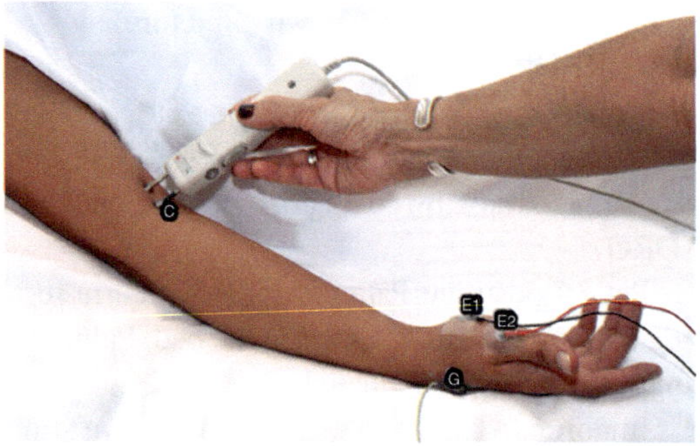

Fig. 2.12 Median motor response recording the abductor pollicis brevis, proximal stimulation at the elbow. C = Cathode; G = Ground

Ground: Between stimulation and recording sites—usually proximal dorsum of hand. Proximal palm may be used instead.

Stimulation:

Distal site: At the wrist between the tendons of the flexor carpi radialis (FCR) and palmaris longus (PL), 5 cm proximal from E1 (See Fig. 2.11).

Proximal site: Antecubital fossa over pulse of brachial artery, just medial to the biceps tendon (See Fig. 2.12).

Caveats/Notes: If the recorded response when stimulating at the antecubital fossa is larger in amplitude than that recorded when stimulating at the wrist, an anatomical variant/anomalous innervation such as a Martin-Gruber anastomosis

(MGA) must be considered (this type of MGA would involve cross-over median fibers innervating nearby thenar muscles which would typically be ulnar-innervated, like the deep head of flexor pollicis brevis and the adductor pollicis).

Ulnar Motor Recording at Abductor Digiti Minimi (ADM)

Anatomy/Innervation: ulnar nerve ← medial cord ← lower trunk ← C8–T1 spinal nerve roots.

Position: Patient supine with forearm supinated extended at the elbow and resting completely on the bed.

Recording electrode location:

E1: Motor point, belly of the ADM.
E2: Mid-portion proximal phalanx fifth finger.

Ground: Between stimulation and recording sites—usually proximal dorsum of hand. Proximal palm may be used instead.

Stimulation:

Distal site: At the wrist medial to the tendon of the flexor carpi ulnaris (FCU), 5 cm proximal from E1 (See Fig. 2.13).

Proximal sites:

- Below elbow: 4 cm distal to the ulnar groove/medial epicondyle on the medial forearm (See Fig. 2.14).
- Above elbow: 6 cm proximal to the ulnar groove/medial epicondyle, at the medial arm between biceps and triceps muscles (See Fig. 2.15).

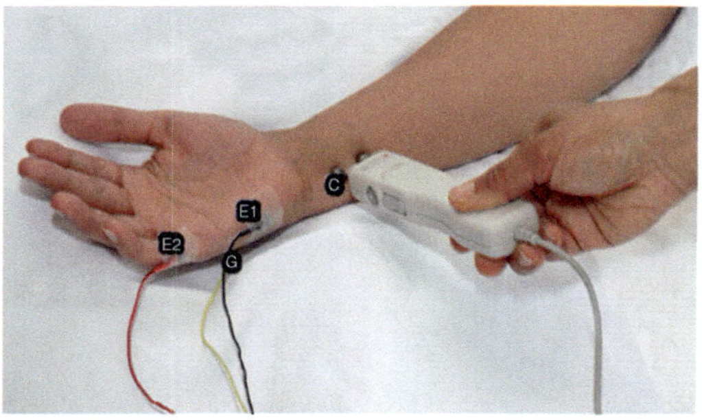

Fig. 2.13 Ulnar motor recording abductor digiti minimi, with distal stimulation at wrist. C = Cathode; G = Ground

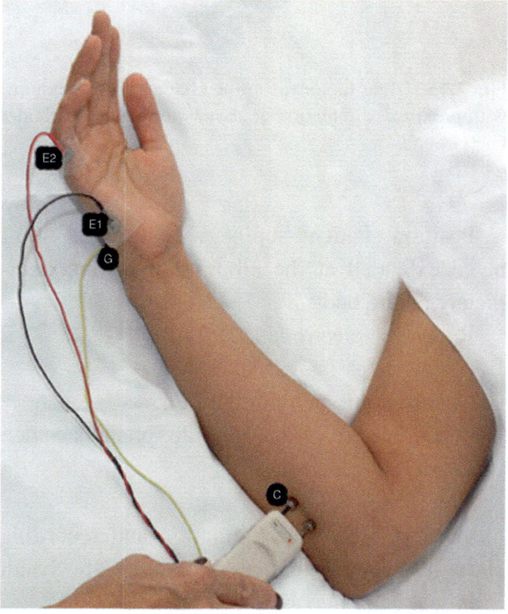

Fig. 2.14 Ulnar motor recording abductor digiti minimi, with proximal stimulation at below-elbow. C = Cathode; G = Ground

Accordingly, the total distance is 10 cm across the elbow between these two proximal stimulation sites. This measurement must be done following the contour of the medial aspect of the forearm and arm, and the elbow must be in a 90 degrees flexed position. This is done to avoid "bunching up" or redundancy of the ulnar nerve if the arm is extended, which could artifactually produce a decreased distance measurement (since this is done on the surface), resulting in spuriously reduced motor conduction velocity.

Caveats/Notes: If the recorded response when stimulating at the elbow suggest a conduction block between the elbow and the wrist, an anatomical variant/anomalous innervation such as a Martin-Gruber anastomosis must be considered (in this scenario, the crossover median-to-ulnar fibers are stimulated at the wrist, but not at the elbow sites).

Ulnar Motor Recording at First Dorsal Interosseous (FDI)

Anatony/Innervation: ulnar nerve ← medial cord ← lower trunk ← C8-T1 spinal nerve roots.

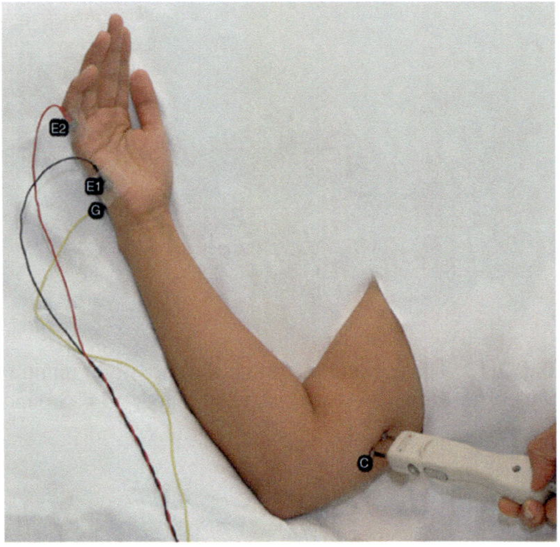

Fig. 2.15 Ulnar motor recording abductor digiti minimi, with proximal stimulation at above-elbow. C = Cathode; G = Ground

Position: Patient supine with forearm supinated extended at the elbow and resting completely on the bed.

Recording electrode location:

E1: Motor point, belly of the FDI.
E2: Midportion of the middle phalanx index finger.

Ground: Between stimulation and recording sites—usually proximal dorsum of hand. Proximal palm may be used instead.

Stimulation:

Distal site: At the wrist slightly radial to the tendon of the flexor carpi ulnaris (FCU), otherwise site similar to that used when recording the ADM (See Fig. 2.16).
Proximal sites:
Below elbow: 4 cm distal to the ulnar groove/medial epicondyle on the medial forearm (See Fig. 2.14—i.e. same stimulation site as when recording ADM).
Above elbow: 6 cm proximal to the ulnar groove/medial epicondyle, at the medial arm between biceps and triceps muscles (See Fig. 2.15—i.e. same stimulation site as when recording ADM).

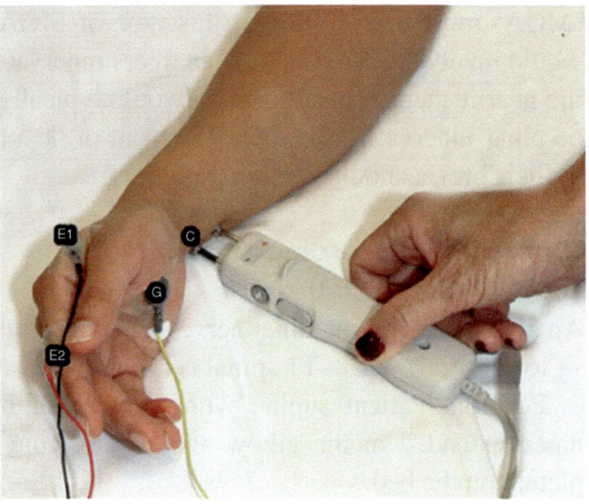

Fig. 2.16 Ulnar motor recording first dorsal interosseous, with distal stimulation at wrist. C = Cathode; G = Ground

Accordingly, the total distance is 10 cm across the elbow between these two proximal stimulation sites. This measurement must be done following the contour of the medial aspect of the forearm and arm, and the elbow must be in a 90 degrees flexed position. This is done to avoid "bunching up" or redundancy of the ulnar nerve if the arm is extended, which could artifactually produce a decreased distance measurement (since this is done on the surface), resulting in spuriously reduced motor conduction velocity.

Caveats/Notes: If the recorded response when stimulating at the elbow suggest a conduction block between the elbow and the wrist, an anatomical variant/anomalous innervation such as a Martin-Gruber anastomosis must be considered (in this scenario, the crossover median-to-ulnar fibers are stimulated at the wrist, but not at the elbow sites).

Radial Motor Recording at Extensor Digitorum (Communis) [ED/EDC]

Anatomy/Innervation: posterior interosseous nerve ← radial nerve, posterior cord ← middle and lower trunks ← C7–C8 spinal nerve roots.

Position: Patient supine with forearm pronated and elbow flexed and arm resting completely on the bed.

Recording electrode location:

E1: Motor point, belly of the EDC.
E2: posterior forearm about 5 cm proximal to dorsum of wrist or ulnar styloid.

Ground: on the forearm between the recording and stimulating sites.

Stimulation:

Distal site: At the elbow, at the groove between biceps and brachioradialis muscles (See Fig. 2.17).

Proximal sites:

Below the spiral groove: between the biceps and triceps muscles, usually performed only if there is a significant drop in amplitude when stimulating above the spiral groove recording EDC (See Fig. 2.18).

Above the spiral groove, between the medial and lateral heads of the triceps (See Fig. 2.19).

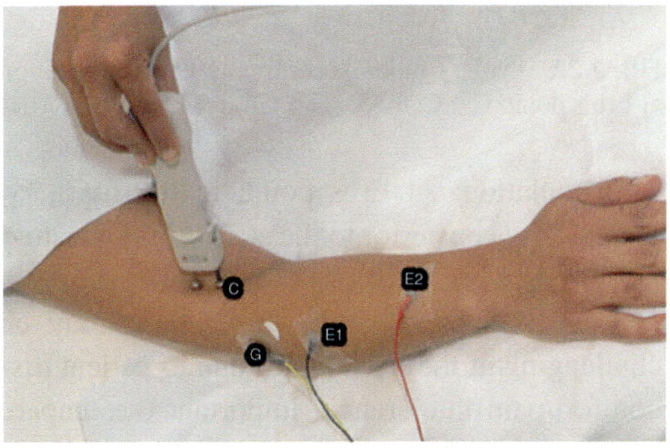

Fig. 2.17 Radial motor recording extensor digitorum, distal stimulation at elbow. C = Cathode; G = Ground

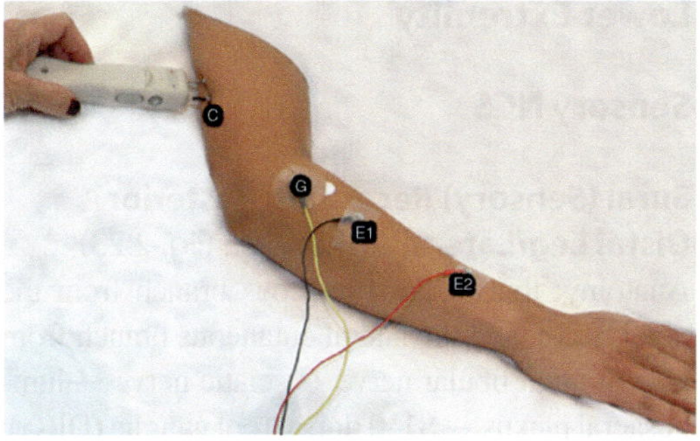

Fig. 2.18 Radial motor recording extensor digitorum, proximal stimulation at below-spiral groove. C = Cathode; G = Ground

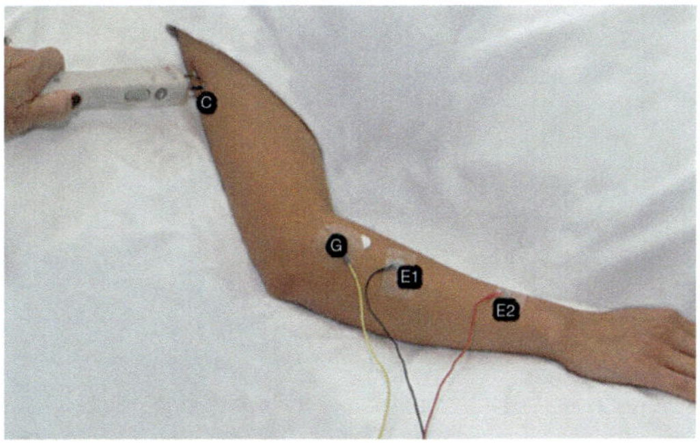

Fig. 2.19 Radial motor recording extensor digitorum, proximal stimulation at above-spiral groove. C = Cathode; G = Ground

Caveats/Notes: Do above spiral groove stimulation site first, and then do the below spiral groove stimulation site, only if there is a significant drop in amplitude (suggesting conduction block).

Musculocutaneous Recording at Biceps Brachii

Anatomy/Innervation: musculocutaneous nerve ← lateral cord ← upper trunk ← C5–C6 spinal nerve roots.

Position: Patient supine with forearm supinated and extended at the elbow and resting completely on the bed.

Recording electrode location:

E1: Motor point, belly of the biceps.
E2: distal upper arm over the biceps tendon and antecubital fossa.

Ground: Between stimulation and recording sites.

Stimulation:

Distal: At the axilla beneath the tendon of the short head of the biceps (See Fig. 2.20).

Proximal: At Erbs point, in the supraclavicular fossa posterior to the sternocleidomastoid muscle (See Fig. 2.21).

Caveat: Supramaximal stimulations may be challenging at the Erb's point due to patient discomfort/pain intolerance. Important to compare

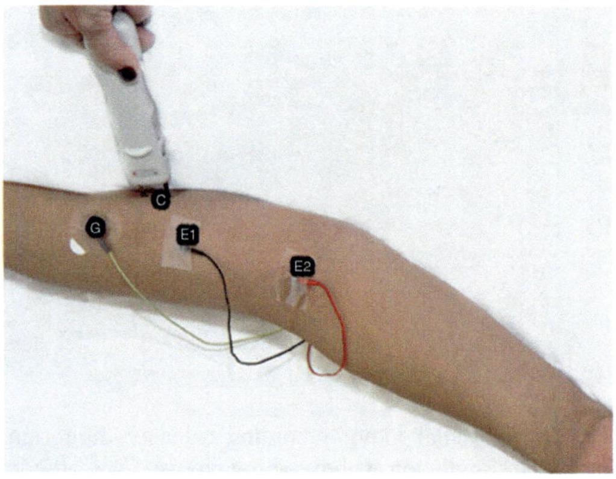

Fig. 2.20 Musculocutaneous motor recording biceps brachii, distal stimulation at axilla. C = Cathode; G = Ground

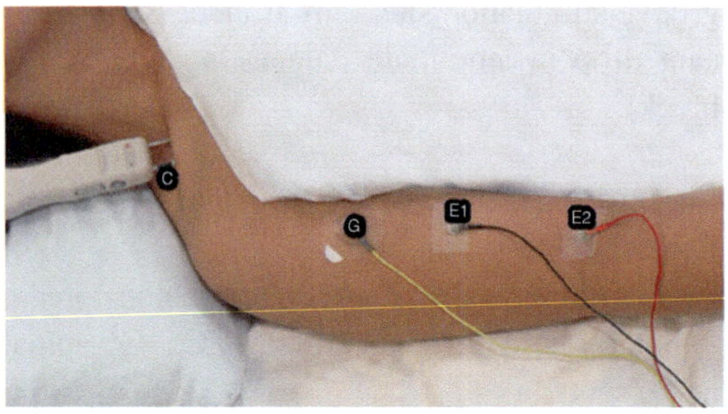

Fig. 2.21 Musculocutaneous motor recording biceps brachii, proximal stimulation at Erb's point. C = Cathode; G = Ground

amplitude and latency of response to the contralateral side.

Axillary Recording at Deltoid Muscle

Anatomy/Innervation: Axillary nerve ← posterior cord ← upper trunk ← C5-C6 spinal nerve roots.

Position: Patient is supine with forearm supinated, resting completely on the bed.

Recording electrode location:

E1: Motor point, belly of the deltoid (lateral head).
E2: distal upper arm, above elbow.

Ground: Between stimulation and recording sites, usually at the shoulder joint.

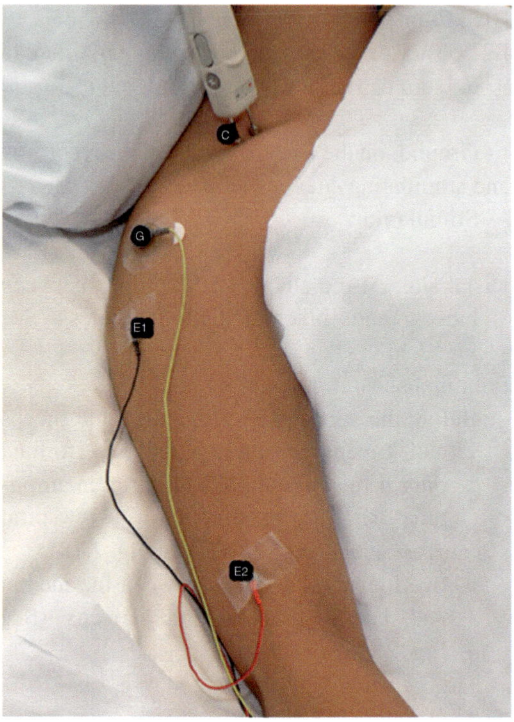

Fig. 2.22 Axillary motor recording deltoid, stimulation at Erb's point. C = Cathode; G = Ground

Stimulation: At Erbs point, in the supraclavicular fossa posterior to the sternocleidomastoid muscle (See Fig. 2.22).

Caveat: Supramaximal stimulations may be challenging at the Erb's point due to patient discomfort/pain intolerance. Important to compare amplitude and latency of response to the contralateral side.

Lower Extremity

Sensory NCS

Sural (Sensory) Recording Posterior Distal Leg/Lateral Ankle (See Fig. 2.23)

Anatomy: the medial cutaneous branch from the tibial nerve, and the lateral cutaneous branch from the common fibular nerve ← sciatic nerve ← lumbosacral plexus ← S1–2 dorsal root ganglia (DRG).

Patient position: Patient in a lateral decubitus position (contralateral limb down), with the knee

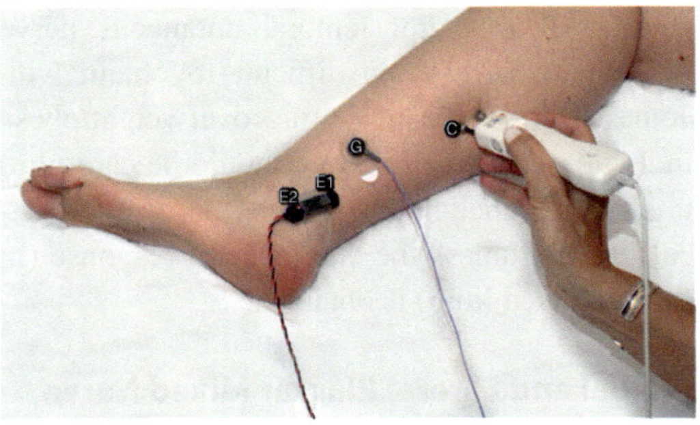

Fig. 2.23 Sural (sensory) recording at ankle/lateral malleolus, stimulating at distal calf. C = Cathode; G = Ground

slightly flexed and leg resting comfortably, completely on the bed.

Recording electrode location:

E1: postero-inferior to the lateral malleolus.
E2: placed on the side of the foot 3 cm distal to E1.

Ground: Lateral lower leg, between stimulation and recording sites.

Stimulation: Posterior aspect of distal leg, with stimulation electrode 14 cm proximal to the E1.

Caveats/Notes: some laboratories use a standardized recording bar electrode (shown in picture).

Superficial Peroneal (Fibular) Sensory Recording Dorsolateral Aspect of Ankle/Proximal Foot (See Fig. 2.24)

Anatomy: peroneal (fibular) nerve ← sciatic nerve ← lumbosacral plexus, L5 (>S1) dorsal root ganglion (DRG).

Patient position: Patient in supine with the leg resting comfortably, completely on the bed.

Recording electrode location:

E1: lower lateral leg, dorsum of ankle with E1 located halfway between lateral malleolus and extensor digitorum longus tendon.
E2: placed 3 cm distal to E1.

Ground: Distal lower leg, between stimulation and recording sites.

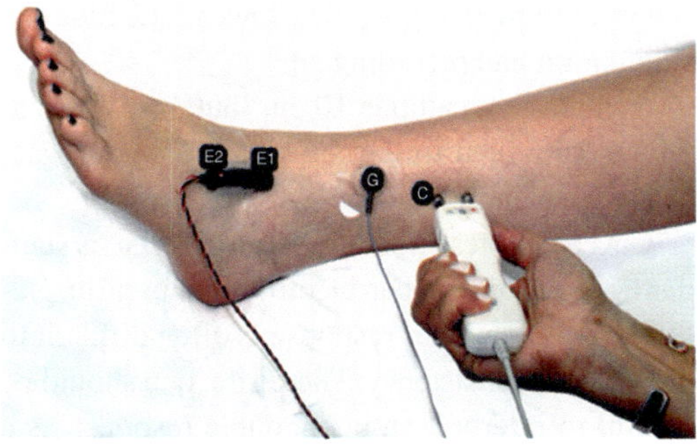

Fig. 2.24 Superficial peroneal (fibular) sensory recording dorsolateral aspect of ankle/proximal foot, stimulating lateral distal leg. C = Cathode; G = Ground

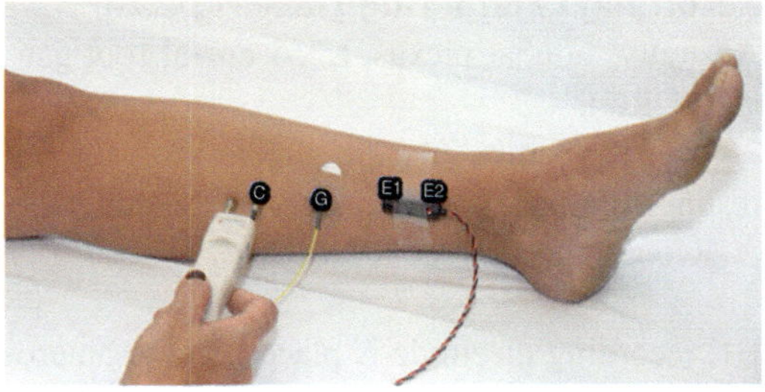

Fig. 2.25 Saphenous (sensory) nerve recording medial distal leg, stimulation at medial calf. C = Cathode; G = Ground

Stimulation: Placing stimulating electrode (cathode) in a straight line 10 cm (but may be up to 14 cm) proximal to E1.

Caveats/Notes: Some laboratories use a standardized recording bar electrode (shown in picture).

Saphenous Nerve Recording Medial Distal Leg (See Fig. 2.25)

Anatomy: femoral nerve ← lumbar plexus ← L3–L4 dorsal root ganglia (DRG).

Patient position: patient supine with the leg resting comfortably, completely on the bed.

Recording electrode location.

E1: medial leg/lower calf at ankle medial to the tibialis anterior tendon.
E2: 3 cm distal to E1, in the space between the medial malleolus and the tibialis anterior muscle tendon.

Ground: medial lower leg/lower calf, between stimulation and recording sites.

Stimulation: cathode 10 cm (but may be up to 14 cm) proximal to E1 between the medial gastrocnemius and the tibia.

Caveats/Notes: Some laboratories use a standardized recording bar electrode (shown in picture). The saphenous response is often difficult to obtain with consistency. Therefore, one should be careful to interpret an unelicitable response as a pathological finding, unless the contralateral response (in an unaffected limb) is obtained.

Lateral Femoral Cutaneous Nerve Recording Lateral Thigh (See Fig. 2.26)

Anatomy: lumbar plexus, L2–3 dorsal root ganglia (DRG).

Patient position: patient supine with the leg resting comfortably, completely on the bed.

Recording electrode location:

E1: recording electrode is placed on the anterolateral aspect of the thigh 12 cm distal to the stimulation site.

E2: 3 cm distal to E1.

Ground: lateral thigh, between stimulation and recording sites.

Stimulation: cathode is placed superior to the inguinal ligament about 1 cm medial to the anterior superior iliac spine (ASIS).

Caveats/Notes: Some laboratories use a standardized recording bar electrode (shown in picture). The lateral femoral cutaneous nerve response is also often difficult to obtain with consistency (especially in overweight/obese individuals). Therefore, one should be careful to interpret an unelicitable response as a pathological finding, unless the contralateral response (in an unaffected limb) is obtained.

Medial and Lateral Plantar Mixed Nerve Response Recording the Medial Ankle (See Figs. 2.27 and 2.28)

Anatomy: tibial nerve ← sciatic nerve ← lumbosacral plexus, S1 (>S2, L4–5) dorsal root ganglia (DRG).

Patient position: Patient supine with the leg resting comfortably, completely on the bed.

Orthodromic stimulation.

Recording electrode location:

E1: recording electrode is placed on the posteromedial aspect of the distal leg/medial malleolus in the hollow between the Achilles tendon and medial malleolus.

E2: 3 cm proximal to E1.

Ground: dorsum of foot, between stimulation and recording sites.

Stimulation:

Medial Plantar: cathode is placed 11–14 cm distal to E1 on the medial aspect of the sole of the foot.

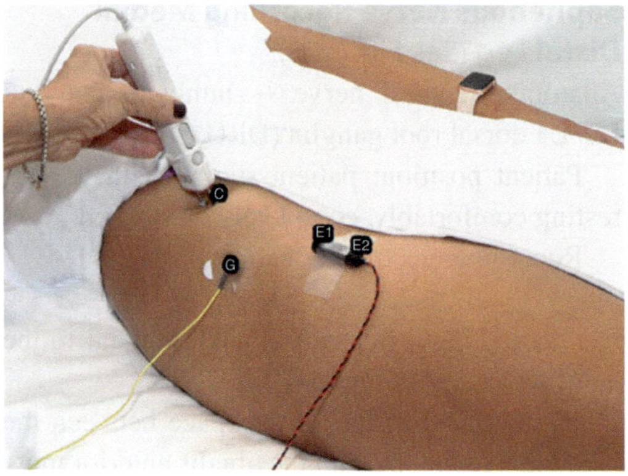

Fig. 2.26 Lateral femoral cutaneous nerve recording lateral thigh, with stimulation above inguinal ligament. C = Cathode; G = Ground

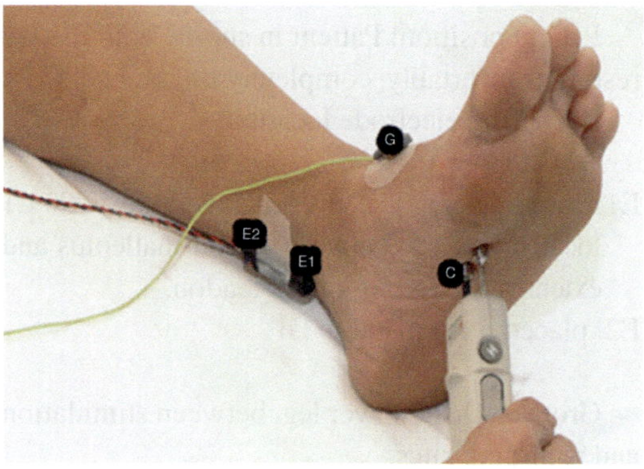

Fig. 2.27 Medial plantar mixed nerve response recording the medial ankle, stimulation at the medial sole. C = Cathode; G = Ground

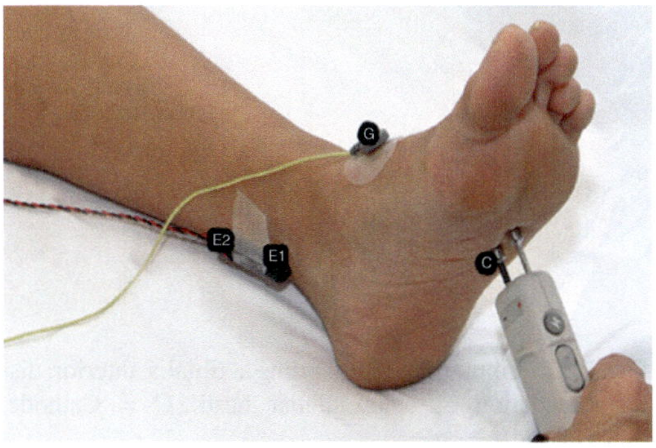

Fig. 2.28 Lateral plantar mixed nerve response recording the medial ankle, stimulation at the lateral sole. C = Cathode; G = Ground

Lateral Plantar: cathode is placed 13–14 cm distal to E1 on the lateral aspect of the sole of the foot.

Caveats/Notes: Some laboratories use a standardized recording bar electrode (shown in picture). Commonly, the plantar mixed nerve responses (especially the lateral response) may be unobtainable secondary to technical factors, especially if the patient is older than 50 years and/or has evidence of thickened skin of the sole of the foot. Therefore, one should be careful to interpret an unelicitable response as a pathological finding, unless the contralateral response (in an unaffected limb) is obtained. When these technical factors are less likely (especially in those less than 50 years old), absent plantar mixed nerve responses may be the earliest electrodiagnostic manifestation of a length-dependent large fiber polyneuropathy. However, the complete set of routine lower extremity studies should be performed and plantar mixed nerve responses interpreted in the context of other electrodiagnostic findings obtained and the clinical presentation.

Motor NCS

Peroneal (Fibular) Motor Recording at Extensor Digitorum Brevis (EDB)

Anatomy/Innervation: Deep Peroneal (fibular) nerve ← Common Peroneal (fibular) nerve ← Sciatic nerve ← Lumbosacral trunk and Posterior division of the Sacral Plexus ← L5-S1 spinal nerve roots.

Patient position: Patient supine with the leg resting comfortably, completely on the bed.

Recording electrode location:

E1: recording electrode is placed on the motor point, belly of the extensor digitorum brevis.

E2: distal to E1, at the fifth metatarsophalangeal joint.

Ground: dorsum of foot, between stimulation and recording sites.

Stimulation:

Distal Site: cathode is place on a straight line up 6–8 cm (usually 7 cm) proximal to E1, stimulating at the distal ankle crease over the peroneal (fibular) nerve (See Fig. 2.29).

Proximal stimulation is performed at two sites:

Below the fibular head: 2–4 cm below the fibular head in the lateral calf (See Fig. 2.30).

Above the fibular head: in the lateral popliteal fossa adjacent to the biceps femoris tendon, about 10–12 cm proximal to the below-fibular head stimulation site (See Fig. 2.31).

Caveats/Notes: Some laboratories only perform a below-fibular head site stimulation when there is evidence of a conduction block between the ankle and above-fibular head stimulation sites.

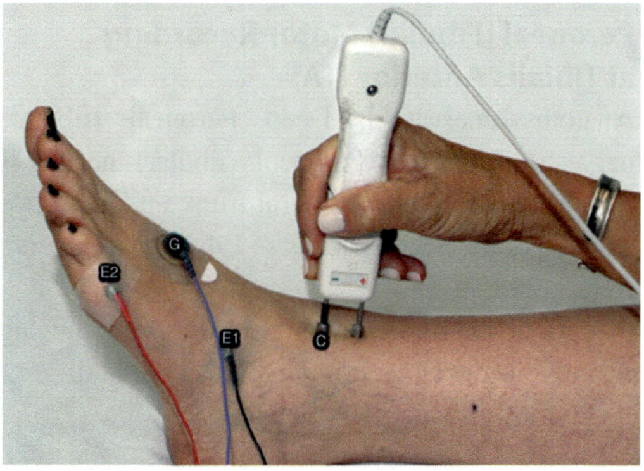

Fig. 2.29 Fibular motor recording at extensor digitorum brevis, distal stimulation at ankle. C = Cathode; G = Ground

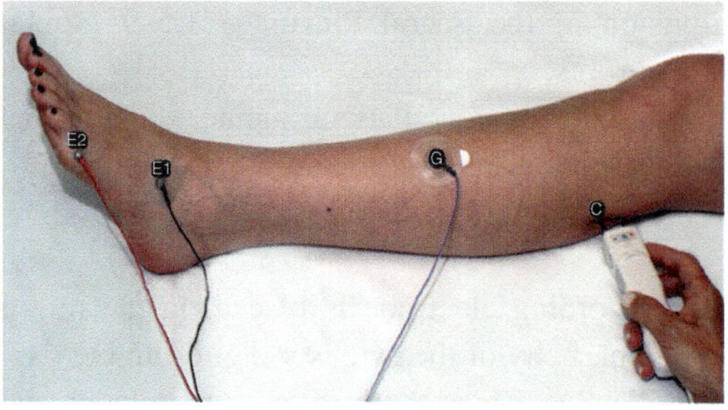

Fig. 2.30 Fibular motor recording at extensor digitorum brevis, proximal stimulation at below-fibular head. C = Cathode; G = Ground

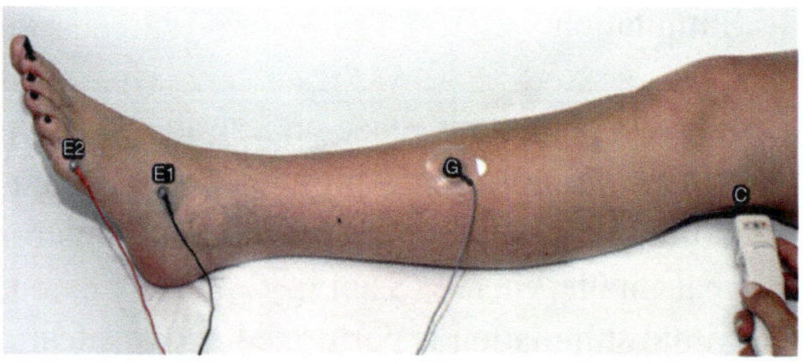

Fig. 2.31 Fibular motor recording at extensor digitorum brevis, proximal stimulation at above-fibular head. C = Cathode; G = Ground

If the amplitude of the CMAP is reproducibly higher at the below and above-fibular head stimulation sites (compared to that at the distal ankle stimulation site), then an accessory peroneal (fibular) nerve variant must be considered. This is typically confirmed by eliciting a significant response with stimulation at the posterior aspect of the lateral malleolus, while recording the EDB.

Peroneal (Fibular) Motor Recording at Tibialis Anterior (TA)

Anatomy/Innervation: Deep Peroneal (fibular) nerve ← Common Peroneal (fibular) nerve ← Sciatic nerve ← Lumbosacral trunk and Posterior division of the Sacral Plexus ← L4, L5 spinal nerve roots.

Patient position: Patient supine with the leg resting comfortably, completely on the bed.

Recording electrode location:

E1: recording electrode is placed on the muscle belly of the tibialis anterior muscle.

E2: placed anterior/top of ankle.

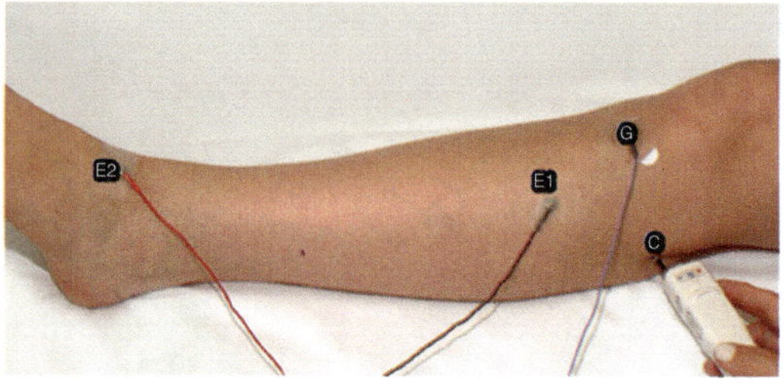

Fig. 2.32 Fibular motor recording at tibialis anterior, distal stimulation at below-fibular head. C = Cathode; G = Ground

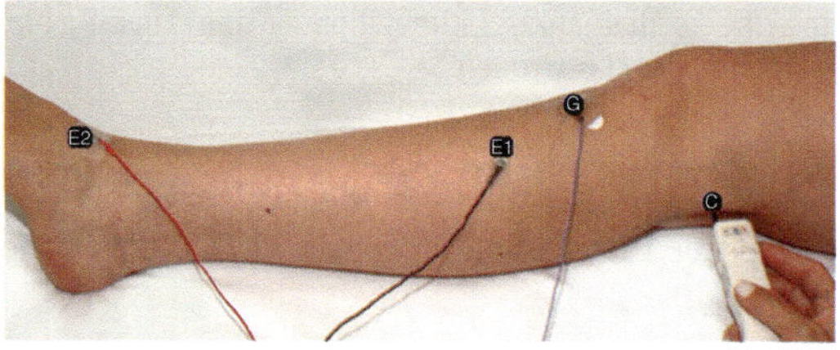

Fig. 2.33 Fibular motor recording at tibialis anterior, proximal stimulation at popliteal fossa/above-fibular head. C = Cathode; G = Ground

Ground: between stimulation and recording sites.

Stimulation:

Stimulation is performed at two sites:

Distal stimulation: 2–4 cm below the fibular head in the lateral calf (See Fig. 2.32).

Proximal stimulation: in the lateral popliteal fossa adjacent to the biceps femoris tendon, about 10–12 cm proximal to the below-fibular head stimulation site (See Fig. 2.33).

Caveats/Notes: Amplitude and configuration of the motor response may vary considerably depending on location of E1. Unless there is evidence of conduction block between the standard distal and proximal stimulation sites outlined, there is usually no need to stimulate further between these sites in the popliteal fossa.

Tibial Motor Recording at Abductor Hallucis (AH)

Anatomy/Innervation: Medial Plantar nerve ← Tibial nerve ← Sciatic nerve ← Anterior division of the Sacral Plexus, S1 > S2 spinal nerve roots.

Patient position: patient supine with the leg resting comfortably, completely on the bed.

Recording electrode location:

E1: recording electrode is placed on AH muscle belly on the medial aspect of the plantar arch, 1 cm distal to the prominence of the navicular bone.
E2: base of great toe, at the first metatarsophalangeal joint.

Ground: dorsum of foot, between stimulation and recording sites.

Stimulation:

Distal site: 8 cm proximal to E1 at the hollow space between the medial malleolus and Achilles tendon (See Fig. 2.34).
Proximal site: lateral aspect of the popliteal fossa, at the level that corresponds to the lower border of the kneecap (See Fig. 2.35).

Caveats/Notes: Proximal stimulation may be difficult to perform in some individuals with an abundant popliteal fat pad, hence firm pressure and higher stimulation intensity may be needed (sometimes associated with marked discomfort). Commonly, a significant drop in amplitude from the proximal stimulation site (compared to that obtained at the distal/ankle stimulation site) is noted. Accordingly, caution must be applied to not overcall a partial/incomplete conduction block in this scenario (typically, an amplitude drop of up to 50% may be dismissed).

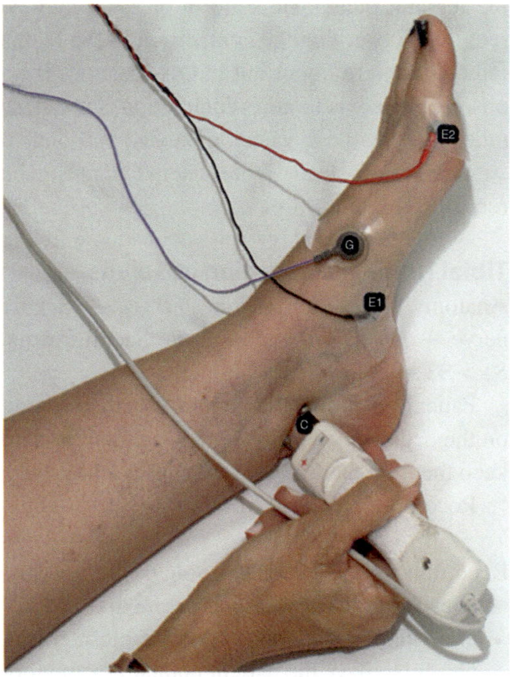

Fig. 2.34 Tibial motor recording abductor hallucis, distal stimulation at medial ankle. C = Cathode; G = Ground

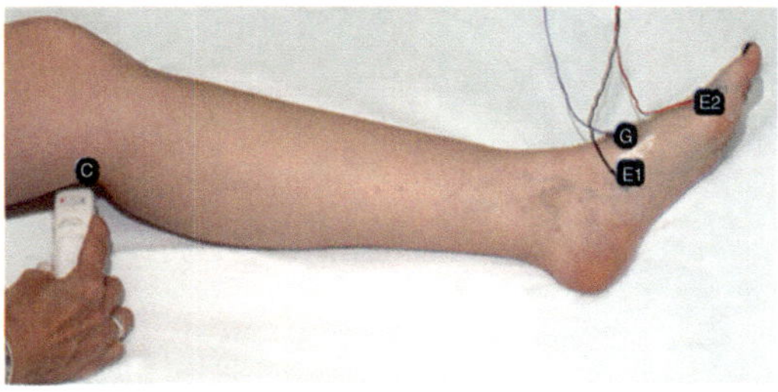

Fig. 2.35 Tibial motor recording abductor hallucis, proximal stimulation at popliteal fossa. C = Cathode; G = Ground

Tibial Motor Recording at Abductor Digiti Quinti Pedis (ADQP)

Anatomy/Innervation: Lateral Plantar nerve ← Tibial nerve ← Sciatic nerve ← Anterior division of the Sacral Plexus, S1 > S2 spinal nerve roots.

Patient position: Patient supine with the leg resting comfortably, completely on the bed.

Recording electrode location:

E1: recording electrode is placed on ADQP muscle belly—about mid-distance between the lower edge of the lateral malleolus and the lateral border of the foot.
E2: little toe, at the fifth metatarsophalangeal joint.

Ground: dorsum of foot, between stimulation and recording sites.

Stimulation:

Distal site: 8 cm proximal to E1 at the hollow space between the medial malleolus and Achilles tendon (See Fig. 2.36).
Proximal site: lateral aspect of the popliteal fossa, at the level that corresponds to the lower bor-

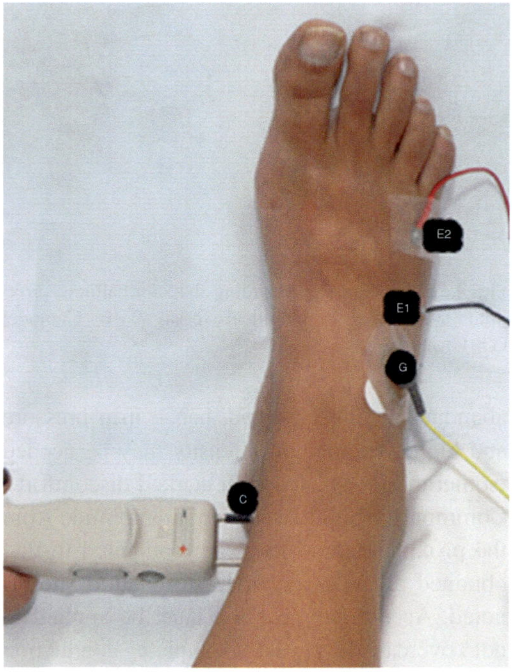

Fig. 2.36 Tibial motor recording abductor digiti quinti pedis, distal stimulation at medial ankle (proximal stimulation at popliteal fossa is identical to that for abductor hallucis). C = Cathode; G = Ground

der of the kneecap (See Fig. 2.35—i.e. same proximal stimulation site when recording AH).

Caveats/Notes: Proximal stimulation may be difficult to perform in some individuals with an abundant popliteal fat pad, hence firm pressure and higher stimulation intensity may be needed (sometimes associated with marked discomfort).

Femoral Motor Recording at Rectus Femoris

Anatomy/Innervation: Femoral nerve ← Posterior division of the Lumbar Plexus ← (L2)L3-L4 spinal nerve roots.

Patient position: Patient supine with the leg resting comfortably, completely on the bed.

Recording electrode location:

E1: recording electrode is placed over the belly of the rectus femoris in the anterior thigh, approximately at mid-point between the hip and knee joints.

E2: tendinous portion just above the knee.

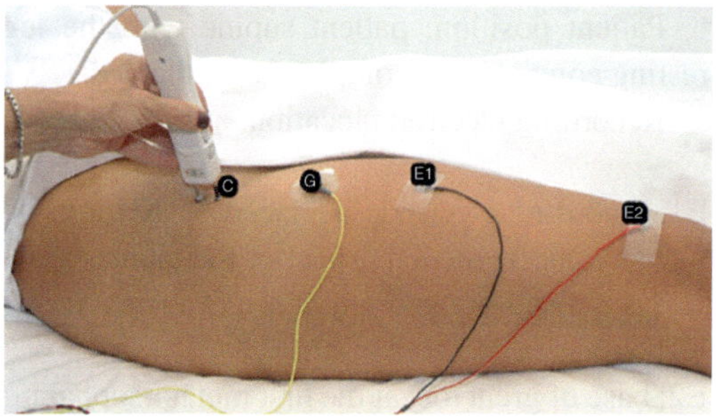

Fig. 2.37 Femoral motor recording at rectus femoris, stimulation at just below inguinal ligament. C = Cathode; G = Ground

Ground: proximal thigh, between stimulation and recording sites.

Stimulation: cathode is place below the inguinal ligament at the inguinal crease, just lateral to the femoral pulse point (See Fig. 2.37).

Caveat: Effective stimulation may be difficult to perform in some larger individuals due to tissue impediment (including difficulty palpating the femoral pulse). Hence firm pressure may be required. Observing the contraction of the rectus femoris is more important in this scenario. If no observable rectus femoris contraction is noted, or other muscles (e.g. vastus medialis) respond to stimulation instead, the cathode must be repositioned.

Tibial H-Reflex Recording at Soleus

Anatomy/Innervation: Tibial nerve ← Sciatic nerve ← Anterior division of the Sacral Plexus, S1 > S2 spinal nerve roots.

Patient position: The patient should be prone on the bed, using a pillow or similar item to help keep the limb comfortable during the study.

Recording electrode location:

Recording: E1 is placed at soleus muscle, just over the point in between the medial and lateral heads of the gastrocnemius muscle. It is helpful to have the patient plantar flex the foot to help with delineating space just below the separation of the two heads of the gastrocnemius muscle. The E1 electrode must be placed over this space.

Reference: E2 is placed in distal leg, typically above or at the Achilles tendon (usually 10–15 cm distal to E1).

Ground: Proximal to E1 on the leg below the knee, between stimulation and recording sites.

Stimulating: mid-popliteal fossa (over the popliteal pulse), with the cathode positioning reversed/polarity of the stimulator reversed, so that the cathode is effectively proximal to the anode in the popliteal fossa (See Fig. 2.38).

Caveats/Notes: The tibial H-reflex response usually has a latency between 25 and 35 ms.

The H-response/reflex begins to be observed before the "M" or muscle response.

As the intensity of the H-reflex stimulation increases, the M response increases and the H-response decreases until the H-response is no longer obtainable.

The tibial H-reflex is commonly absent after age 60, after lumbosacral spine surgeries, proximal (e.g. root-level) demyelination injury, axon-loss radiculopathies, and large fiber polyneuropathies [loss of the sensory (afferent) and/or motor (efferent) volley]. Therefore, this response provides a very sensitive evaluation of those S1 > S2/tibial sensory fibers that pass through the popliteal fossa.

The tibial H-reflex is affected by both axon loss and demyelination processes along the S1 > S2/tibial nerve fiber pathway from the popliteal fossa to the spinal cord, including the preganglionic sensory root segment.

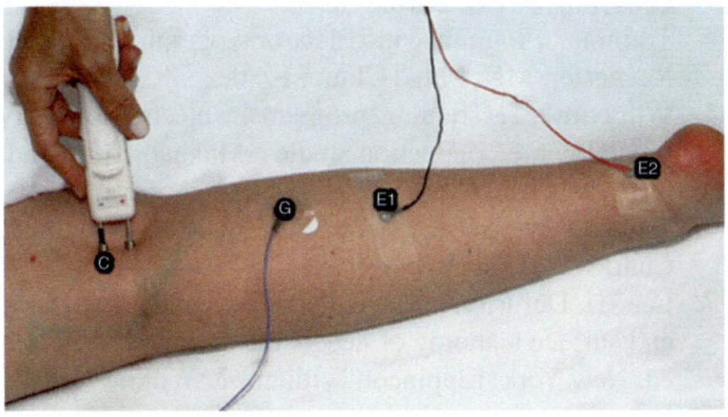

Fig. 2.38 Tibial H-Reflex recording at Soleus. C = Cathode; G = Ground

Although a bilaterally absent tibial H-reflex response may confer less diagnostic yield in the work-up of a focal lesion/process, reduction or absence of the response with preservation on the contralateral/unaffected side is diagnostically valuable.

The lack of proper positioning and patient relaxation commonly results in an absent/suboptimal response.

Spinal Accessory Motor Recording at Trapezius

Anatomy/Innervation: spinal accessory nerve ← C3&C4 spinal nerves.

Patient position: Patient supine with arm resting comfortably, completely on the bed.

Recording electrode location:

E1: Belly of the (upper) trapezius muscle.

E2: placed on top of the shoulder (over glenohumeral joint).

Ground: upper back, between stimulation and recording sites.

Stimulation: lateral to the sternocleidomastoid muscle.

This setup can be used during the repetitive nerve stimulation protocol, in the work-up of a neuromuscular junction transmission disorder (See Fig. 2.39).

Caveats/Notes: Some laboratories may use a standardized bar electrode connected to the hand-held stimulator prongs via an adapter (shown in picture).

Facial Motor Recording at Nasalis

Anatomy/Innervation: Facial nerve (cranial nerve VII) originates from the union of the axons coming from the facial motor nucleus (primarily motor fibers for facial expression muscles) and the nervus intermedius (giving parasympathetic, taste, and non-taste sensory fibers). The zygomatic branch innervates the nasalis muscle.

Patient position: Patient supine, semi-recumbent.

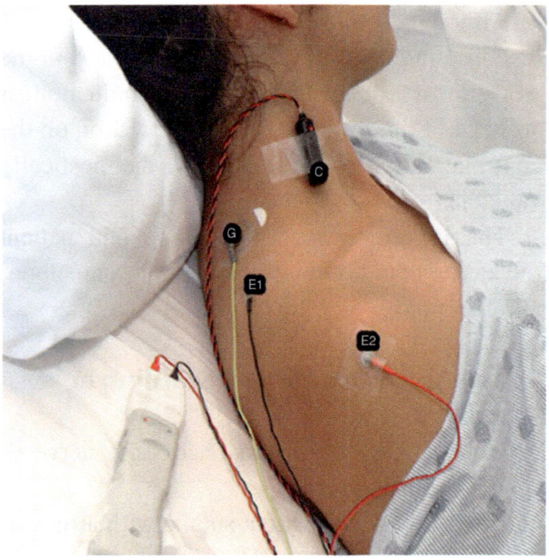

Fig. 2.39 Spinal accessory motor recording at trapezius, stimulation lateral to the sternocleidomastoid muscle. C = Cathode; G = Ground

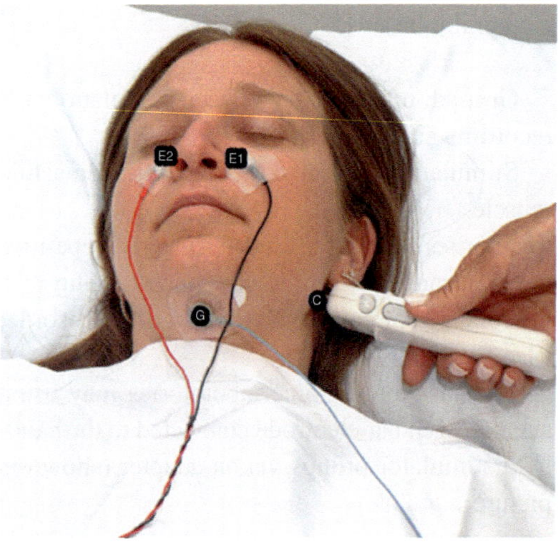

Fig. 2.40 Facial motor recording at nasalis, stimulation at anterior mastoid process. C = Cathode; G = Ground

Recording electrode location:

E1: recording electrode is placed on the nasalis muscle (immediately lateral to mid-nose) bilaterally.
E2: placed at the same location contralaterally.

Ground: under the chin (shown in picture), or forehead.

Stimulation: cathode is place just below the ear and anterior to the mastoid process (See Fig. 2.40).

Caveat: Disposable electrodes may be used for facial nerve conduction studies. In a similar manner, other facial muscles may be used for recording purposes. However, each laboratory must ensure technique consistency for results reliability, reproducibility, and comparison purposes.

The nasalis (shown), frontalis, zygomaticus, orbicularis oris, orbicularis oculi, buccinators or quadratus labii superioris (levator labii superioris), and mentalis muscles may all be target muscles from which the facial CMAP response may be recorded.

The chosen muscle will depend on the clinical context and indication, determined on a case-by-case basis.

Suboptimal placement of the stimulating electrode may result in an initial positive deflection in the motor response. The appropriate motor response consists of an initial negative deflection.

Suggested Reading

1. Kubhare D, Robinson L, Buschbacher R, editors. Buschbacher's manual of nerve conduction studies. 3rd ed. New York: Demos Medical; 2016.
2. Neal PJ, Katirji B. Nerve conduction studies. Practical guide and diagnostic protocols. AANEM. 2011.
3. Ferrante M. Comprehensive electromyography with clinical correlations. Cambridge: Cambridge University Press; 2018.
4. Training Programs in Electromyography Manual. Rochester, MN: Mayo Clinic; 1980.
5. Wilbourn AJ. Training program in electromography special nerve conduction studies. Manual. Cleveland, OH: Cleveland Clinic; 1992.
6. Hammer K. Nerve conduction studies. Springfield: Charles C. Thomas Pub; 1981.
7. Lee HJ, DeLisa JA. Manual of nerve conduction study and surface anatomy of needle electromyography. 4th ed. New York: Lippincott Williams & Wilkins; 2005.

3 Atlas of Needle Electrode Examination (NEE)

Nestor Galvez-Jimenez, John A. Morren, and Alexandra Soriano

The needle electrode examination (NEE) requires that electromyographers employ a bedside manner and skill set that minimize patient anxiety and discomfort, as well as maximize patient cooperation. With experience and the appropriate diligence, the NEE will model a successful combination of art and science in electrodiagnostic medicine.

It is necessary to have a replete knowledge of musculoskeletal anatomy as it pertains to "surface localization" which facilitates correct needle insertion point positions (using several surface landmarks, including bony prominences). However it is also important to be versed in cross-sectional anatomy to aid in the safe and adequate placement of the needle (particularly the recording tip) during the study. Providing clear, precise instructions to the patient, with appropriate body and limb positioning are also key to successful NEE, as are several measures to reduce complications like appropriate skin cleaning/antisepsis, electrical grounding, and puncture site compression post needle removal. Depending on the muscle being studied, there may be several specific caveats, confounders, precautions and tips to keep in mind to ensure successful examination.

Upper Extremity

Abductor Pollicis Brevis (APB)

Innervation: Median nerve ← medial cord ← lower trunk ← C8–**T1** spinal nerve roots.

Activation: With forearm and hand supinated have patient abduct the thumb.

Needle placement: Into the thenar eminence, anterolateral to the mid-point of first metacarpal (See Fig. 3.1).

Indications include: Carpal tunnel syndrome, proximal median neuropathies, lower trunk/ medial cord plexopathy, thoracic outlet syndrome, C8–T1 radiculopathy.

Notes and precautions/confounders: Best muscle to sample distal to the carpal tunnel. This

N. Galvez-Jimenez (✉) · A. Soriano
Braathen Neurological Center, Cleveland Clinic Florida, Weston, FL, USA

Cleveland Clinic Lerner College of Medicine of Case Western Reserve University, Cleveland, OH, USA
e-mail: galvezn@ccf.org; soriana@ccf.org

J. A. Morren
Neuromuscular Center, Neurological Institute, Cleveland Clinic, and Cleveland Clinic Lerner College of Medicine of Case Western Reserve University, Cleveland, OH, USA
e-mail: morrenj@ccf.org

N. Galvez-Jimenez et al. (eds.), *Electrodiagnostic Medicine*,
https://doi.org/10.1007/978-3-030-74997-2_3

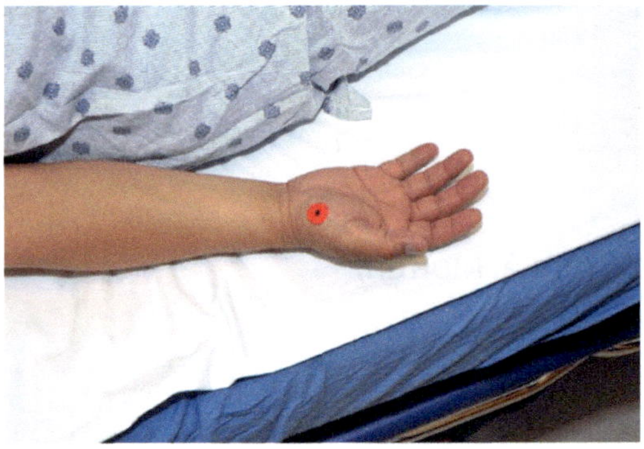

Fig. 3.1 Needle insertion site (black dot in center of red circle) for needle electrode examination of the abductor pollicis brevis

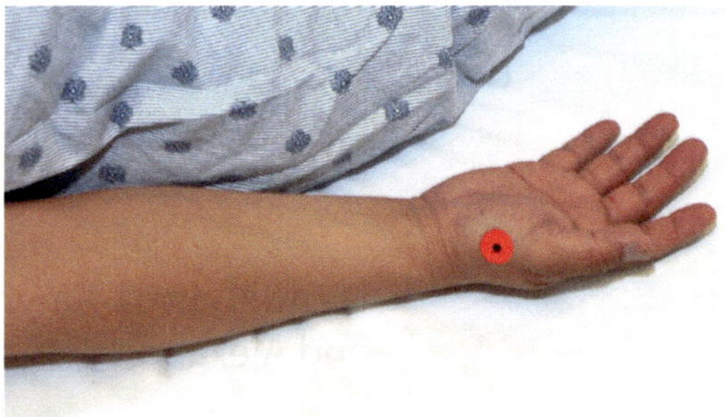

Fig. 3.2 Needle insertion site (black dot in center of red circle) for needle electrode examination of the opponens pollicis

muscle is spared in anterior interosseous syndrome. Tends to be difficult to tolerate due to exquisite tenderness in some.

Opponens Pollicis

Innervation: Median nerve ← medial cord ← lower trunk ← C8–T1 spinal nerve roots.

Activation: With forearm and hand supinated have patient oppose the thumb to the little finger.

Needle placement: Into the lateral thenar eminence (lateral to the site for abductor pollicis brevis), with oblique needle insertion, almost parallel to the palm (See Fig. 3.2).

Indications include: Carpal tunnel syndrome, proximal median neuropathies, lower trunk or medial cord plexopathies, thoracic outlet syndrome, or C8–T1 radiculopathy.

Notes and precautions/confounders: This muscle is right below (deep to) the abductor pollicis brevis muscle, so avoid inserting needle too superficially.

Flexor Pollicis Brevis

Innervation: Median (superficial head) and ulnar (deep head) nerves ← medial cord ← lower trunk ← C8–T1 spinal nerve roots.

Activation: Flexion of thumb at the metacarpophalangeal joint.

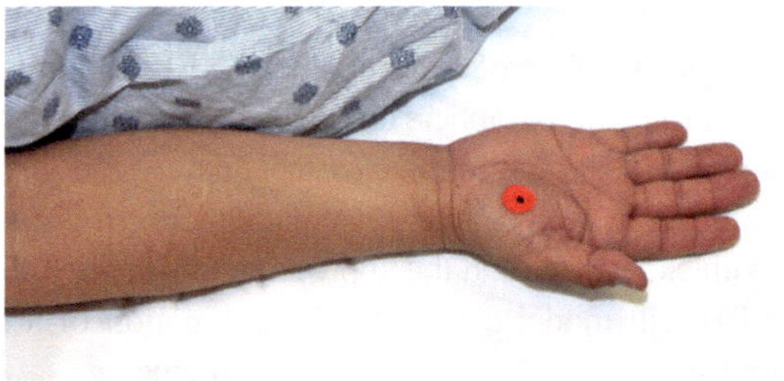

Fig. 3.3 Needle insertion site (black dot in center of red circle) for needle electrode examination of the flexor pollicis brevis

Needle placement: Just lateral (superficial head) or just medial (deep head) to the mid-point of the first metacarpal bone in the thenar eminence (See Fig. 3.3).

Indications include: Generally avoided in most routine work-ups (especially due to dual innervation). May have some utility in cases of lower trunk or medial cord plexopathies, or C8–T1 radiculopathy.

Notes and precautions/confounders: Has mixed ulnar (deep head) and median (superficial head) innervation, with potential variability in normal subjects. Accordingly, interpretation of abnormalities should be done with caution.

Pronator Quadratus (PQ)

Innervation: Anterior interosseous nerve (branch) ← median nerve ← lateral and medial cords, middle ← lower trunk ← C7–C8–T1 spinal nerve roots.

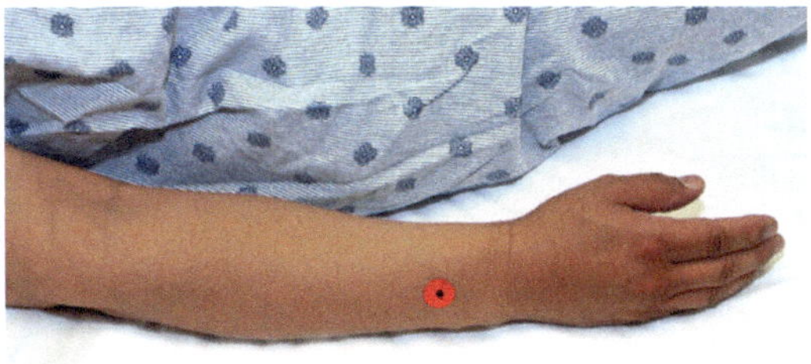

Fig. 3.4 Needle insertion site (black dot in center of red circle) for needle electrode examination of the pronator quadratus

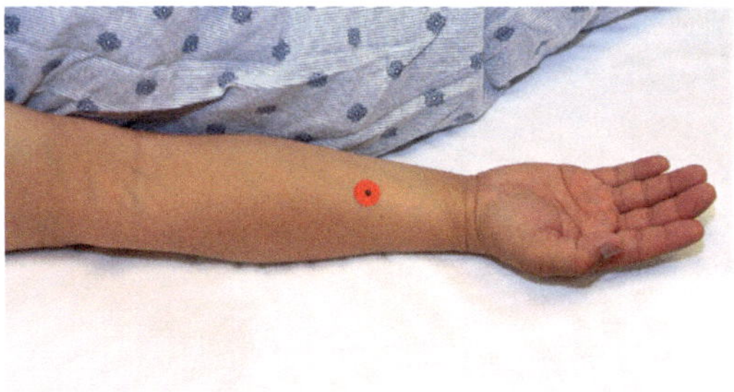

Fig. 3.5 Needle insertion site (black dot in center of red circle) for needle electrode examination of the flexor pollicis longus

Activation: with elbow slightly flexed, have the patient pronate the hand.

Needle placement: Three fingerbreadths proximal to the mid-point of an imaginary line drawn from the ulnar to radial styloid, insertion via the dorsal forearm with slight angulation of the needle laterally (towards radius) ensuring depth sufficient to pierce interosseous membrane, this with hand in mid-position between supination and pronation (See Fig. 3.4).

Indications include: Anterior interosseous nerve syndrome, proximal median neuropathies.

Notes and precautions/confounders: The muscle is deep to the finger and thumb extensor tendons and muscles, and the needle must be inserted sufficiently deep, through the interosseous membrane (usually one detects confirmatory tissue resistance changes from the needle when this is achieved).

Flexor Pollicis Longus

Innervation: anterior interosseous nerve (branch) ← median nerve ← lateral and medial cords ← middle and lower trunks ← (C7)**C8**–T1 spinal nerve roots.

Activation: Flexion of the thumb at the interphalangeal joint.

Needle placement: with hand supinated, over the radius and proximally one third the distance up from the lateral wrist toward the lateral elbow (see Fig. 3.5).

Indications include: Anterior interosseous nerve syndrome or proximal median neuropathies, C8–T1 radiculopathy.

Notes and precautions/confounders: If the needle is inserted or oriented too medially, it may enter the radial artery and potentially lead to a large hematoma from arterial (high-pressure) blood loss.

Flexor Digitorum Profundus to Digits 2,3 (FDP)

Innervation: anterior interosseous nerve (branch) ← median nerve ← lateral and medial cord ← middle and lower trunk ← C7–**C8** spinal nerve roots.

Activation: flexion of digits 2 or 3 at the distal interphalangeal (DIP) joint.

Needle placement: three to four fingerbreadths distal to the olecranon and about 1 fingerbreadth medial to the ulna. The penetration depth should be about 3–4 cm (twice as deep as the ulnar-innervated counterpart of this muscle going to digits 4,5). (see Fig. 3.6)

Indications include: Anterior interosseous nerve syndrome or proximal median neuropathies.

Notes and precautions/confounders: Due to the depth of this muscle, the needle tip may come

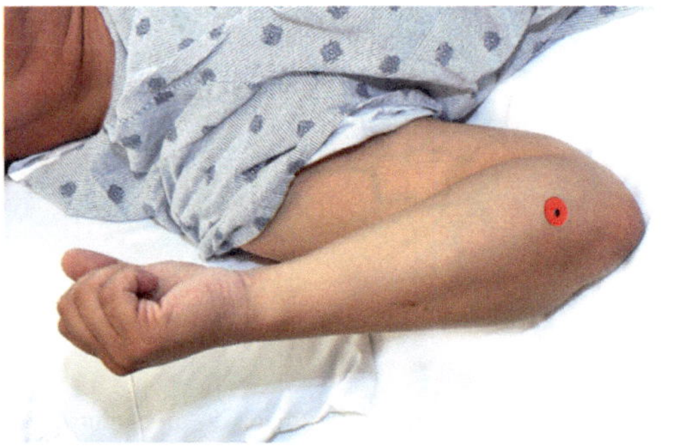

Fig. 3.6 Needle insertion site (black dot in center of red circle) for needle electrode examination of the flexor digitorum profundus to digits 2,3

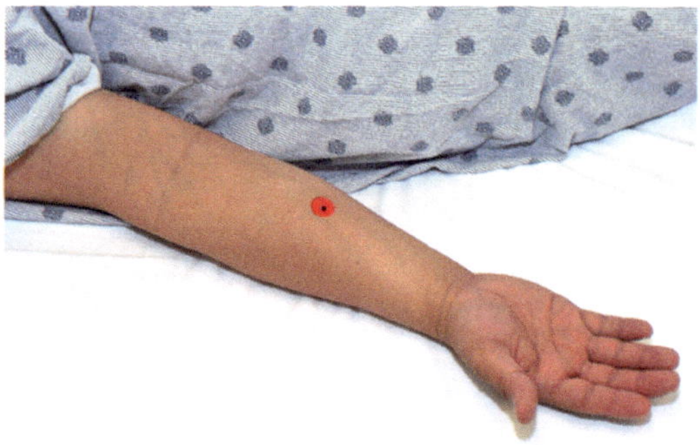

Fig. 3.7 Needle insertion site (black dot in center of red circle) for needle electrode examination of the flexor digitorum superficialis

quite close to the main trunk of the ulnar nerve, so insertion while the patient is gently activating the muscle may provide assurance that adequate depth is attained and not surpassed. If insertion is too superficial, the FDP to digits 4,5 (ulnar-innervated) will be sampled erroneously.

Flexor Digitorum Superficialis (Sublimis)

Innervation: median nerve ← medial and lateral cord ← middle and lower trunks ← C7–C8–(T1) spinal nerve roots.

Activation: flexion of the digits at the proximal interphalangeal (PIP) joints.

Needle placement: Volar aspect, about 2–3 cm medial to the mid-point between the biceps tendon and the mid-wrist, with the forearm supinated (see Fig. 3.7).

Indications include: Proximal median neuropathies, but not in the anterior interosseous nerve syndrome.

Notes and precautions/confounders: This muscle is more superficial than the FDP. The median nerve can be close if needle is inserted in the midline and too deep. If insertion is too lateral, the needle may enter the flexor carpi radialis (also median-innervated).

Flexor Carpi Radialis (FCR)

Innervation: median nerve ← lateral cord ← upper and middle trunks, C6–C7 spinal nerve roots.

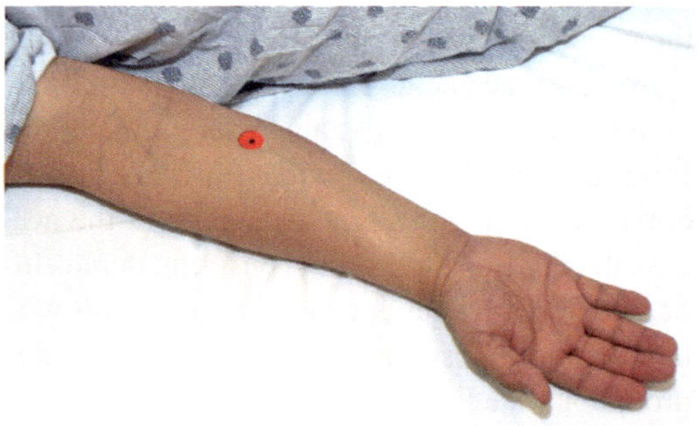

Fig. 3.8 Needle insertion site (black dot in center of red circle) for needle electrode examination of the flexor carpi radialis

Activation: flexion of the wrist with radial deviation.

Needle placement: About four fingerbreadths distal to the mid-point between the biceps tendon and medial epicondyle, with forearm supinated.

Indications include: Proximal median neuropathies, pronator teres syndrome, but not in anterior interosseous nerve syndrome. Also used in the demonstration of a C6–C7 radiculopathy or a brachial plexopathy affecting the lateral cord (see Fig. 3.8).

Notes and precautions/confounders: If needle is placed too deeply it can inadvertently contact the median nerve. Insertion too laterally may encounter the brachioradialis (radial-innervated); insertion too laterally and proximally may encounter the pronator teres (also median-innervated); insertion too medially may encoun-

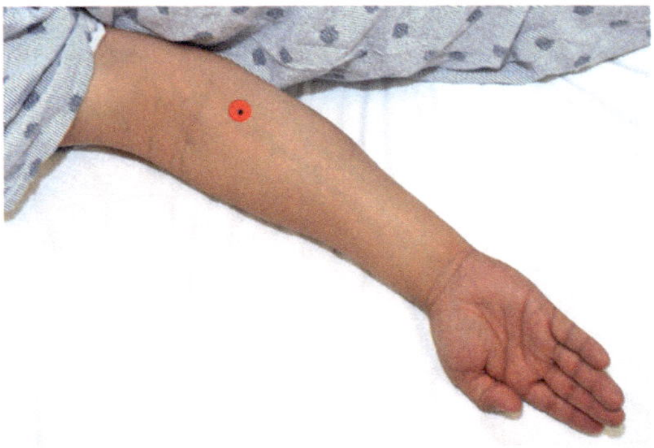

Fig. 3.9 Needle insertion site (black dot in center of red circle) for needle electrode examination of the pronator teres

ter the palmaris longus or flexor digitorum superficialis (both median-innervated).

Pronator Teres (PT)

Innervation: median nerve ← lateral cord ← upper and middle trunks ← C6–C7 spinal nerve roots.

Activation: With elbow extended, have patient pronate the hand ("like turning a door knob") against some resistance from the examiner.

Needle placement: about three fingerbreadths distal to the mid-point between biceps tendon and medial epicondyle, with forearm supinated (see Fig. 3.9).

Indications include: Proximal median neuropathies, but typically spared in pronator teres syndrome; also spared in the anterior interosseous nerve syndrome. Also used to demonstrate involvement in C6–C7 radiculopathy.

Notes and precautions/confounders: If needle is placed too deeply it can inadvertently contact the median nerve. Needle insertion too laterally may penetrate the brachioradialis (radial-innervated); insertion too medially may penetrate the flexor carpi radialis (median-innervated as well); insertion too deeply may penetrate the flexor digitorum superficialis (median-innervated as well).

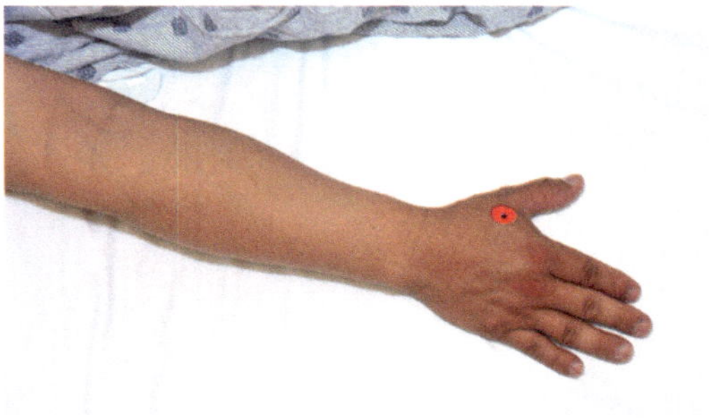

Fig. 3.10 Needle insertion site (black dot in center of red circle) for needle electrode examination of the first dorsal interosseous

First Dorsal Interosseous (FDI)

Innervation: ulnar nerve ← medial cord ← lower trunk ← C8–T1 spinal nerve roots.

Activation: Abduction of index finger (e.g. asking the patient to make a fist, then have index finger point upwards).

Needle placement: in the dorsal hand, halfway between the first and second metacarpophalangeal (MCP) joints, with the needle inserted obliquely more towards the second MCP joint (Fig. 3.10).

Indications include: Ulnar neuropathy, lower trunk or medial cord brachial plexopathy, thoracic outlet syndrome or C8–T1 radiculopathy.

Notes and precautions/confounders: Generally easy muscle to access reliably by needle examination, without significant potential for errors or confounders.

Abductor Digiti Minimi (ADM)

Innervation: ulnar nerve ← medial cord ← lower trunk ← C8–T1 spinal nerve roots.

Activation: Abduction of the little finger (for ease, the patient may spread all fingers during activation).

Needle placement: In the medial aspect of the hand (hypothenar eminence), mid-point of the fifth metacarpal (See Fig. 3.11).

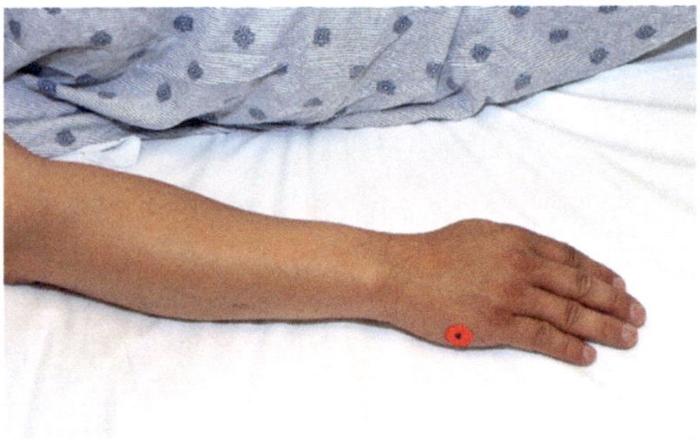

Fig. 3.11 Needle insertion site (black dot in center of red circle) for needle electrode examination of the abductor digiti minimi

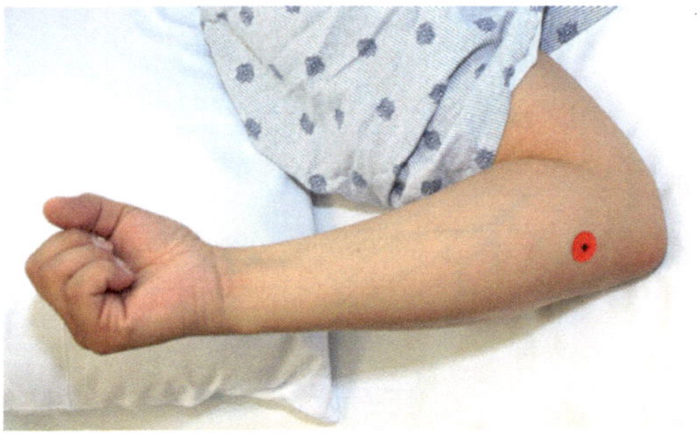

Fig. 3.12 Needle insertion site (black dot in center of red circle) for needle electrode examination of the flexor digitorum profundus to digits 4,5

Indications include: ulnar neuropathy (may be spared in some ulnar lesions at Guyon's canal), lower trunk or medial cord brachial plexopathy, thoracic outlet syndrome, C8–T1 radiculopathy.

Flexor Digitorum Profundus (FDP) to Digits 4,5

Innervation: ulnar nerve ← medial cord ← lower trunk ← C8–T1 spinal nerve roots.

Activation: flexion of digits 4,5 at the distal interphalangeal joints.

Needle placement: three to four fingerbreadths distal to the olecranon and about 1 fingerbreadth medial to the ulna. The penetration depth should be about 1.5 to 2 cm (half as deep as the median-innervated counterpart of this muscle going to digits 2,3) (See Fig. 3.12).

Indications include: ulnar neuropathy at the elbow; lower trunk or medial cord brachial plexopathy, thoracic outlet syndrome, C8–T1 radiculopathy.

Notes and precautions/confounders: The more superficial muscle (to digits 4,5) is the one innervated by the ulnar nerve, which makes it relatively easy to study (compared to the median-innervated FDP to digits 2,3, which is deeper).

Flexor Carpi Ulnaris (FCU)

Innervation: ulnar nerve ← medial cord ← lower trunk ← C8–T1 spinal nerve roots.

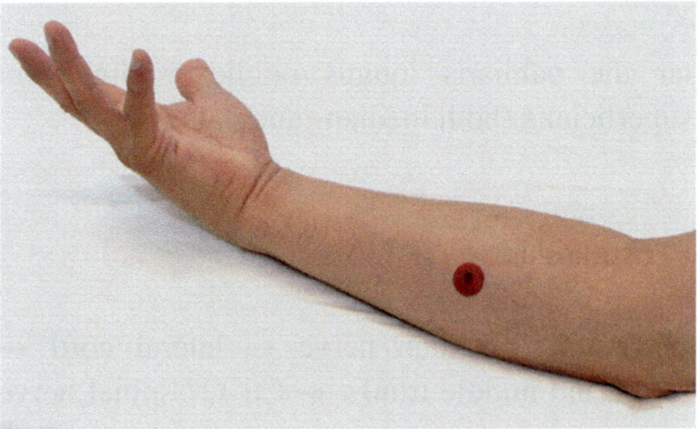

Fig. 3.13 Needle insertion site (black dot in center of red circle) for needle electrode examination of the flexor carpi ulnaris

Activation: flexion or wrist with ulnar deviation.

Needle placement: with the forearm supinated, the needle is inserted at about 4–5 fingerbreadths distal to the medial epicondyle, along the medial aspect of the ulna (see Fig. 3.13).

Indications include: ulnar neuropathy at the elbow (though fascicular sparing may be seen); lower trunk or medial cord brachial plexopathy, thoracic outlet syndrome, C8–T1 radiculopathy.

Notes and precautions/confounders: insert the needle superficially as the muscle tends to be very thin. Deeper insertions may penetrate the flexor digitorum superficialis (median-innervated), or even flexor digitorum profundus (median- and ulnar-innervated). Too lateral an insertion may end up in the palmaris longus or flexor carpi radialis (both of these being median-innervated).

Extensor Indicis [Proprius] (EI/EIP)

Innervation: posterior interosseous nerve ← radial nerve, posterior cord ← middle and lower trunks ← C7–C8 spinal nerve roots.

Activation: extension of index finger.

Needle placement: towards the radial (lateral) aspect of the ulna, three to four fingerbreadths proximal to the ulnar styloid, with forearm and hand pronated (see Fig. 3.14).

Indications include: radial neuropathy including posterior interosseous (branch) neuropathy, lower > middle trunk or posterior cord brachial plexopathy, thoracic outlet syndrome, C8 > C7 radiculopathy.

Notes and precautions/confounders: If the needle is inserted too superficially and/or too proximally it may be in the extensor carpi ulnaris, extensor digiti minimi, or extensor digitorum (all radial/posterior interosseous-innervated). If insertion is performed too laterally, it may penetrate the extensor pollicis longus (still radial/posterior interosseous-innervated).

Extensor Carpi Ulnaris (ECU)

Innervation: posterior interosseous nerve ← radial nerve ← posterior cord ← middle and lower trunks ← C7–C8 spinal nerve roots.

Activation: extension of wrist with ulnar deviation.

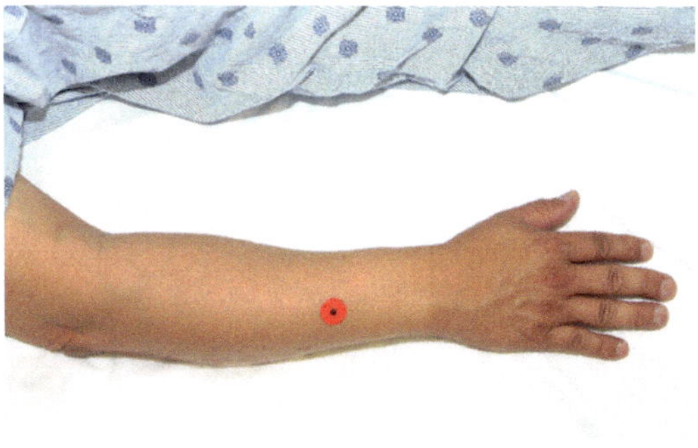

Fig. 3.14 Needle insertion site (black dot in center of red circle) for needle electrode examination of the extensor indicis

Needle placement: on the lateral aspect (radial side) of the mid-point of the ulnar, with forearm pronated (see Fig. 3.15).

Indications include: radial neuropathy including posterior interosseous neuropathy, lower trunk or posterior cord brachial plexopathy, thoracic outlet syndrome, C7–C8 radiculopathy.

Notes and precautions/confounders: too lateral an insertion may lead to penetrating the extensor digiti minimi (quinti) or extensor digitorum (both radial/posterior interosseous-innervated).

Extensor Digitorum [Communis] (ED/ EDC)

Innervation: posterior interosseous nerve ← radial nerve, posterior cord ← middle and lower trunks ← **C7**–C8 spinal nerve roots.

Activation: extension of the middle finger (see Fig. 3.16).

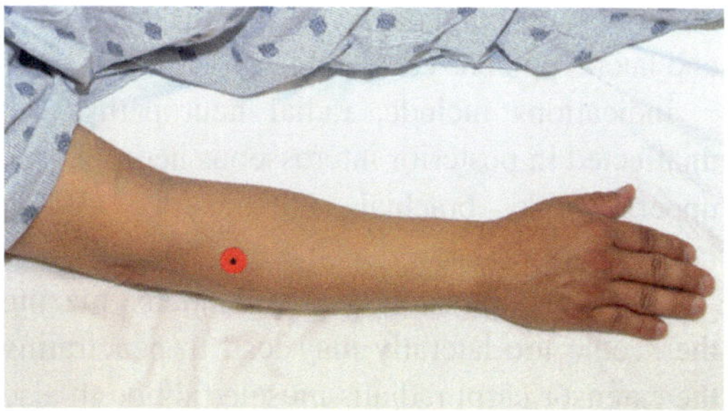

Fig. 3.15 Needle insertion site (black dot in center of red circle) for needle electrode examination of the extensor carpi ulnaris

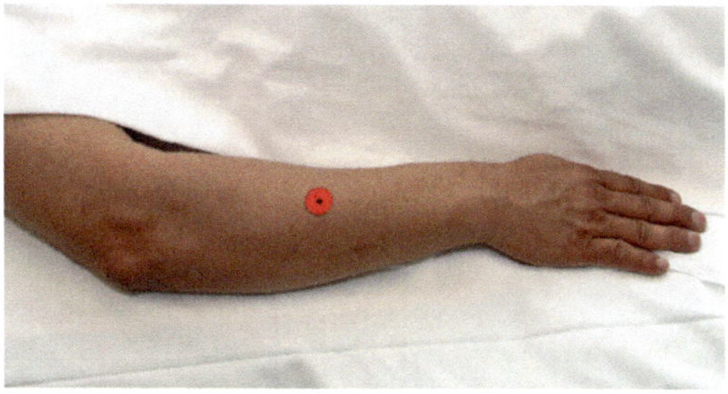

Fig. 3.16 Needle insertion site (black dot in center of red circle) for needle electrode examination of the extensor indicis

Needle placement: with the forearm pronated, the needle is inserted mid-forearm, at the mid-point between the ulna and radius.

Indications include: radial neuropathy including posterior interosseous neuropathy, **C7**–8 radiculopathy.

Notes and precautions/confounders: If needle is inserted too medially, it may enter the extensor digiti minimi or the extensor carpi ulnaris (both posterior interosseous-innervated); insertion too laterally may penetrate the extensor carpi radialis (radial-innervated). This muscle is commonly sampled during single fiber EMG studies.

Brachioradialis

Innervation: radial nerve ← posterior cord ← upper trunk ← C5–C6 spinal nerve roots.

Activation: flexion of elbow with wrist in mid position between pronation and supination.

Needle placement: three to four fingerbreadths distal to mid-point between the biceps tendon and lateral epicondyle (see Fig. 3.17).

Indications include: radial neuropathy (but unaffected in posterior interosseous neuropathy), upper trunk brachial plexopathy, C5–C6 radiculopathy.

Notes and precautions/confounders: placing the needle too laterally may lead to penetrating the extensor carpi radialis muscle (although also radial-innervated).

Anconeus

Innervation: radial nerve ← posterior cord ← upper, middle and lower trunks ← C6–**C7**–C8 spinal nerve roots.

Activation: Extension of the elbow.

Needle placement: Two to three fingerbreadths distal to the olecranon, on the radial aspect of the ulna, with the forearm pronated (see Fig. 3.18).

Indications include: radial neuropathies above the spiral grove, since it is the only muscle in the forearm that receives its radial innervation from above the spiral grove. Accordingly, the anconeus is spared in radial neuropathy at (or distal to) the spiral grove.

Notes and precautions/confounders: placing the needle on the medial aspect of the ulna may lead to inadvertently recording the flexor digitorum profundus (mixed median and ulnar innervation). If insertion is too lateral, it may penetrate the extensor carpi ulnaris (posterior interosseous-innervated).

Triceps Brachii

Innervation: Radial nerve ← posterior cord ← upper, **middle** and lower trunks ← C6–**C7**–C8 spinal nerve roots.

Activation: Elbow extension.

Needle placement: Mid-point between lateral epicondyle and shoulder (to access the lateral

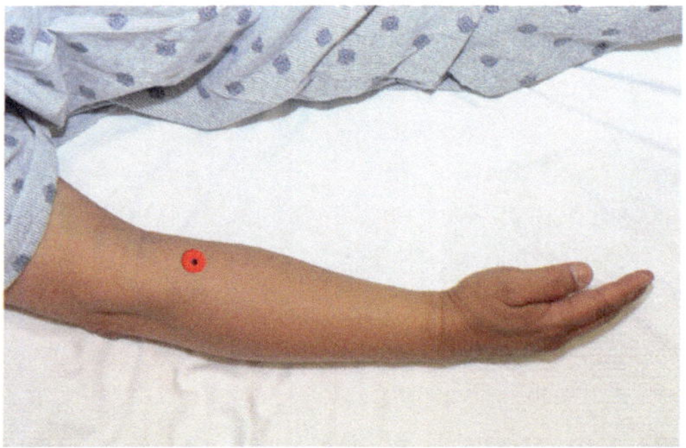

Fig. 3.17 Needle insertion site (black dot in center of red circle) for needle electrode examination of the brachioradialis

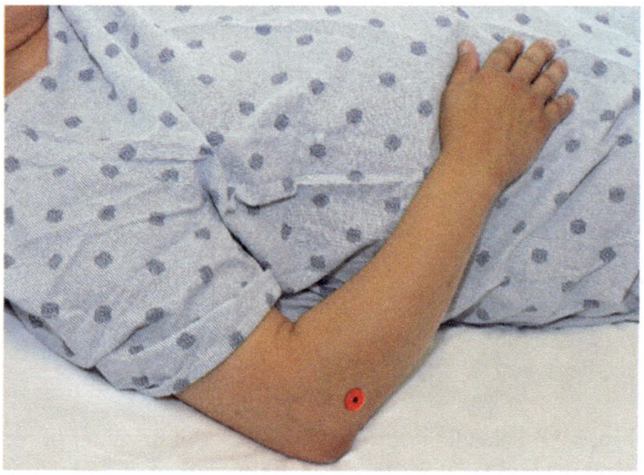

Fig. 3.18 Needle insertion site (black dot in center of red circle) for needle electrode examination of the anconeus

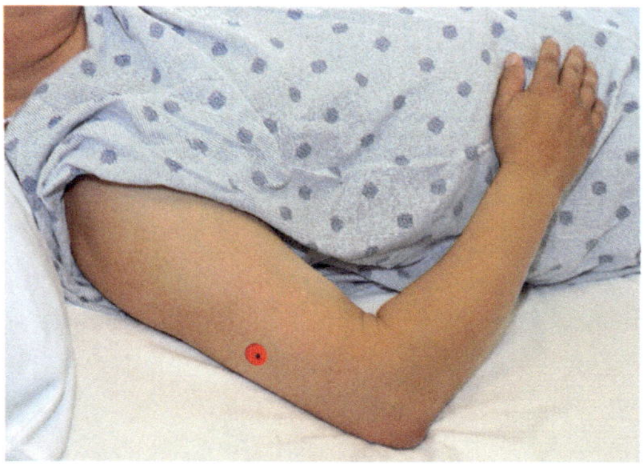

Fig. 3.19 Needle insertion site (black dot in center of red circle) for needle electrode examination of the triceps brachii

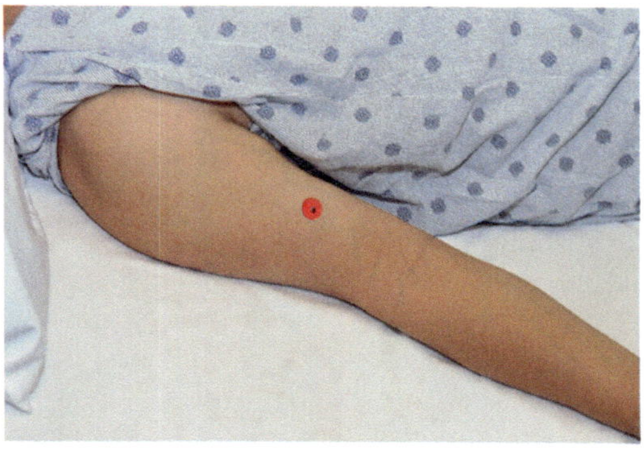

Fig. 3.20 Needle insertion site (black dot in center of red circle) for needle electrode examination of the biceps brachii

head of the triceps), with forearm pronated and elbow flexed (see Fig. 3.19).

Indications include: **C7(>C6,C8)** radiculopathy. Not typically affected in radial neuropathy at the spiral groove as it receives its innervation from above this segment.

Notes and precautions/confounders: Approach from the lateral head will minimize risk of inadvertently contacting vascular and nervous structures (e.g. the brachial artery and the radial nerve trunk) in the area. If the needle is inserted too anteriorly, it may encroach onto the biceps brachii or the brachialis muscle (musculocutaneous-innervated); insertion too proximally runs the risk of entering the deltoid muscle (axillary-innervated).

Biceps Brachii

Innervation: musculocutaneous nerve ← lateral cord ← upper trunk ← C5–C6 spinal nerve roots.

Activation: flexion of the elbow with hand supinated.

Needle placement: just lateral to the mid-point in the muscle between the anterior shoulder and biceps tendon/mid-antecubital fossa (see Fig. 3.20).

Indications include: C5 or C6 radiculopathies, brachial plexopathies involving upper trunk or lateral cord.

Notes and precautions/confounders: inserting the needle on the medial side of the muscle can encroach the brachial artery, the median or ulnar nerve and major veins (e.g. basilic vein) in the area. Needle insertion too deeply may enter the brachialis (also musculocutaneous-innervated); insertion too proximally may enter the anterior head of the deltoid (axillary-innervated), or the pectoralis major (medial and lateral pectoral-innervated).

Pectoralis Major

Innervation: Medial and lateral pectoral nerves ← medial and lateral cords ← upper-middle and lower trunks ← C5–C6 spinal nerve roots (clavicular portion) and C7–C8–T1 spinal nerve roots (sternocostal portion).

Activation: Shoulder adduction.

Needle placement: In the anterior lower shoulder, at the anterior axillary line, just medial to the anterior axillary fold (see Fig. 3.21).

Indications: infrequently studied (isolated lateral or medial pectoral neuropathy is very rare), but may be abnormal in brachial plexopathy or cervical radiculopathy at multiple levels-C5–C6 if testing clavicular portion, or C7–C8–T1 if testing sternocostal portion.

Notes and precautions/confounders: Placing the needle more medially and deeply may inadvertently penetrate the intercostal space and pleura,

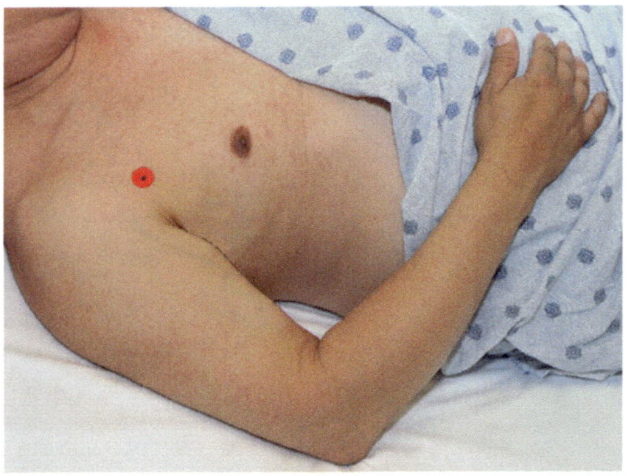

Fig. 3.21 Needle insertion site (black dot in center of red circle) for needle electrode examination of the pectoralis major

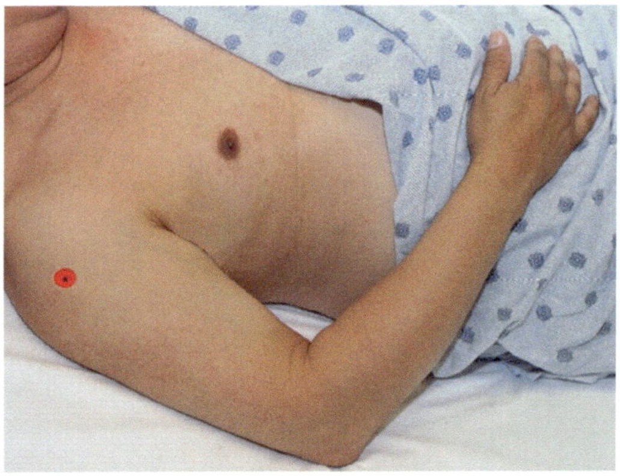

Fig. 3.22 Needle insertion site (black dot in center of red circle) for needle electrode examination of the deltoid

with risk of pneumothorax, or the needle may cause penetration injury to components of the brachial plexus, or major blood vessels (e.g. subclavian artery) in the area. Placing the needle too laterally may misdirect it into the deltoid muscle.

Deltoid

Innervation: Axillary nerve ← posterior cord ← upper trunk ← C5–C6 spinal nerve roots.

Activation: Shoulder abduction.

Needle placement: (for middle head) Outer aspect of the shoulder, about three to four fingerbreadths below the lateral aspect of the acromion (see Fig. 3.22).

Indications include: Axillary neuropathy, upper trunk or posterior cord brachial plexopathy, C5–C6 radiculopathy.

Notes and precautions/confounders: Fairly easy muscle to sample and away from major nerves and vessels, especially if the medial head is examined.

Teres Minor

Innervation: axillary nerve ← posterior cord ← upper trunk ← C5–C6 spinal nerve roots.

Activation: external rotation of the arm.

Needle placement: With the patient in the lateral decubitus position (contralateral side down), the needle is placed about one fingerbreadth lateral to the outer border of the middle third of the scapula (see Fig. 3.23).

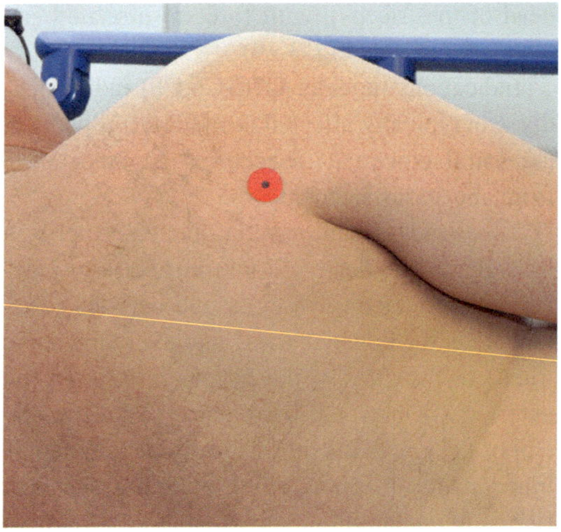

Fig. 3.23 Needle insertion site (black dot in center of red circle) for needle electrode examination of the teres minor

Indications include: axillary neuropathy, upper trunk and posterior cord brachial plexopathy, C5–C6 radiculopathy.

Notes and precautions/confounders: placing the needle too medially and/or superiorly can get it into the infraspinatus (suprascapular-innervated), and placing the needle too laterally and/or superiorly may get it into the posterior head of the deltoid (also axillary-innervated).

Upper Trapezius

Innervation: spinal accessory nerve ← C3–C4 spinal nerve roots.

Activation: Shrugging/elevating of the shoulder.

Needle placement: With the patient in the lateral decubitus position (contralateral side down), the needle is inserted just lateral to the junction of the shoulder and the neck (see Fig. 3.24).

Indications include: spinal accessory nerve injury, C3–4 radiculopathy.

Notes and precautions/confounders: Insert the needle superficially, as going too deep may place it in the rhomboids or paraspinal muscles (especially if too medial as well), or it may enter the apical pleura (risk for pneumothorax).

Sternocleidomastoid

Innervation: spinal accessory nerve ← C3–C4 spinal nerve roots.

Activation: Turning head and neck to the contralateral side.

Needle placement: mid-point of the muscle (between the mastoid process and sternal head), ensuring the muscle is well-delineated by palpation as well. The needle should enter the muscle at an angle so that it is almost parallel to its fibers when being advanced (see Fig. 3.25).

Indications include: spinal accessory nerve injury, C3–4 radiculopathy.

Notes and precautions/confounders: If the needle insertion is too anteriorly and/or medially, it may cause penetration injury to the carotid artery or jugular vein. Unlike the trapezius, this muscle is often spared in iatrogenic injury of the spinal accessory nerve with lymph node dissection in the posterior triangle of the neck.

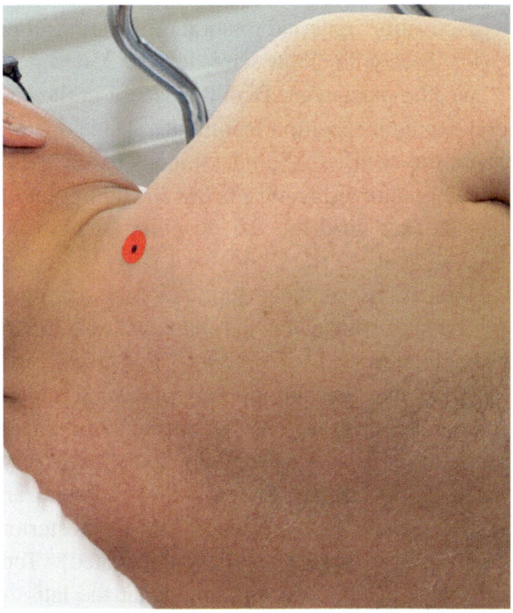

Fig. 3.24 Needle insertion site (black dot in center of red circle) for needle electrode examination of the upper trapezius

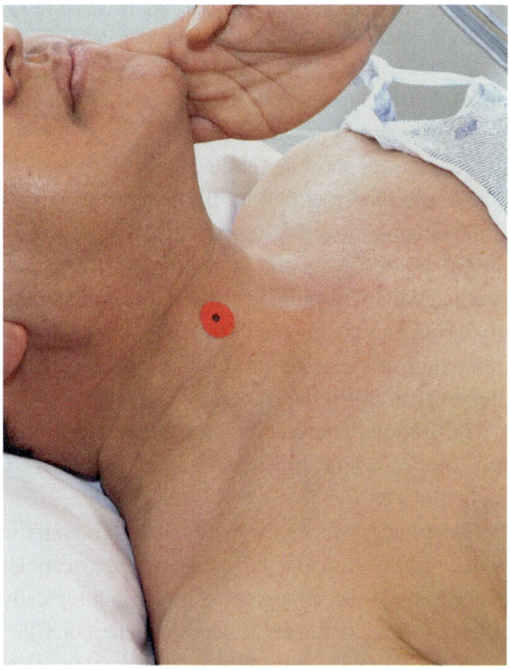

Fig. 3.25 Needle insertion site (black dot in center of red circle) for needle electrode examination of the sternocleidomastoid

Supraspinatus

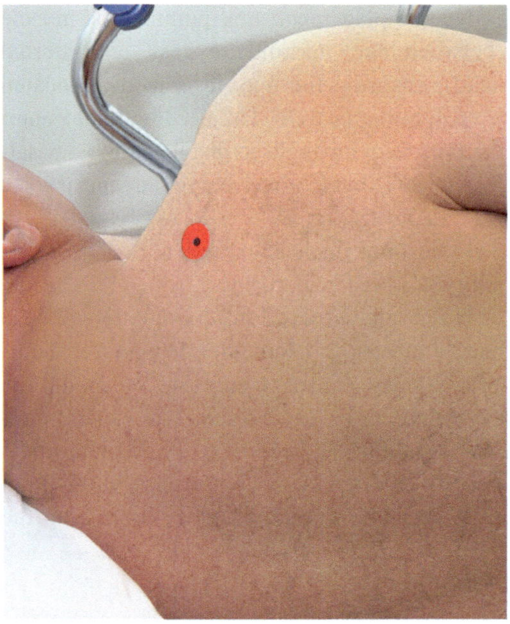

Fig. 3.26 Needle insertion site (black dot in center of red circle) for needle electrode examination of the supraspinatus

Innervation: suprascapular nerve ← upper trunk ← C5–C6 spinal nerve roots.

Activation: shoulder abduction.

Needle placement: With the patient in the lateral decubitus position (contralateral side down), insert the needle in the supraspinous fossa, just medial to the mid-point of the scapular spine, gently advancing the needle to the bone, then slightly retracting the needle to ensure penetration is deeper than overlying trapezius (see Fig. 3.26).

Indications include: suprascapular neuropathy, upper trunk brachial plexopathy, C5–C6 radiculopathy.

Notes and precautions/confounders: The muscle will typically be unaffected in cases of suprascapular neuropathy at the spinoglenoid notch (but typically affected with a lesion at the suprascapular notch).

A superficial needle insertion may place it at the trapezius muscle (innervated by the spinal accessory nerve, C3–4 spinal nerve roots).

Infraspinatus

Innervation: supra-scapular nerve ← upper trunk ← C5–C6 spinal nerve roots.

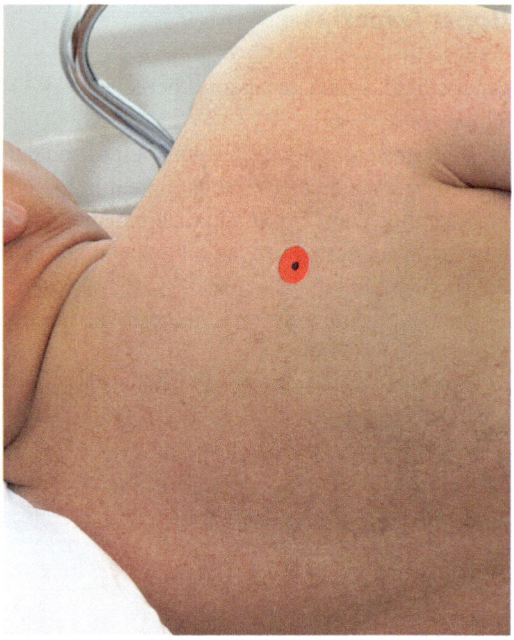

Fig. 3.27 Needle insertion site (black dot in center of red circle) for needle electrode examination of the infraspinatus

Activation: external rotation of the arm (more easily done with elbow semi-flexed).

Needle placement: With the patient in the lateral decubitus position (contralateral side down), insert the needle in the infraspinous fossa, about one to two fingerbreadths below the mid-point of the medial third of the scapular spine (see Fig. 3.27).

Indications include: suprascapular neuropathy, upper trunk brachial plexopathy, C5–C6 radiculopathy.

Notes and precautions/confounders: A superficial insertion may place the needle in the trapezius muscle (innervated by the spinal accessory nerve, C3–4 spinal nerve roots). Too lateral an insertion may place the needle into the posterior head of the deltoid (axillary-innervated). Too inferior a needle insertion may enter the latissimus dorsi (thoracodorsal-innervated).

Rhomboids

Innervation: Dorsal scapular nerve ← **C5** spinal nerve root (pre-brachial plexus).

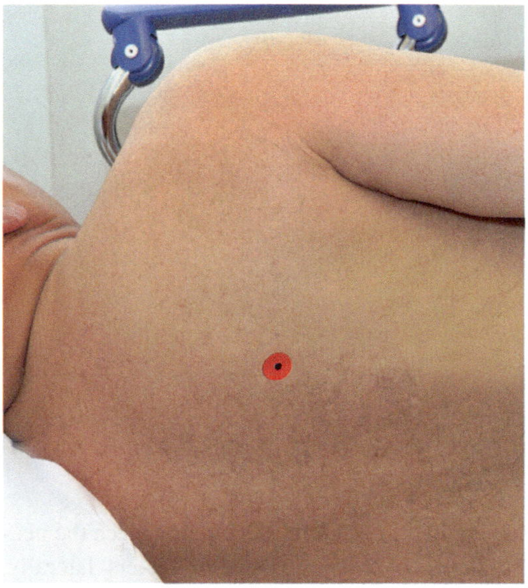

Fig. 3.28 Needle insertion site (black dot in center of red circle) for needle electrode examination of the rhomboid major

Activation: Ask the patient to retract (draw back) the shoulder blade toward the spine.

Needle placement: With the patient in the lateral decubitus position (contralateral side down).

Rhomboid major (illustrated in Fig. 3.28 below): about one to two fingerbreadths medial to the medial border of the scapula, at the midpoint between the scapular spine and the inferior angle.

Rhomboid minor: about one to two fingerbreadths medial to the medial border of the scapular spine.

Indications include: C5 radiculopathy.

Notes and precautions/confounders: Avoid deep needle insertion due to risk of pneumothorax if the needle traverses a posterior intercostal space.

However, too superficial an insertion will put the needle in the trapezius muscle (innervated by the spinal accessory nerve, C3–4 spinal nerve roots). Too inferior a needle insertion (for the rhomboid major) may enter the latissimus dorsi (thoracodorsal-innervated).

The rhomboids are typically not involved in brachial plexopathies of the upper trunk (innervated directly by **C5** spinal nerve roots).

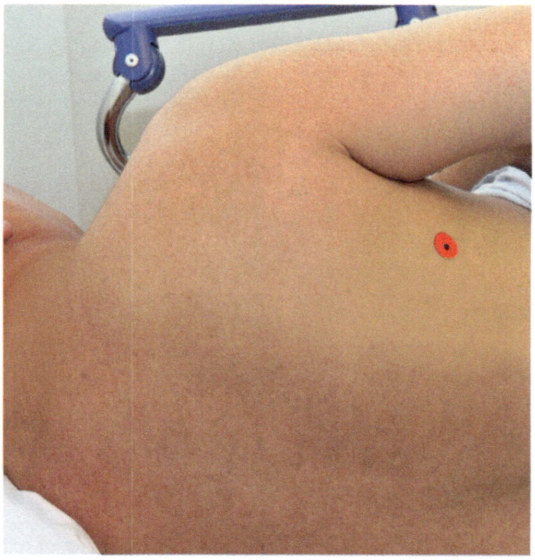

Fig. 3.29 Needle insertion site (black dot in center of red circle) for needle electrode examination of the latissimus dorsi

Latissimus Dorsi

Innervation: thoracodorsal nerve ← posterior cord ← upper, middle and lower trunks ← C6–C7–C8 spinal nerve roots.

Activation: Extension (pushing back) of the arm, with the arm also being internally rotated and abducted.

Needle placement: With the patient in the lateral decubitus position (contralateral side down), insert the needle about one fingerbreadth lateral to the inferior angle of the scapula, within the posterior axillary fold (see Fig. 3.29).

Indications include: brachial plexopathy, C6–C7–C8 radiculopathies.

Notes and precautions/confounders: Too superior a needle insertion runs the risk of inadvertently sampling the teres major (lower subscapular-innervated).

Serratus Anterior

- Innervation: Long thoracic nerve ← C5–C6–C7 spinal nerve roots
- Activation: Forward flexion of the arm, reaching anteriorly, then pushing forward (e.g. against a wall)

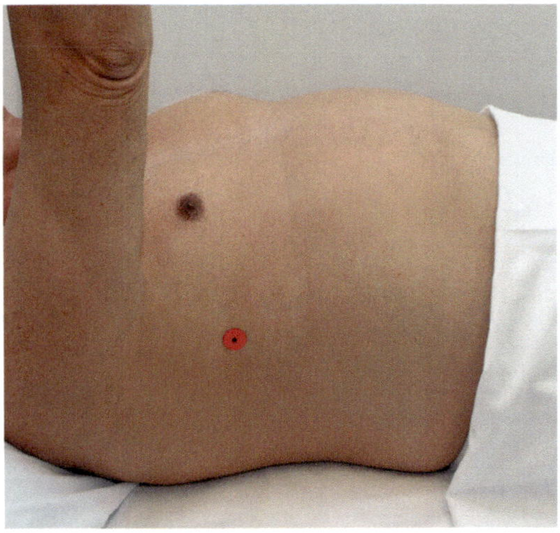

Fig. 3.30 Needle insertion site (black dot in center of red circle) for needle electrode examination of the serratus anterior

- Needle placement: In the mid-axillary line, identify and isolate a rib at about the mid-thoracic level, placing two fingers in between adjacent intercostal spaces, and then inserting the needle perpendicular to the skin until gently abutting the bony rib (see Fig. 3.30).
- Indications include: Long thoracic neuropathy, brachial plexopathy, C5–C7 radiculopathy (especially in conditions associated with medial scapular winging)
- Notes and precautions/confounders: If the needle is inserted in the intercostal space, it may pierce the pleura and lead to pneumothorax. If the needle insertion is too close to the inferior border of the rib, it may injure the adjacent neurovascular bundle.

Cervical Paraspinal Muscles

- Innervation: Posterior/dorsal rami of the cervical spinal nerves. Overlap innervation of C4 through C8/T1 spinal nerve root segments (overlap may occur for up to 4–6 contiguous segments/levels).
- Activation: Neck extension (e.g. pushing head back against the examiner's hand).
- Needle placement: Identify the spinous process at the level of interest [the vertebra prominens (C7) at the base of the neck may be useful as a reference level], and place the needle about two to four centimeters laterally, with the tip of the electrode oriented medially towards the deeper muscle layers (the vertebral lamina being deep to this) (see Fig. 3.31).

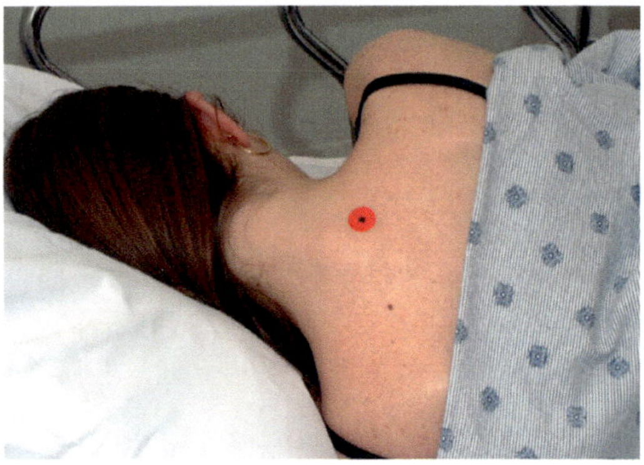

Fig. 3.31 Needle insertion site (black dot in center of red circle) for needle electrode examination of the (low) cervical paraspinal muscles

- Indications include: To differentiate between an intraspinal canal process (e.g. radiculopathy or anterior horn cell disorder) versus a lesion distal to the dorsal root ganglia (which will affect corresponding sensory nerve action potentials as well). These muscles may also be affected in many proximal myopathies, having high diagnostic yield for certain disorders (e.g. Pompe disease).
- Notes and precautions/confounders: Needle examination that is too deep may irritate the bony vertebral laminae with resultant excessive pain. It is not necessary to always have the patient activate these muscles, as it is generally uncomfortable/difficult to execute and the evaluation of recruitment and motor unit morphology is seldom further helpful in most studies, except in patients with myopathies, and motor neuron diseases.

Lower Extremity

Extensor Digitorum Brevis

Innervation: Deep Peroneal (fibular) nerve ← Common Peroneal (fibular) nerve ← Sciatic nerve ← Lumbosacral trunk and Posterior division of the Sacral Plexus ← L5–S1 spinal nerve roots.

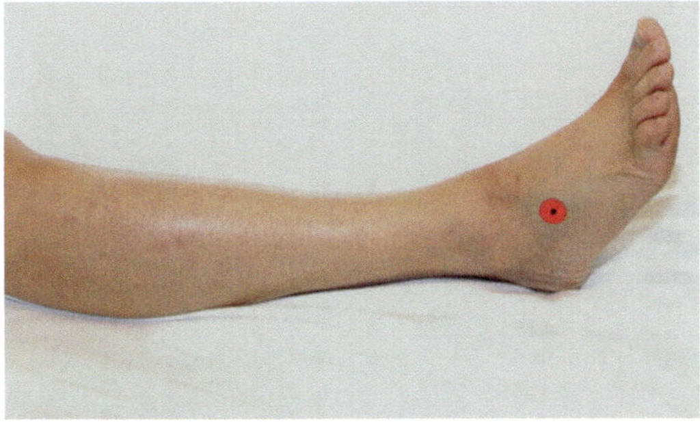

Fig. 3.32 Needle insertion site (black dot in center of red circle) for needle electrode examination of the extensor digitorum brevis

Activation: Patient to extend the toes.

Needle placement: Three finger breadths distal to the lower border of the lateral malleolus parallel to the border of the foot (see Fig. 3.32).

Indications include: entrapment/injury of the common peroneal (fibular) nerve (e.g. at the fibular head), Anterior tarsal tunnel syndrome, L5, S1 radiculopathies.

Potential Confounders: Interpretation of abnormalities from this muscle needs to be taken with care as it is common to find features of chronic denervation in normal subjects without any symptoms. This may be attributable to the effects of chronic local trauma, as can be seen with footwear/shoewear.

Extensor Hallucis Longus

Innervation: Deep Peroneal (fibular) nerve ← Common Peroneal (fibular) nerve ← Sciatic nerve, Lumbosacral trunk and Posterior division of the Sacral Plexus, L5 > S1 spinal nerve roots.

Activation: Patient to extend the big toe.

Needle placement: Three to five fingerbreadths above the bimalleolar line of the ankle just lateral to the crest of the tibia (see Fig. 3.33).

Indications include: **L5** > S1 radiculopathies, deep or common peroneal (fibular) nerves, often abnormal in peripheral neuropathies.

Potential Confounders: If electrode inserted too superficially and too proximal, it will be in the tibialis anterior; if inserted too laterally it will be in the peroneus tertius.

Peroneus Tertius

Innervation: Deep Peroneal (fibular) nerve ← Common Peroneal (fibular) nerve ← Sciatic nerve, Lumbosacral trunk and Posterior division of the Sacral Plexus, L5 > S1 spinal nerve roots.

Activation: Patient to dorsiflex and evert the foot.

Needle placement: one handbreadth above the bimalleolar line of the ankle and two finger breaths lateral to the tibia (see Fig. 3.34).

Indications include: **L5** > S1 radiculopathies, deep or common peroneal (fibular) neuropathy.

Potential Confounders: If electrode inserted too medially will be in the extensor hallucis longus, if inserted too proximally it will be in the tibialis anterior, or the extensor digitorum longus.

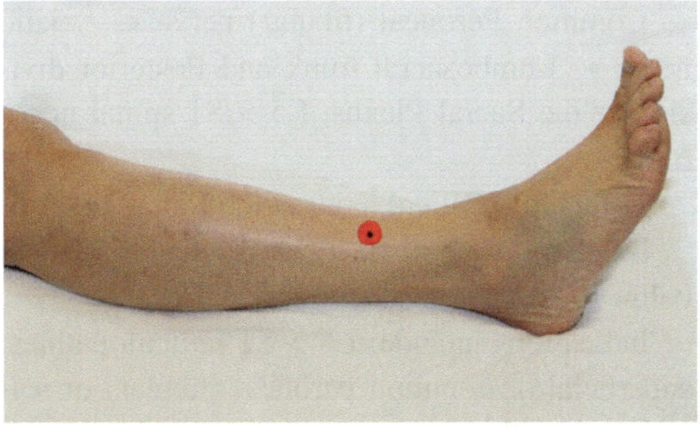

Fig. 3.33 Needle insertion site (black dot in center of red circle) for needle electrode examination of the extensor hallucis longus

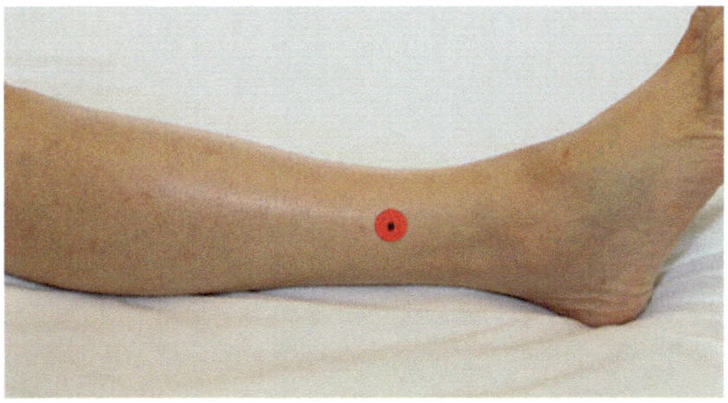

Fig. 3.34 Needle insertion site (black dot in center of red circle) for needle electrode examination of the peroneus tertius

Tibialis Anterior

Innervation: Deep Peroneal (fibular) nerve ← Common Peroneal (fibular) nerve ← Sciatic nerve ← Lumbosacral trunk and Posterior division of the Sacral Plexus ← L4, **L5** spinal nerve roots.

Activation: Patient to dorsiflex the foot.

Needle placement: Four fingerbreadths below the tibial tuberosity and one fingerbreadth lateral to the tibial crest (see Fig. 3.35).

Indications include: L4, L5 radiculopathies, deep or common peroneal (fibular) or sciatic neuropathies.

Potential Confounders: If electrode inserted too laterally and to deeply will be in the extensor digitorum longus.

Peroneus Longus

Innervation: Superficial Peroneal (fibular) nerve ← Common Peroneal (fibular) nerve ← Sciatic nerve ← Lumbosacral trunk and Posterior division of the Sacral Plexus, L5 > S1 spinal nerve roots.

Activation: Patient to evert the foot.

Needle placement: Three fingerbreadths below the fibular head (see Fig. 3.36).

Indications include: L5 > S1 radiculopathies, superficial or common peroneal (fibular) or sciatic neuropathies.

Potential Confounders: If electrode inserted too posterior it will be in the soleus, if inserted too anteriorly it will be in the extensor digitorum longus.

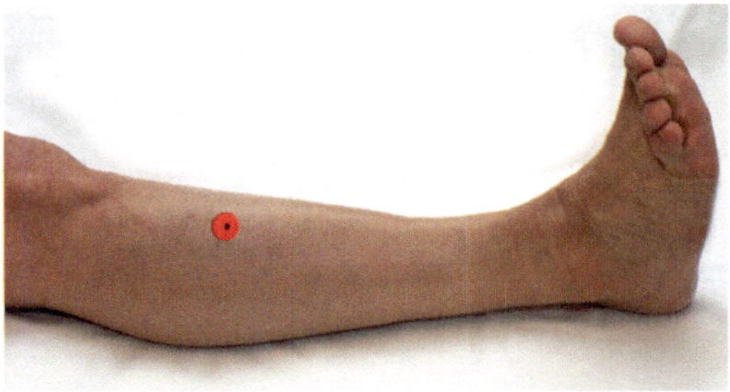

Fig. 3.35 Needle insertion site (black dot in center of red circle) for needle electrode examination of the tibialis anterior

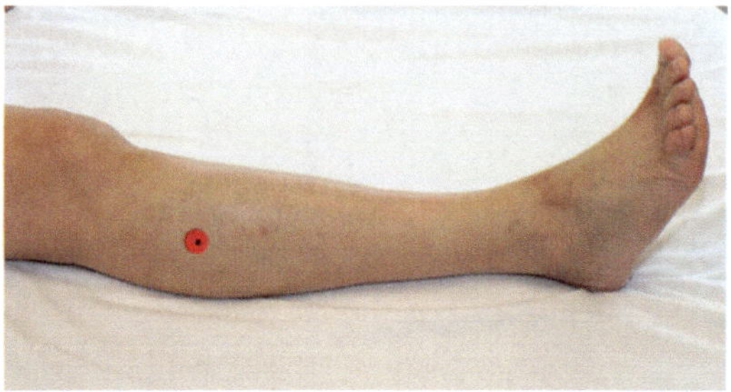

Fig. 3.36 Needle insertion site (black dot in center of red circle) for needle electrode examination of the peroneus longus

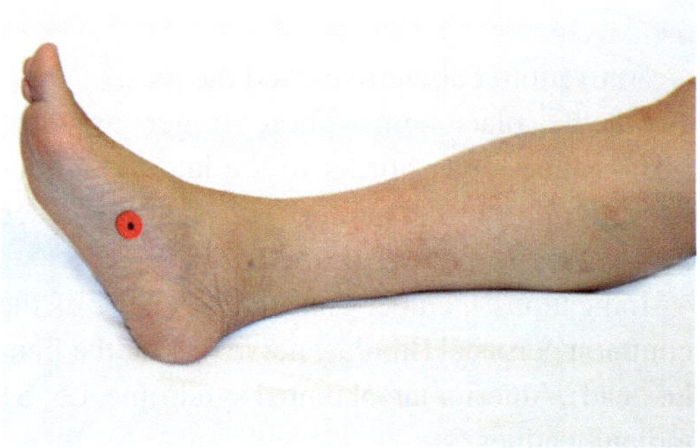

Fig. 3.37 Needle insertion site (black dot in center of red circle) for needle electrode examination of the abductor hallucis

Abductor Hallucis

Innervation: Medial Plantar nerve ← Tibial nerve ← Sciatic nerve ← Anterior division of the Sacral Plexus, S1 > S2 spinal nerve roots.

Activation: Patient to spread the toes.

Needle placement: One fingerbreadth below the navicular bone on mid portion of the medial aspect of the foot (see Fig. 3.37).

Indications include: peripheral neuropathy, medial plantar nerve lesions, tarsal tunnel syndrome, other tibial neuropathies, sciatic neuropathy, sacral plexopathy, S1 > S2 radiculopathies.

Potential Confounders: If electrode inserted too distally it will be in the flexor hallucis brevis, if inserted too deep it will be in the flexor digitorum brevis. Interpretation of abnormalities from this muscle needs to be taken with care as it is common to find features of chronic denervation in normal subjects without any symptoms. This may be attributable to the effects of chronic local trauma, as can be seen with footwear/shoewear.

Flexor Hallucis Brevis

Innervation: Medial Plantar nerve ← Tibial nerve ← Sciatic nerve ← Anterior division of the Sacral Plexus, S1, S2 spinal nerve roots.

Activation: Patient to flex the great toe.

Needle placement: Proximal and medial to the tendon of the flexor hallucis longus (see Fig. 3.38).

Indications include: peripheral neuropathy, medial plantar nerve lesions, tarsal tunnel syndrome, other tibial neuropathies, sciatic neuropathy, sacral plexopathy, S1, S2 radiculopathies.

Potential Confounders: If electrode inserted too laterally it will be in the adductor hallucis, if inserted too medially it will be in the abductor hallucis. Interpretation of abnormalities from this muscle needs to be taken with care as it is common to find features of chronic denervation in normal subjects without any symptoms. This may be attributable to the effects of chronic local trauma, as can be seen with footwear/shoewear.

Flexor Digitorum Longus

Innervation: Tibial nerve ← Sciatic nerve ← Anterior division of the Sacral Plexus, L5 > S1 spinal nerve roots.

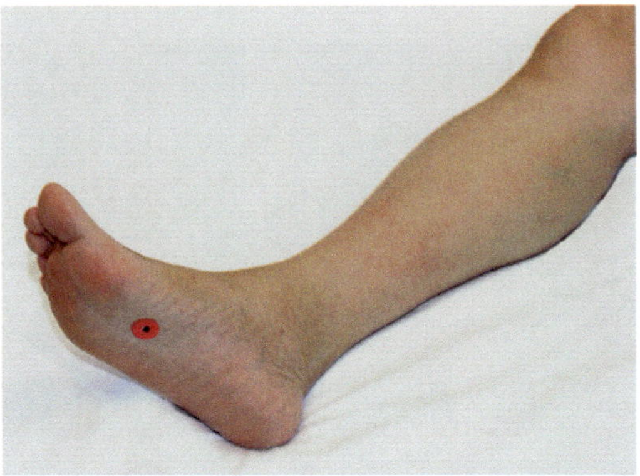

Fig. 3.38 Needle insertion site (black dot in center of red circle) for needle electrode examination of the flexor hallucis brevis

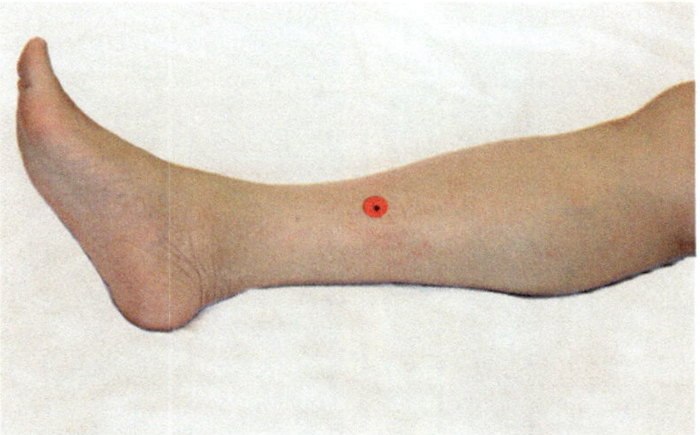

Fig. 3.39 Needle insertion site (black dot in center of red circle) for needle electrode examination of the flexor digitorum longus

Activation: Patient to flex the toes without flexing the ankle.

Needle placement: Just posterior of the medial edge of the tibia at midpoint (see Fig. 3.39).

Indications include: tibial neuropathy, sciatic neuropathy, sacral plexopathy, L5 > S1 radiculopathies. Useful in the evaluation of a foot drop to differentiate either a sciatic neuropathy or an intraspinal process (particularly at L5) from a peroneal (fibular) neuropathy.

Potential Confounders: If electrode inserted too superficial it will be in the soleus, if inserted too deep it will be in the tibialis posterior (although this is also tibial/L5 > S1-innervated).

Iliopsoas or Iliacus

Innervation: Femoral nerve ← Posterior division of the Lumbar Plexus ← L2, L3 (L4) spinal nerve roots.

Activation: Patient to flex the hip.

Needle placement: Two fingerbreadths lateral from the femoral artery pulse and one to two fingerbreadths below the inguinal ligament (see Fig. 3.40).

Indications include: high/proximal femoral neuropathy, posterior division lumbar plexopathy, L2, L3, L4 radiculopathies, myopathies (proximal muscle typically with high yield for myopathic changes in affected patients).

Potential Confounders: If electrode inserted too medially it will contact the neurovascular bundle, if inserted too laterally it will be in the sartorius.

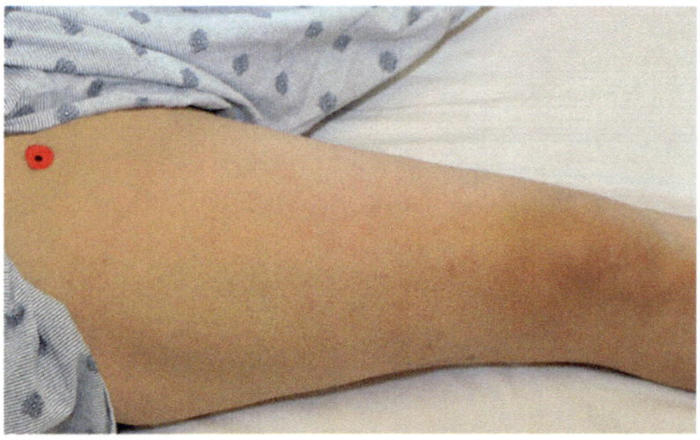

Fig. 3.40 Needle insertion site (black dot in center of red circle) for needle electrode examination of the iliopsoas/iliacus

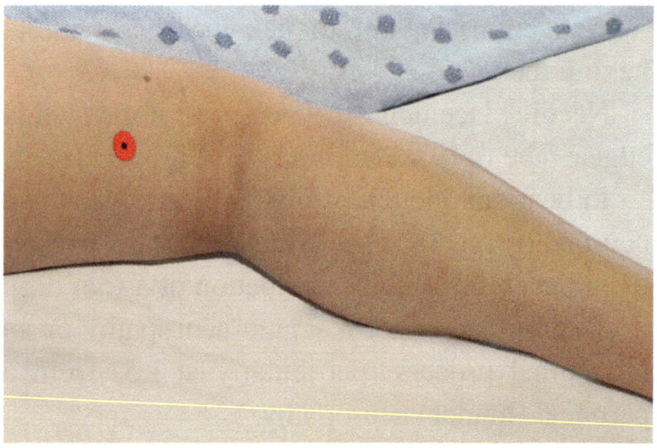

Fig. 3.41 Needle insertion site (black dot in center of red circle) for needle electrode examination of the short head of biceps femoris

Short Head of Biceps Femoris

Innervation: Sciatic nerve (Peroneal (fibular) division) ← Posterior division of the Sacral Plexus ← S1 > L5 spinal nerve roots.

Activation: Patient to flex the knee.

Needle placement: Three finger breadths proximal to the lateral knee and medial to the long head of biceps femoris tendon (see Fig. 3.41).

Indications include: sciatic neuropathy, S1 > L5 radiculopathies.

Of note, this is considered the only muscle above the knee innervated by the peroneal (fibular) division of the sciatic nerve. Important to check in suspected peroneal (fibular) neuropathy.

Potential Confounders: If electrode inserted too medially it will be in the semimembranosus, if inserted too laterally it will be in the long head of the biceps femoris.

Long Head of Biceps Femoris

Innervation: Sciatic nerve (Tibial division) ← Anterior division of the Sacral Plexus ← S1 > L5 spinal nerve roots.

Activation: Patient to flex the knee.

Needle placement: Insert the needle at midpoint between the lateral knee and the ischial tuberosity (see Fig. 3.42).

Indications include: sciatic neuropathy, Anterior division sacral plexopathy, S1 > L5 radiculopathies.

Potential Confounders: if needle electrode is inserted too medially, it will be in the short head of the biceps femoris.

Semimembranosus

Innervation: Sciatic nerve (Tibial division) ← Anterior division of the Sacral Plexus ← L5 > S1 spinal nerve roots.

Activation: Patient to flex the knee and internally rotate the tibia.

Needle placement: Three finger breadths proximal to the medial knee and medial (though can be lateral as well) to the semitendinosus tendon (see Fig. 3.43).

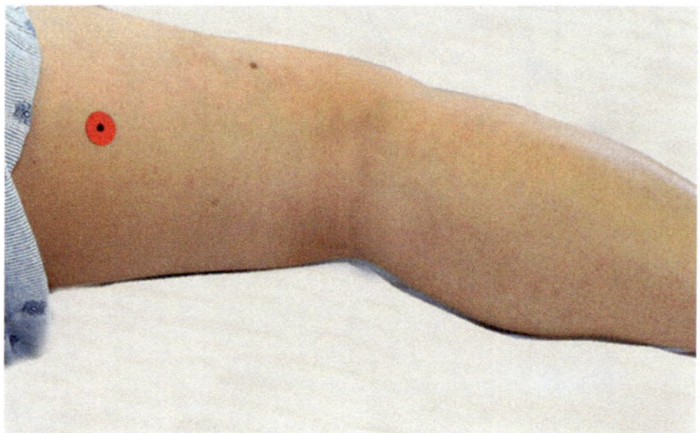

Fig. 3.42 Needle insertion site (black dot in center of red circle) for needle electrode examination of the long head of biceps femoris

Indications Include: sciatic neuropathy, Anterior division sacral plexopathy, L5 > S1 radiculopathies.

Potential Confounders: If electrode inserted too laterally it will be in the semitendinosus and if inserted further laterally it will be in the short head of the biceps femoris; if inserted too deeply will be in the adductor magnus.

Semitendinosus

Innervation: Sciatic nerve (Tibial division) ← Anterior division of the Sacral Plexus ← L5 > S1 spinal nerve roots.

Activation: Patient to flex the knee and internally rotate the tibia.

Needle placement: Midpoint between the ischial tuberosity and the medial knee (superficial to the semimembranosus) (see Fig. 3.44).

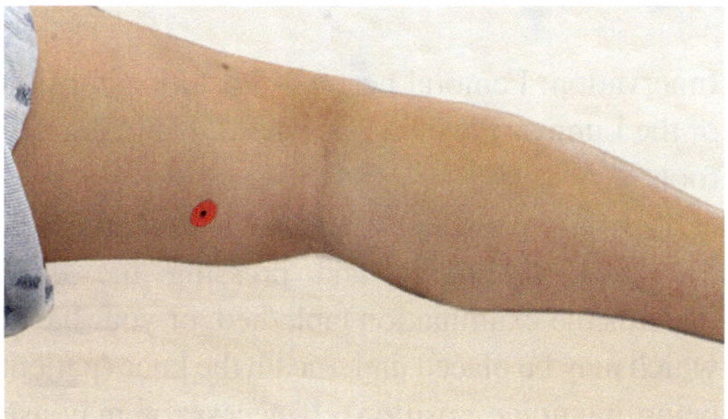

Fig. 3.43 Needle insertion site (black dot in center of red circle) for needle electrode examination of the semimembranosus

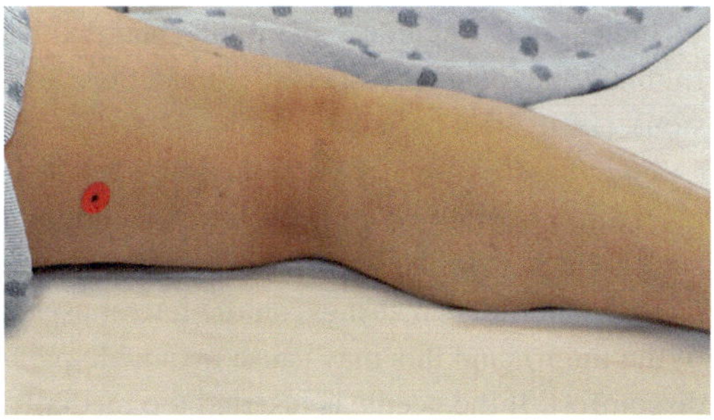

Fig. 3.44 Needle insertion site (black dot in center of red circle) for needle electrode examination of the semitendinosus

Indications include: sciatic neuropathy, Anterior division sacral plexopathy, L5 > S1 radiculopathies.

Potential Confounders: If electrode inserted too lateral it will be in the long head of biceps femoris, if inserted too medial or too deep it will be in the semimembranosus.

Tensor Fascia Lata

Innervation: Superior gluteal nerve ← Posterior division of the Sacral Plexus ← L5 > S1 spinal nerve roots.

Activation: Patient to internally rotate thigh (this muscle is also a weak hip abductor).

Needle placement: Two finger breadths anterior to the greater trochanter (see Fig. 3.45).

Indications include: Superior gluteal neuropathy, Posterior division sacral plexopathy, L5 > S1 radiculopathies.

Potential Confounders: If electrode inserted too anterior it will be in the sartorius or rectus femoris, if inserted too deep it will be in the vastus lateralis, if inserted too posteriorly it will be in the gluteus medius (although this is also superior gluteal/L5 > S1-innervated).

Gluteus Medius

Innervation: Superior gluteal nerve ← Posterior division of the Sacral Plexus ← L5 > S1 spinal nerve roots.

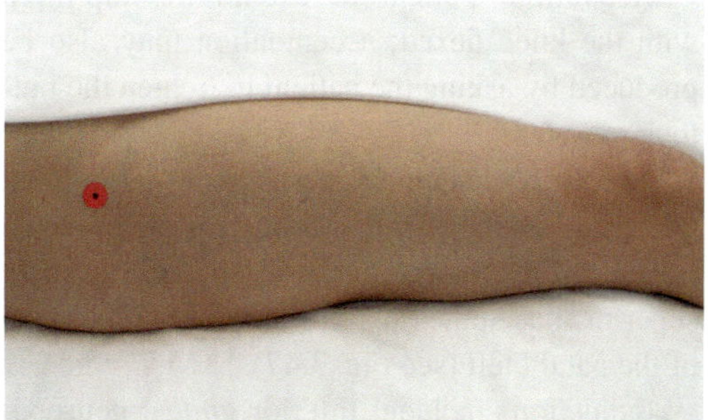

Fig. 3.45 Needle insertion site (black dot in center of red circle) for needle electrode examination of the tensor fascia lata

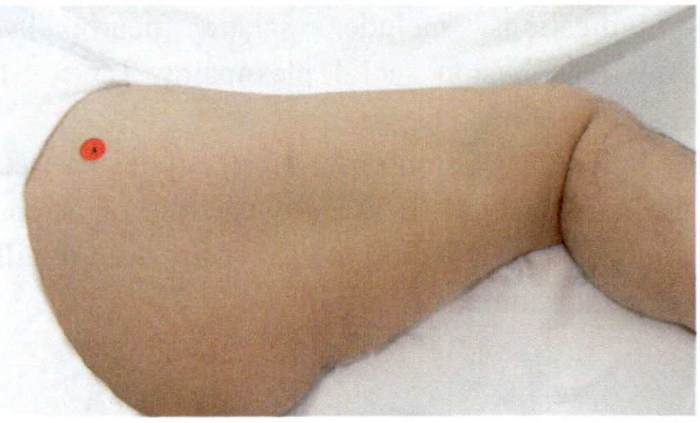

Fig. 3.46 Needle insertion site (black dot in center of red circle) for needle electrode examination of the gluteus medius

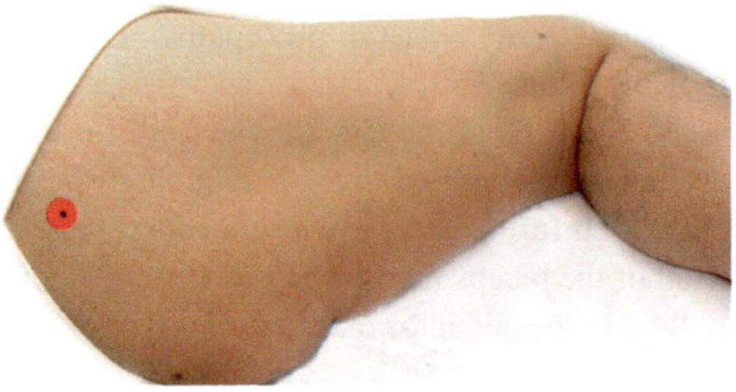

Fig. 3.47 Needle insertion site (black dot in center of red circle) for needle electrode examination of the gluteus maximus

Activation: Patient to abduct the thigh.

Needle placement: With the patient in the lateral decubitus position, contralateral side down, the needle is inserted about two finger breadths posterior to the mid-point between the summit of the iliac crest and the greater trochanter (see Fig. 3.46).

Indications include: Superior gluteal neuropathy, Posterior division sacral plexopathy, L5 > S1 radiculopathies.

Potential Confounders: If the needle is inserted too anteriorly, it may be in the tensor fascia lata (although this is also superior gluteal/ L5 > S1-innervated).

Gluteus Maximus

Innervation: Inferior gluteal nerve ← Posterior division of the Sacral Plexus ← S1(S2) > L5 spinal nerve roots.

Activation: Patient to extend the hip/thigh with the knee flexed; accentuation may also be produced by asking the patient to tighten the buttock muscles.

Needle placement: Superior external buttock quadrant (as shown), or about 2 finger breadths lateral to the midpoint between the posterior superior iliac spine (at sacral dimple) and the top of the natal cleft (see Fig. 3.47).

Indications include: Inferior gluteal neuropathy, Posterior division sacral plexopathy, S1 > L5 radiculopathies.

Potential Confounders/Pitfalls: Iatrogenic injury to the sciatic nerve is the major issue to avoid. This tends to occur if needle insertion is too lateral or inferior to the site recommended above.

Vastus Lateralis

Innervation: Femoral nerve ← Posterior division of the Lumbar Plexus ← (L2)L3–L4 spinal nerve roots.

Activation: Patient to extend and gently lock the knee, tightening and pressing the knee towards the examination table/bed, or your hand, which may be placed underneath the knee (patient being in supine position). If necessary, may ask the patient to elevate the heel off the bed.

Needle placement: lateral aspect of the upper thigh, anterior to the groove formed between the outer portion of the hamstrings and vastus lateralis (see Fig. 3.48).

Indications include: Femoral neuropathy, Lumbar plexopathy (especially posterior division), (L2)L3–L4 radiculopathies.

Potential Confounders/Pitfalls: If the needle is placed too laterally, it may go into the iliotibial band (which is in the groove between the vastus lateralis and the hamstrings, on the lateral aspect of the thigh), and this may cause avoidable pain/ discomfort. If the needle is inserted too medially, it may enter the rectus femoris (although this is also femoral/(L2)L3–4-innervated).

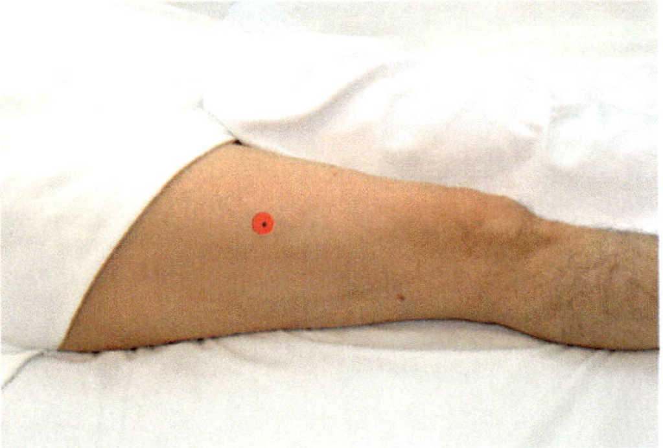

Fig. 3.48 Needle insertion site (black dot in center of red circle) for needle electrode examination of the vastus lateralis

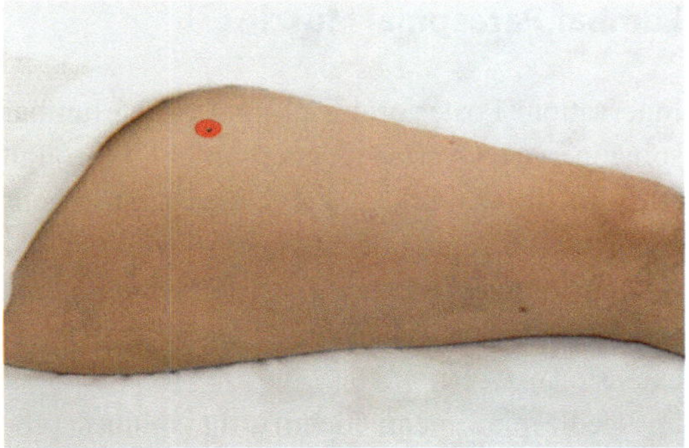

Fig. 3.49 Needle insertion site (black dot in center of red circle) for needle electrode examination of the rectus femoris

Rectus Femoris

Innervation: Femoral nerve ← Posterior division of the Lumbar Plexus ← (L2)L3–L4 spinal nerve roots.

Activation: Patient to extend the knee and flex at the hip (this muscle spans both the knee and hip joints.

Needle placement: Anterior aspect of the thigh, at the midpoint between the knee and anterior superior iliac spine (see Fig. 3.49).

Indications include: Femoral neuropathy, Lumbar plexopathy (especially posterior division), (L2)L3–L4 radiculopathies.

Confounders: If too distal of a needle insertion, the muscle become thin and more tendinous and tends to be painful, with risk of abutting the distal femoral bone/periosteum. If needle insertion is too lateral or too medial, the vastus lateralis or vastus medialis (respectively) may be entered—although both are also femoral/(L2)L3–4-innervated.

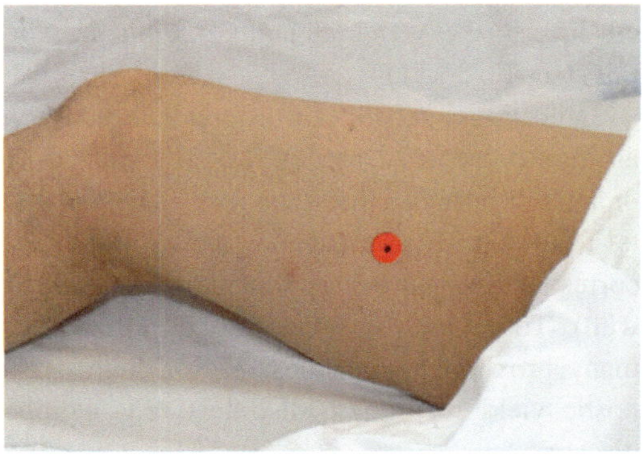

Fig. 3.50 Needle insertion site (black dot in center of red circle) for needle electrode examination of the adductor longus

Adductor Longus

Innervation: Obturator nerve ← Anterior division of the Lumbar Plexus ← L2–L4 spinal nerve roots.

Note: Needle examination of this muscle is often helpful in differentiating a lumbar plexopathy (affecting the anterior division) from a femoral mononeuropathy.

Activation: Patient to adduct the thigh.

Needle placement: Proximal medial thigh, about three to four finger breadths distal to the pubic tubercle (see Fig. 3.50).

Indications include: Obturator neuropathy, Lumbar plexopathies (especially anterior division), L2–L4 radiculopathies.

Potential Confounders: If the needle is placed too distally, the adductor longus is no longer superficial, and the adductor magnus may be entered. The latter muscle is partially innervated by the sciatic nerve (tibial division) as well, and may provide misleading data.

Lumbar Paraspinal Muscles

Innervation: Posterior/dorsal rami of the lumbar spinal nerves. Overlap innervation of L1 through S1 spinal nerve root segments (overlap may occur for up to 4–6 contiguous segments/levels).

Activation: Hip extension. Alternatively, may ask the patient to arch the trunk backwards (spine extension).

Needle placement: Identify the spinous process (using as a reference, the L3–L4 level in between the posterior superior iliac crest on either side), and place the needle about two to four centimeters laterally, with the tip of the electrode oriented medially towards the deeper muscle layers (the vertebral lamina being deep to this) (see Fig. 3.51).

Indications include: To differentiate between an intraspinal canal process (e.g. radiculopathy or anterior horn cell disorder) versus a lesion distal to the dorsal root ganglia (which will affect corresponding sensory nerve action potentials as well). These muscles may also be affected in many proximal myopathies, having high diagnostic yield for certain disorders (e.g. Pompe disease).

Potential Confounders/Pitfalls: Needle examination that is too deep may irritate the bony vertebral laminae with resultant excessive pain. It is not necessary to always have the patient activate these muscles as it is generally uncomfortable/difficult to execute and the evaluation of recruitment and motor unit morphology is seldom further helpful in most studies, except in patients with myopathies, and motor neuron diseases.

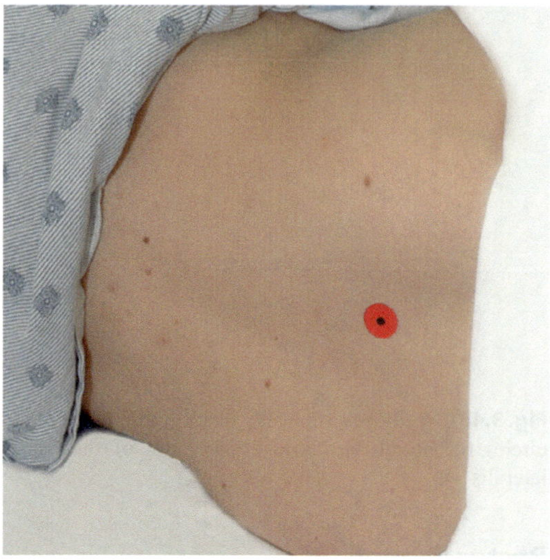

Fig. 3.51 Needle insertion site (black dot in center of red circle) for needle electrode examination of the (low) lumbar paraspinal muscles

Suggested Reading

1. Leis AA, Trapani VC. Atlas of electromyography. Oxford: Oxford University Press; 2000.
2. Perotto A, Delagi EF. Anatomical guide for the electromyographer: the limbs and trunk. 5th ed. Springfield, IL: Charles C. Thomas Publisher; 2011.
3. Lee HJ, DeLisa JA, Lee HJ. Manual of nerve conduction study and surface anatomy for needle electromyography. In: Surface anatomy for clinical needle electromyography. 4th ed. Philadelphia: Lippincott Wilkins and Williams; 2005.

Introduction to Needle Electromyography

4

Bryan Tsao

What Do We Measure with the Needle EMG?

A single motor unit includes one anterior horn cell (AHC), its axon process and terminal branches, neuromuscular junction, and muscle fibers. The electrical activity of motor units recorded with a needle electrode or motor unit action potentials (MUAPs), is the sum of action potentials generated by those muscle fibers that fire singly or in groups near the electrode [1]. In contrast to the NCS which assess both motor and sensory nerves, the needle EMG only assesses the integrity of the motor unit, but is a more quantitative method for doing so (Table 4.1).

The needle EMG search contains two portions: searching at rest for *spontaneous activity* and assessing with muscle activation *MUAP appearance and recruitment*. When the needle is moved within resting muscle, muscle fiber discharges are induced that result in normal *insertional activity*, recognized by its sharp, distinct, and brief sound. Normal insertional activity lasts less than 200–300 μsec after needle movement stops [3–5] (Fig. 4.1).

A benign variant of normal insertional activity comprised of irregularly firing discharges, often in the form of positive sharp waves that typically resolve with 10 s of onset, is termed “snap, crackle, pop”. This is more often found in younger, healthy, muscular males, more frequently in the lower limbs than upper limbs, and most commonly in the medial gastrocnemius muscle [3]. Abnormal increased insertional activity includes trains of positive sharp waves and fibrillation potentials, sometimes irregular in their firing frequency, that last more than 300 μsec but are non-sustained.

Opposite of increased insertional activity is *decreased insertional activity*, identified when the needle is moved through electrically inactive tissue, e.g., subcutaneous adipose, edema, or necrotic or fibrotic muscle. Certain neuromuscular conditions associated with disorders of glycogen metabolism (i.e., myophosphorylase, phosphofructokinase deficiency) as well as ion channel defects during episodes of periodic paralysis can also result in decreased insertional activity or electrical silence [3].

Spontaneous activity is defined as discharges that occur without being triggered by needle movement and continue longer than 200–300 μsec or indefinitely. Normal increased spontaneous activity is seen when the needle tip approximates the neuromuscular junction generating *end-plate spikes* (from the terminal axon) and *end-plate noise* (from the release of mini end-plate potentials); this is interpreted by patients as a particularly strong aching or painful sensation (Figs. 4.2 and 4.3).

B. Tsao (✉)
Department of Neurology, Loma Linda University School of Medicine, Loma Linda, CA, USA
e-mail: btsao@llu.edu

N. Galvez-Jimenez et al. (eds.), *Electrodiagnostic Medicine*,
https://doi.org/10.1007/978-3-030-74997-2_4

Table 4.1 Advantages and limitations of nerve conduction studies and the needle EMG [2]

Nerve conduction studies	
Advantages	Subclinical detection of demyelinating lesions Less uncomfortable, requires less cooperation Highly sensitive in differentiating axon loss from demyelination Can locate focal demyelinating lesions
Limitations	Routine studies primarily assess the distal nerves Certain sensory responses may be lost with age Less sensitive for axon loss
Needle EMG	
Advantages	Subclinical detection of axon loss lesions Allows for more widespread examination of the peripheral nervous system Can diagnose myopathy
Limitations	Requires patient cooperation and is generally more uncomfortable Does not evaluate sensory fibers Insensitive for demyelinating lesions

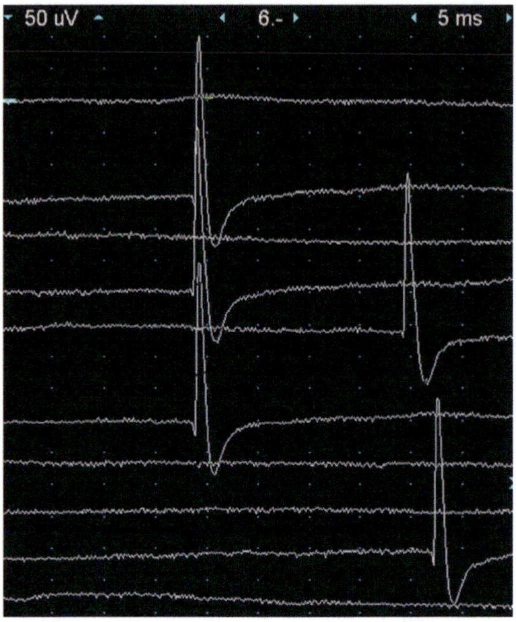

Fig. 4.2 End-plate spikes (raster plot)—the baseline is normal and the initial negative (upward) deflection of the potential distinguishes it from spike fibrillation potentials (which have an initial positive or downward deflection)

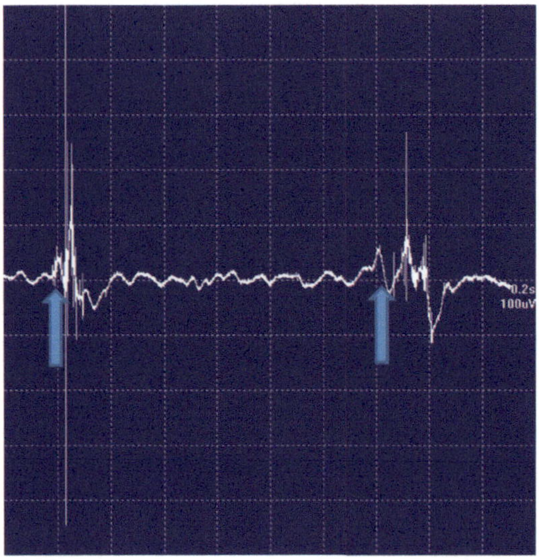

Fig. 4.1 Normal insertional activity—short duration discharges triggered by needle movement (indicated by blue arrows), associated with a sharp, discrete, and brief sound. Normally, this activity lasts less than 200–300 μsec after the cessation of needle movement

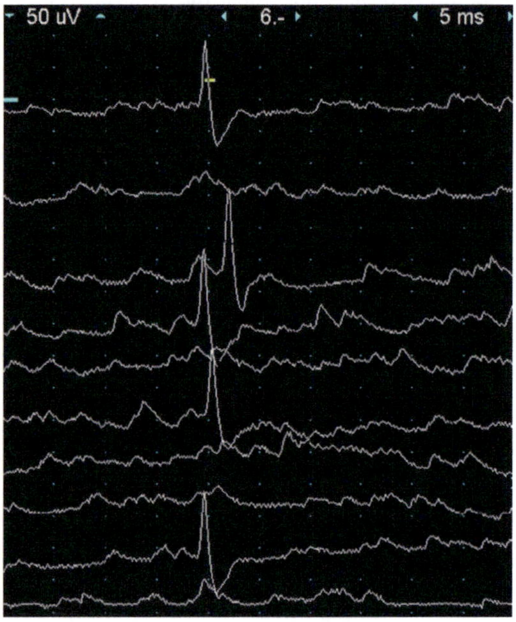

Fig. 4.3 Endplate spikes and endplate noise—note increased baseline "hiss" or low amplitude waveforms compared to a normal smooth baseline as well as the initial negative (upward) deflection of the endplate spike potential

Fasciculation potentials are MUAPs that fire in a spontaneous manner singly or in groups and are characterized by their irregular rate. It is often said that "fasciculations are only as bad as the company they keep". Accordingly, fasciculation potentials are normal when they occur in isolation, and even when abundant are most often seen with benign fasciculation or the benign cramp-fasciculation syndrome. While fasciculations potentials may be the initial manifestation of amyotrophic lateral sclerosis or grouped into myokymic potentials as part of focal or generalized myokymic conditions, it is only when they are accompanied by other abnormal findings in sufficient distribution (such as evidence of widespread denervation and reinnervation), should they be considered abnormal (Fig. 4.4).

Abnormal spontaneous activity spontaneous comes in many forms and includes *fibrillation potentials, positive sharp waves, myotonia, myokymia, neuromyotonia, complex repetitive discharges, cramps, tremor*, and *electrical artifact*, each described in Table 4.2 and illustrated in Figs. 4.5, 4.6, 4.7, 4.8, 4.9, 4.10, 4.11, 4.12 and 4.13.

During low levels of muscle contraction, MUAPs are assessed for amplitude (peak-to-peak), duration, number of phases (baseline crossings plus one; normal is four or less), and serrations or turns (changes in waveform deflection without baseline crossing) (Fig. 4.14a, b). Each muscle has its own morphology or characteristic MUAP appearance related to the ratio of the muscle fibers innervated by a single motor neuron/AHC and to the way the muscle's end plate zone is laid out in the muscle belly [3]. For example, MUAPs in normal gluteus maximus, biceps, brachioradialis, iliacus, frontalis, obicularis oris, obicularis oculi, and paraspinal muscles tend to have MUAPs with shorter mean duration and increased number of phases, with up to 10–30% of normal MUAPs having more than five phases [4]. In contrast, MUAPs in the triceps, vastus lateralis, and tibialis anterior tend to have a slightly longer duration. Normal duration ranges from ≤10–15 msec and MUAP amplitude is typically ≤2–3 millivolts.

Age is another factor that affects MUAP duration such that broad MUAPs of slightly

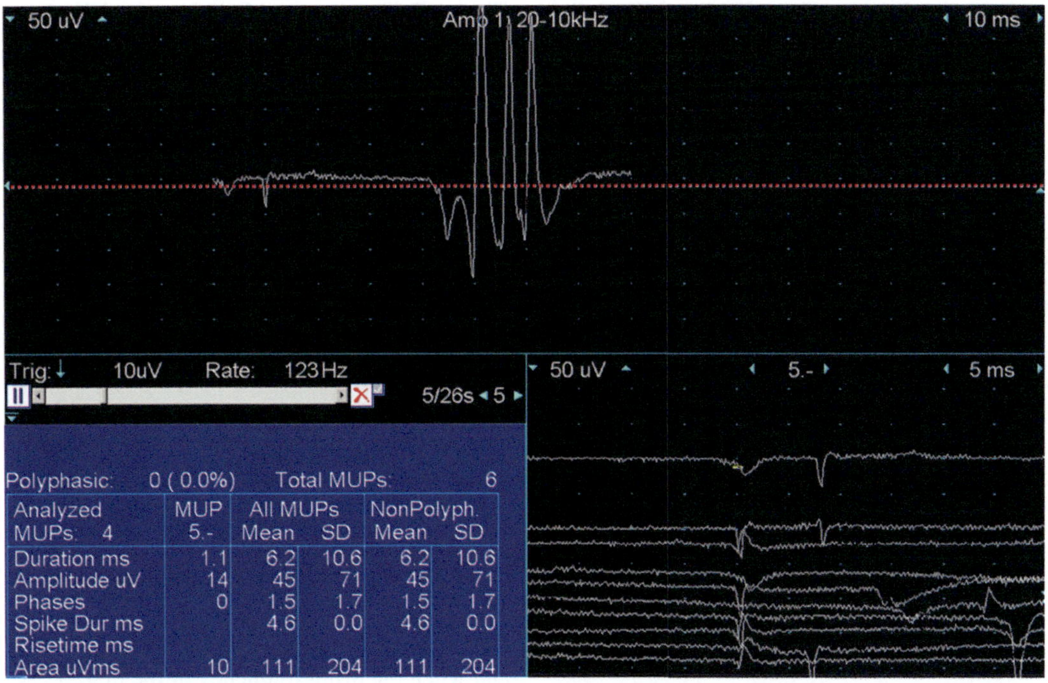

Fig. 4.4 Complex fasciculation potential on a background of small positive sharp wave potentials (shown on the lower right rastered screen)

Table 4.2 Types of spontaneous activity [4]

Type	Generator	Characteristics
End-plate spikes	Terminal axon	Biphasic with initial negative deflection, irregular
End-plate noise	Mini end-plate potentials	High-pitched hissing
Fasciculation potentials	AHC, nerve > muscle	Simple or polyphasic MUAP appearance, irregular/random rates varying from 0.005 Hz to many per minute
Fibrillation potentials	Muscle fiber	Triphasic (positive-negative-positive) potentials. Rarely irregular but not as irregular as end-plate spikes
Positive sharp waves	Muscle fiber	Mono or biphasic wave, fires regularly or irregularly
Myotonia	Muscle fiber	Brief biphasic or triphasic spikes that fire between 20–100 Hz with a waxing and waning (crescendo and decrescendo) pattern; positive sharp positive wave form induced by needle insertion
Myokymia	Groups of motor units	Regular or semi-regular bursts of normal MUAPs at 0.1–10 Hz
Neuromyotonia	Motor units	High frequency (up to 300 Hz) discharges with characteristic 'pinging' sound
CRD	Muscle	Groups of simple or complex spike patterns (via ephaptic transmission) that regularly repeat at 0.3–150 Hz
Cramp	Multiple motor units	Fire synchronously between 40 and 60 Hz, rarely up to 200–300 Hz
Tremor	Motor units/CNS origin	Correlates with the type of tremor
Artifact	Pacemaker (among other types)	Small very regular spikes (pacemaker)

AHC anterior horn cell, *CNS* central nervous system, *CRD* complex repetitive discharge, *MUAP* motor unit action potential

increased duration in a 75 year old may be normal for the patient's age but may be abnormal for a younger patient. The regulation of surface temperature during the EDX study is essential not only for NCSs but also needle EMG. Cooling results in delayed inactivation of sodium channels in nerve and muscle and increased duration of action potentials so that an increase in MUAP amplitude and duration is expected [3]. Cooling of the muscle will increase the amplitude and duration of waveforms while cooling of the nerve may inhibit spontaneous firing and reduce the discharge frequency of spontaneous neuronal discharges [6]. Thus, it is imperative that the limbs be maintained within the same temperature range as desired for NCS (>32 °C for the upper and >30 °C for the lower limbs, per American Association of Neuromuscular and Electrodiagnostic Medicine laboratory accreditation guidelines).

The theory behind MUAP recruitment is straightforward but the ability to consistently judge MUAP recruitment takes considerable experience and is one of the more difficult EDX skills to acquire. MUAPs are recruited in an orderly manner based on the *Henneman size principle* which refers to the orderly successive activation of MUAPs such that small, "weak" type I motor units are activated first in early or minimal contraction, and sequentially larger, "stronger" type II motor units are called up to deliver an increase in muscle power [3]. Initial MUAP recruitment is best assessed with minimal activation when most MUAPs represent the smaller motor units that comprise type I muscle fibers [7] (Fig. 4.15). With minimal volitional contraction, a single MUAP begins to fire at a frequency of around 5 Hz. With increased effort and when the firing frequency of the first MUAP reaches 10 Hz, a second MUAP is recruited. With continued increased effort, when the firing

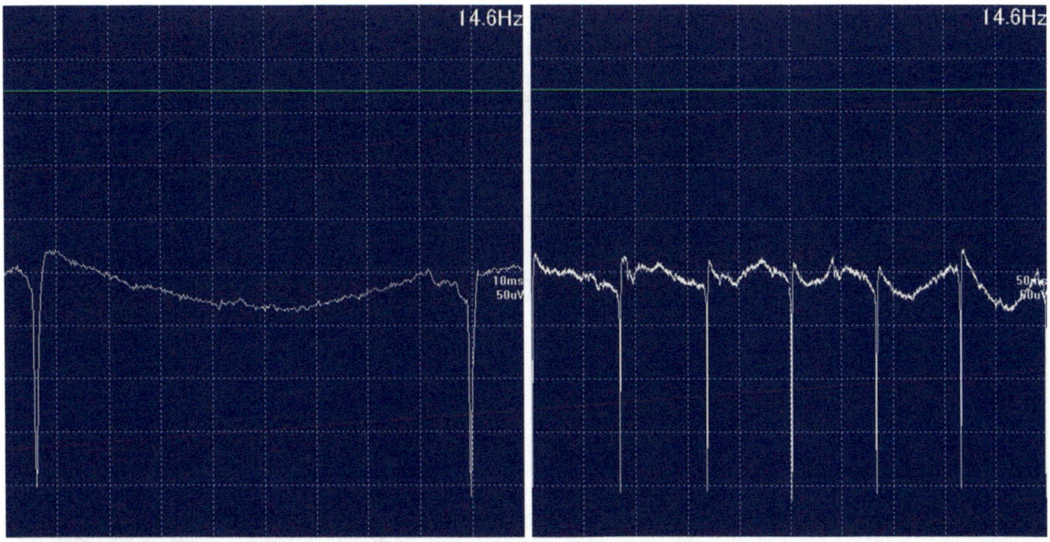

Fig. 4.5 Fibrillation potentials (positive wave form)—note the low amplitude (~200 μV), short duration (~8 ms), regularly-firing potentials

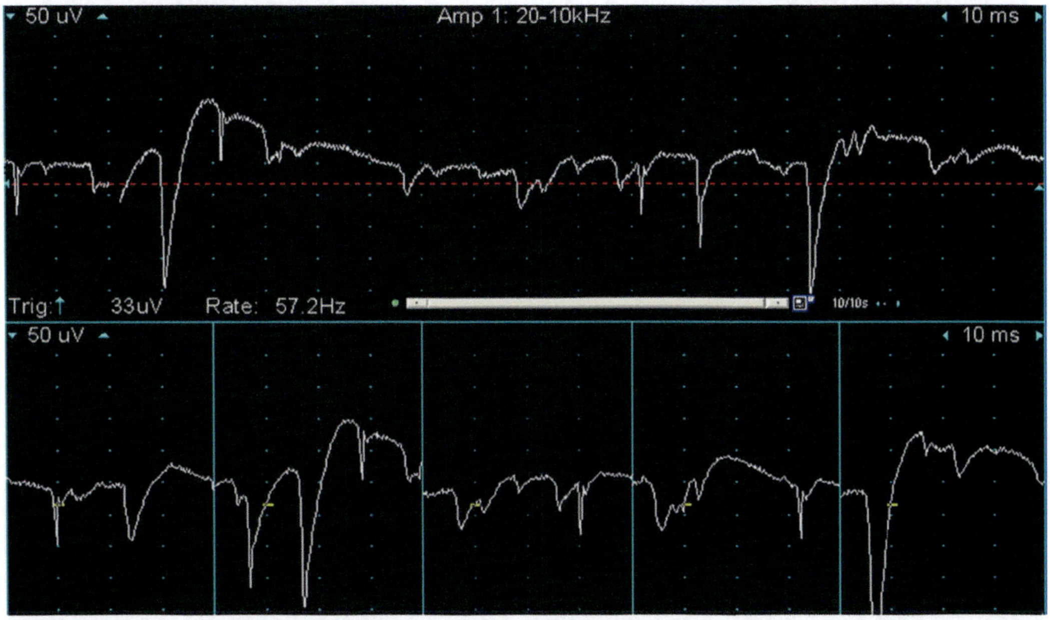

Fig. 4.6 Many positive sharp wave potentials—note the initial positive or downward deflection from baseline

frequency of the first potential reaches 15 Hz, a third MUAP is recruited, and so forth. Thus, for every 5 Hz increase in firing frequency of the original MUAP, an additional MUAP is recruited. This is referred to as the 5:1 recruitment ratio or the rule of 5's. When the recruitment ratio is increased, especially to 10:1, there are too few motor units for the rate of firing frequency and force produced, implying *reduced recruitment*, most commonly due to neurogenic disease in the form of axon loss (Fig. 4.16) or demyelinating conduction block. The sound differences between normal MUAP recruitment or severely reduced recruitment is easily recognized by the

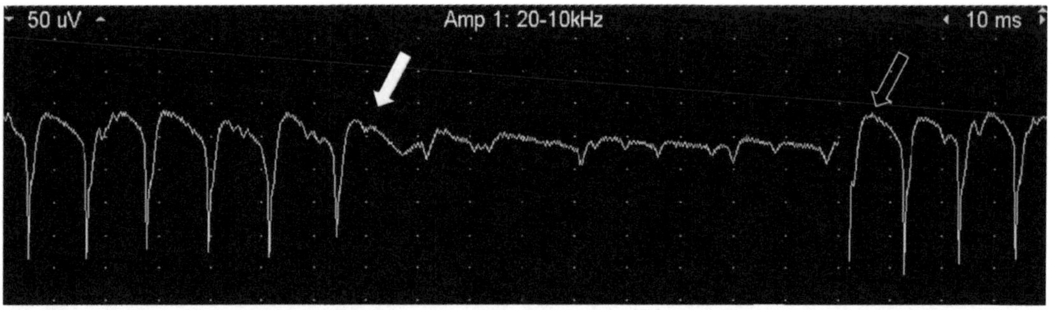

Fig. 4.7 Myotonic potentials—note the positive sharp wave morphology with a transition comprising reduced frequency and amplitude of the waveform (solid white arrow) and then recurrence of myotonic potentials (white outline arrow), hence the typical waxing and waning profile

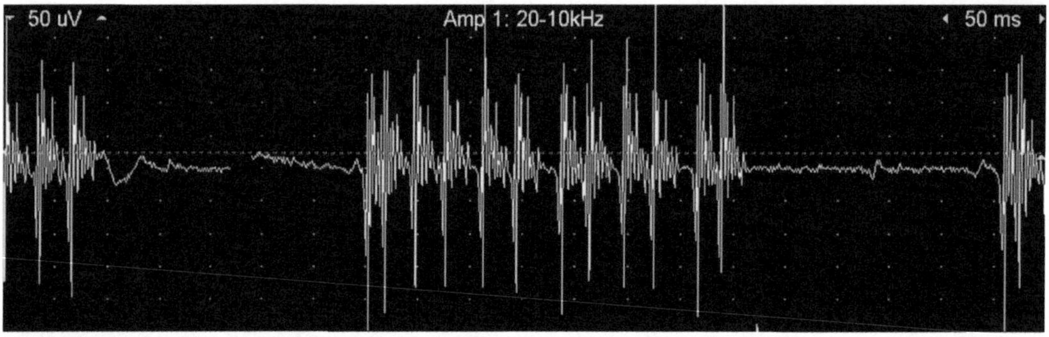

Fig. 4.8 Myokymic potentials—note the semi-rhythmic firing of grouped motor unit potentials occurring in bursts, typically producing a "marching soldiers" sound

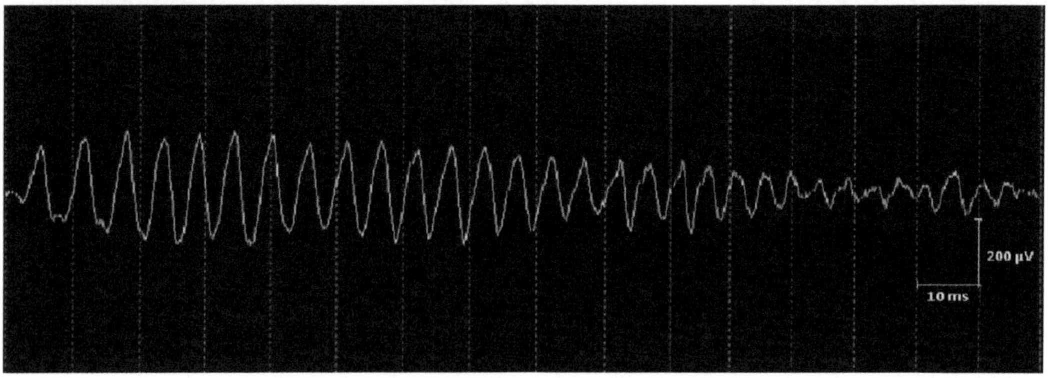

Fig. 4.9 Neuromyotonia—note the spontaneous, brief, very high-frequency discharge (~180 Hz) which tapers off in amplitude to create the characteristic "pinging" sound

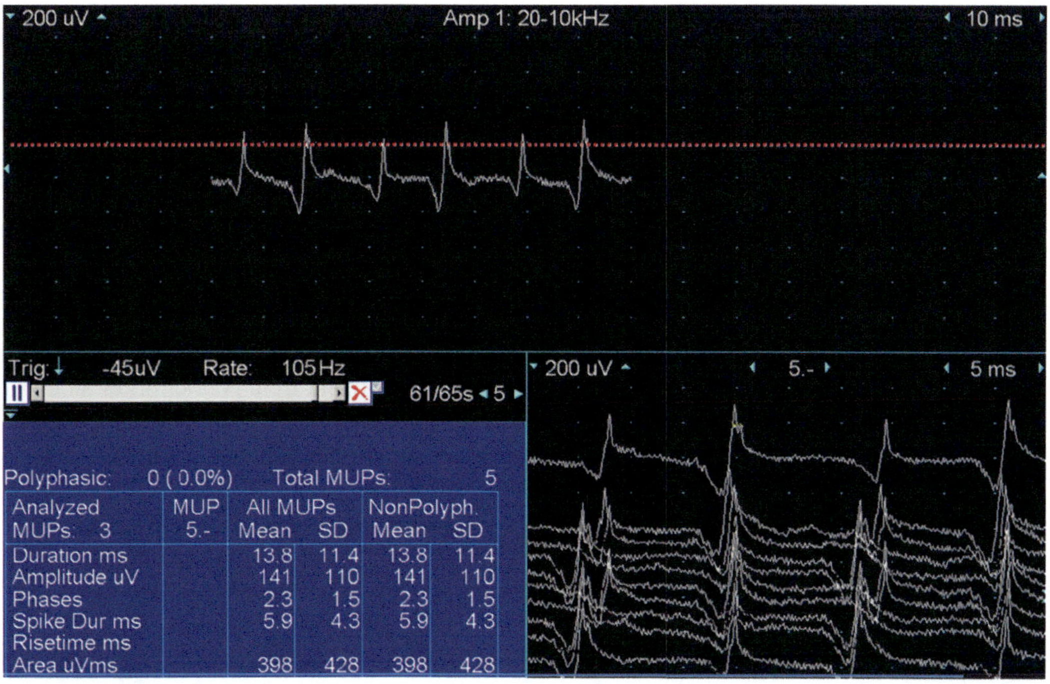

Fig. 4.10 Complex repetitive discharges (CRDs)—note the regularly repeating potentials with inter-potential duration of ~10 ms (~100 Hz frequency, particularly fast in this example). These have typical abrupt onset and cessation

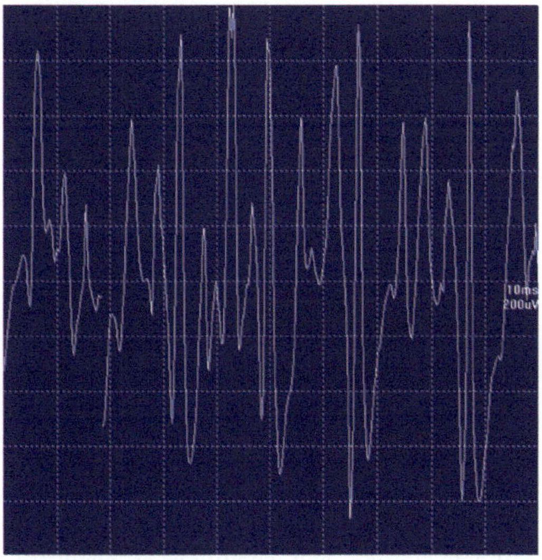

Fig. 4.11 Cramp potentials—note MUAPs firing synchronously (typically 40–60 Hz), correlating with involuntary painful contraction of the muscle being examined

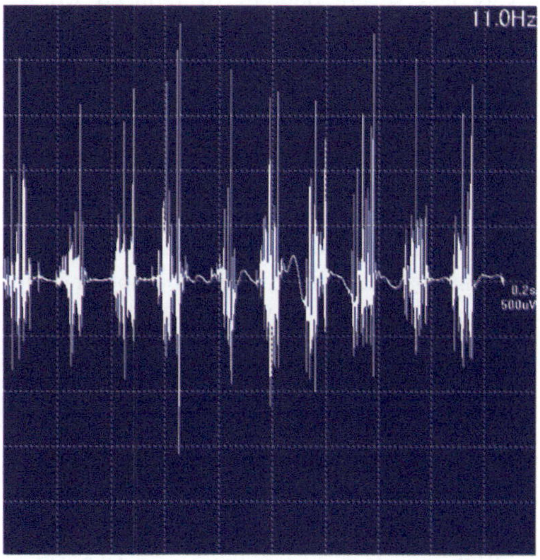

Fig. 4.12 Tremor tracing—normal MUAPs activated in a very intermittent but regular manner, corresponding with the frequency of the underlying tremor

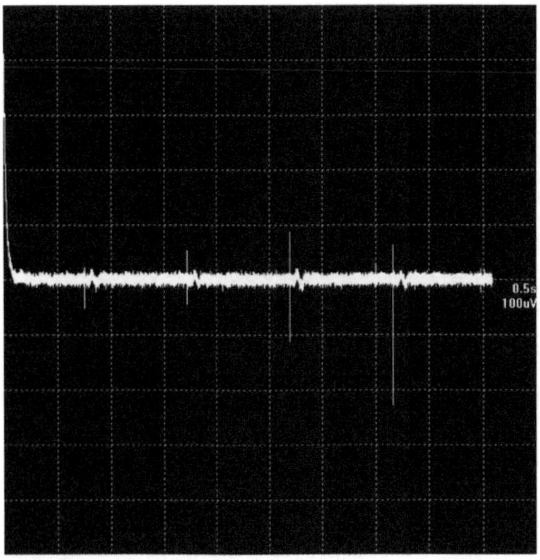

Fig. 4.13 Artifact from an implanted cardiac pacemaker device (detected while recording spontaneous activity in the lumbar paraspinal muscles)—note the small, very regular spikes corresponding to the pacemaker setting of 60 beats per minute

seasoned EDX medicine consultant. However, it becomes increasingly difficult to judge progressively less severe degrees of reduced MUAP recruitment. One commonly used method of MUAP recruitment defines four grades of recruitment, where 4R = only a single MUAP (severely or profoundly reduced); 3R = 2–3 MUAPs (markedly reduced); 2R = 4 or more MUAPs (moderately reduced); and 1R = just less than normal but not as reduced as the 2R designation, i.e., mildly reduced. Another annotation for 4R is single MUAP (SMU). In practice, most EDX medicine consultants do not routinely calculate recruitment ratios or the firing frequency of MUAPS. Instead, the degree of abnormal recruitment is judged by a combination of visual and auditory recognition. Hence the semi-quantitative nature of the needle EMG.

With muscle disorders there is a drop out of muscle fibers and a reduction in contractile force per motor unit. This results in a decreased recruitment ratio (below 4:1) or the activation of too many MUAPs for the degree of muscle contraction, termed *early (sometimes also referred to as "rapid") recruitment* [4] (Fig. 4.17). The best way to determine early recruitment is if the EDX examiner can feel and judge the amount of force that is being sustained by the patient while assessing the number of displayed MUAPs.

Incomplete MUAP recruitment can also result from poor volitional muscle contraction, most often in the setting of pain-limited effort or functional weakness. It can also be seen in the presence of pre-existing upper motor neuron disorders (e.g., with myelopathy, prior stroke, multiple sclerosis, etc.) when patients are unable to activate muscles effectively on command. Incomplete MUAP recruitment from poor effort or an upper motor neuron disorder can be indistinguishable and appear as either intermittent firing, or firing at slow frequencies despite maximal effort, referred to as "slow firing MUAPS". Whenever this is present, the electromyographer can only attest that recruitment of the number of MUAPs present is appropriate to the degree the muscle is activated [8].

How Do We Perform These Measurements?

During needle EMG the typical display sweep speed is set at 10 msec/division. The sensitivity is set to 50 uV/division when searching for spontaneous activity and 200 uV when assessing for MUAP appearance and recruitment. To better visualize abnormally large MUAPs, the sensitivity setting may have to be temporarily adjusted to 1000 uV or 1 mV [4]. Needle EMG may employ either of two types of needles: concentric or monopolar (Table 4.3 and Fig. 4.18a, b). For concentric needles with a range of 23–25 gauge, anywhere from 8 to 20 muscle fibers belonging to same motor unit contribute to the MUAP [3].

The ideal time frame in which to perform NCS and needle EMG depends on the suspected pathophysiology and condition at hand (see Chap. 2). For any peripheral condition causing weakness, the needle EMG can performed from the moment weakness is present. It is, however, unable to differentiate between axon loss and demyelinating conduction block as the causative pathophysiology when done too early. For example, if we perform the needle EMG in a

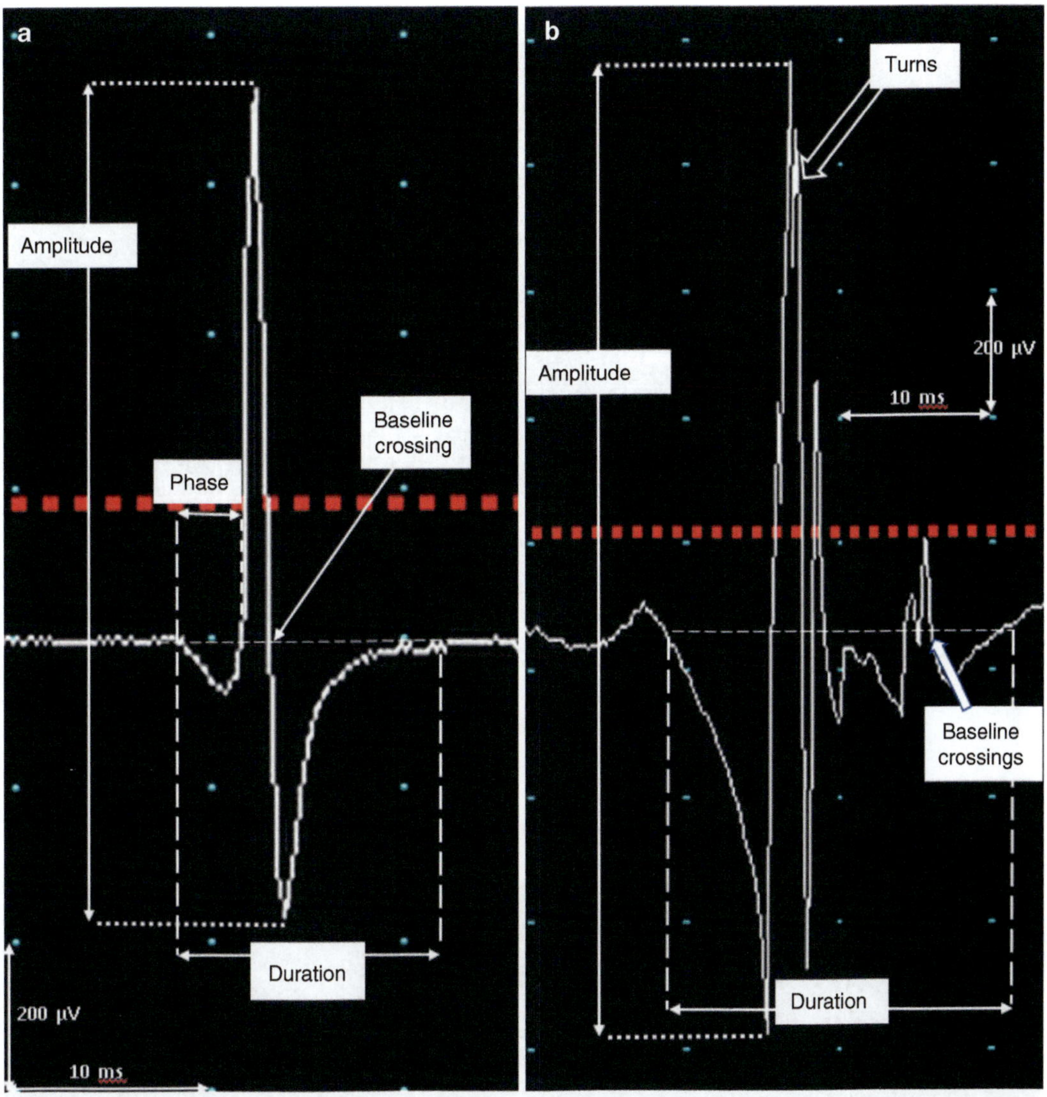

Fig. 4.14 (**a**) Normal motor unit action potential (MUAP) at 200 μV sensitivity and 10 ms sweep speed. Phases equal the number of baseline crossings (single white arrow) +1. In this MUAP, there are 2 baseline crossings +1 = 3 phases. Amplitude measures the entire vertical dimension of the MUAP, and in this illustration spans about just under six boxes or just under 1200 μV or 1.2 mV (normal is <2–3 mV). MUAP duration is measured from the onset of initial baseline deflection to the final return to baseline, measuring about one and a quarter boxes or 10.2–10.3 ms (normal is generally <15 ms). (**b**) Complex MUAP with increased duration and phases, at 200 μV sensitivity and 10 ms sweep speed. The duration is over two boxes wide or >20 ms, while the number of phases is at least six baseline crossings (solid white arrow) +1 = 7 total (normal generally 4 or less). Turns or serrations are changes in deflections without baseline crossings and are seen pointed out with the open arrow. The amplitude of this MUAP spans nearly eight boxes or 1600 μV or 1.6 mV, still within normal limits

muscle immediately after an acute axon lesion or immediately after a focal demyelinating lesion appears, the needle EMG will show a reduction in MUAP recruitment that is proportional to the degree of motor axon loss or conduction block. In this setting, NCS may determine if there is a focal demyelinating conduction block as long as proximal and distal stimulation (with the lesion in between these sites) is possible, and 5–7 days have passed to allow for Wallerian degeneration

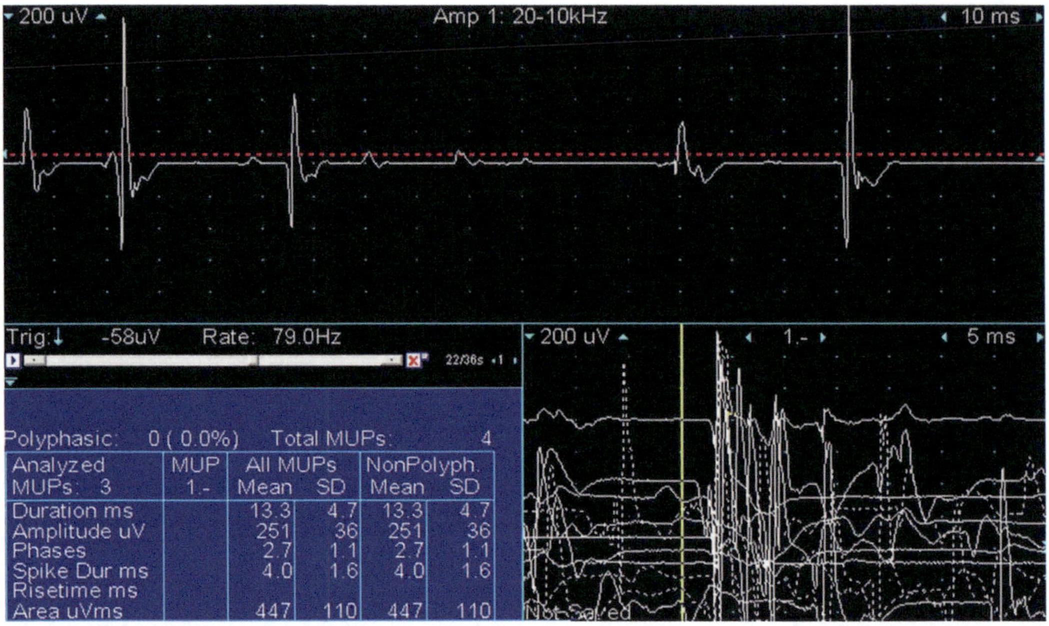

Fig. 4.15 Normal motor unit action potentials (MUAPs) within a normal recruitment pattern

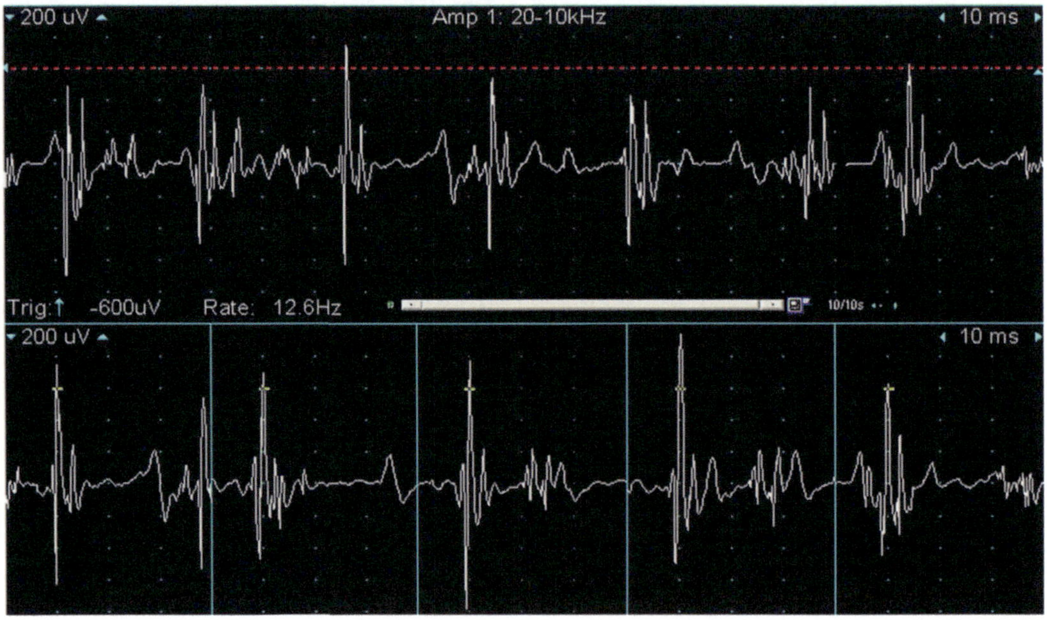

Fig. 4.16 Chronic motor axon loss/neurogenic recruitment pattern with complex MUAPs of increased duration and phases, high firing frequency of >30 Hz, with reduced number of recruited MUAPs (i.e. <4–5 MUAPs total, with recruitment ratio >5)

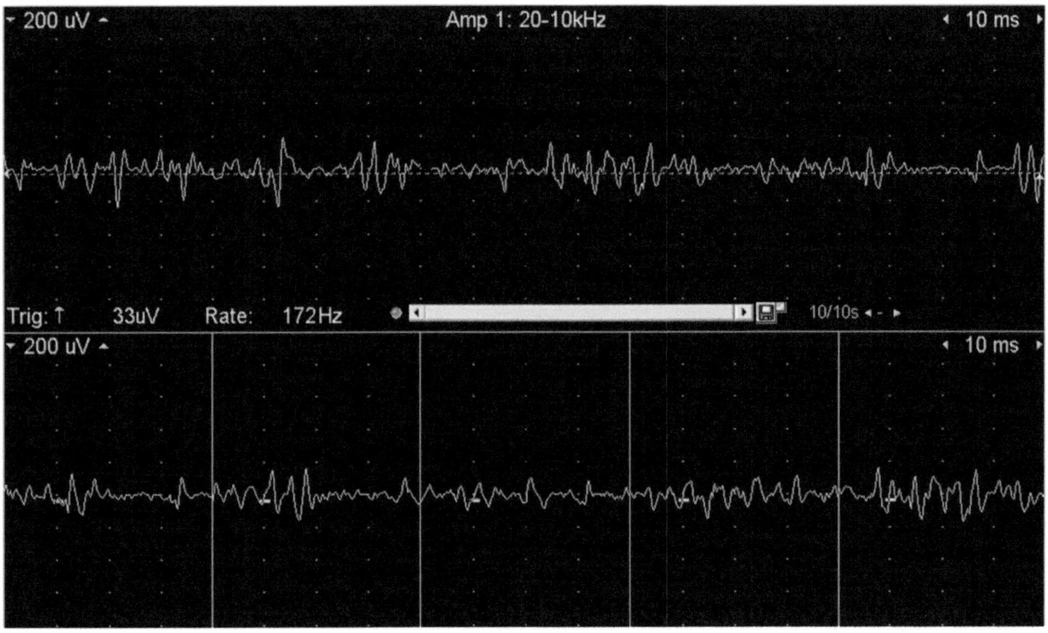

Fig. 4.17 Typical EMG findings in myopathy—note MUAPS of decreased duration, reduced amplitude, and increased phases (polyphasia). The large number of MUAPs at relatively low levels of contraction effort is consistent with "rapid" or "early" MUAP recruitment

Table 4.3 Comparison of concentric and monopolar needle electrodes [9]

	Concentric	Monopolar
Recording surface	20–100 μm^2	100–500 μm^2
Active electrode	On beveled edge of needle tip	Larger needle tip surface
Reference electrode	Needle shaft	Surface electrode
Patient tolerance	Lower	Higher
MUAP amplitude	Lower	Higher
MUAP duration	Shorter	Longer
LFF setting	10 Hz	20 Hz
HFF setting	10–20 kHz	20 kHz
Cost	Higher	Lower

μm micrometers, *MUAP* motor unit action potential, *LFF* low frequency filter (high-pass), *HFF* high frequency filter (low-pass)

to occur. This would exclude acute axon loss effects which may transiently mimic a conduction block (what constitutes a so-called "acute discontinuity lesion"). However, the acute-stage needle EMG alone will not be able to differentiate between acute axon loss and demyelinating conduction block and would have to be repeated after at least 3 weeks has passed in order to appreciate the development of fibrillation potentials. Waiting until 4–5 weeks have passed since the onset of symptoms (in particular weakness) increases the yield of the study as certain patients may not manifest significant fibrillation potentials at precisely 21 days. In short, a few conditions are amendable to needle EMG and NCS in under 3 weeks from target symptoms onset, including acquired demyelinating polyneuropathies and other focal demyelinating conditions, e.g., acute demyelinating polyradiculoneuropathy, radial nerve compression at the spiral groove (and similar entrapment mononeuropathies), and differentiating demyelinating conduction block from axon loss in facial neuropathy due to Bell's palsy.

The art of conducting the needle EMG relies on anticipating whether or not all the muscles that ideally need to be examined can be examined. The EDX consultant must factor patient tolerance

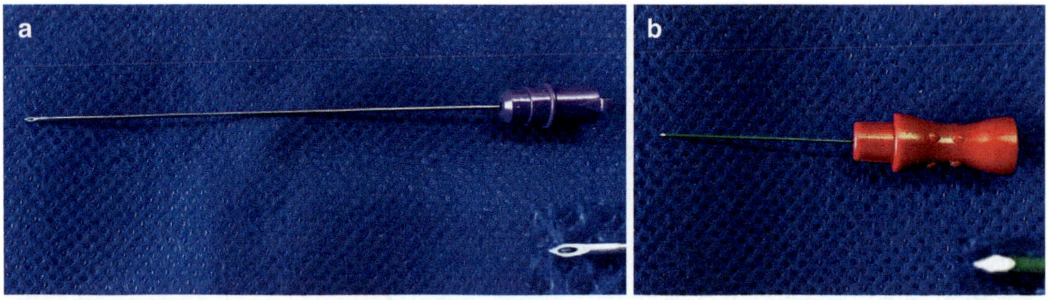

Fig. 4.18 (**a**) Picture of a concentric EMG needle (75 mm × 0.6 mm)—note, as seen in the magnified view in the inset (right lower corner), there is an outer cannula or "sleeve" of metal (E2 electrode) that is the external needle shaft, and the bevel tip discloses an internal metal wire shaft (E1 electrode) separated by an interposed layer of (darker) insulation material. (**b**) Picture of a monopolar EMG needle (25 mm × 0.35 mm)—note, as seen in the magnified view in the inset (right lower corner), there is an outer "sleeve" of green insulation material on the surface of the needle shaft and the "trocar" tip exposes a single metallic electrode (E1) surface

and prioritize which muscles to study based on their diagnostic yield. Here are some guidelines for performing the optimal needle EMG:

1. Educate the patient on what is about to take place, preferably using the term *pin* instead of *needle*.
2. Position the patient comfortably—they may need extra pillows; the room must be warm, slightly darkened, and quiet; and the limb positioned where maximum muscle relaxation can occur.
3. Start with high-yield and accessible muscles e.g., the triceps if cervical radiculopathy is suspected or tibialis anterior if lumbosacral radiculopathy is suspected. It may also be prudent to not start with muscles that are well-known to be rather sensitive/painful (e.g. the abductor pollicis brevis). You may routinely assess various muscles in a specific order, but be ready to adapt the study if it looks like patient tolerance is wearing thin.
4. While inserting the needle, some EDX medicine consultants like to say, "Here comes a little pinch" or other verbal clues to alert the patient and either simultaneously pinch, tap, or stretch the skin as a sensory distraction (pain-gating theory). Avoid having the length of the muscle significantly change (e.g. by having the patient fully contract or relax) while the needle is considerably intramuscular. You may withdraw the needle to the subcutaneous layer and then reinsert into the muscle during contraction and withdraw the needle similarly prior to muscle relaxation.
5. If the muscle is difficult to localize on the surface, first assess for MUAP configuration and recruitment before spontaneous activity so that you know you're in the desired muscle. This method is also preferred when searching muscles near vital structures, e.g., first have the patient activate to reliably localize the serratus anterior (to avoid pneumothorax) or the flexor pollicis longus (to avoid radial arterial puncture/hematoma).
6. Always finish the EDX examination with brief post-study instructions (covering typical post-EMG sequelae, which are usually benign and self-resolving), letting the patient know when results are expected to be posted to the ordering provider, help the patient sit up, and offer to assist with dressing (or call in a gender appropriate assistant) and safe departure.

Additional recommendations are listed in Table 4.4.

The needle EMG examination typically includes a single insertion into the muscle of choice, followed by 4–6 brief needle movements or searches that are divided into four quadrants of each muscle. There should be at least at least 2 s

Table 4.4 Additional guidelines on performing the needle EMG

Upper limb
– For extensor indicis proprius or other finger/wrist extensors, gently support the volar surface of the wrist in pronation to produce a 'limp' hand
– Palpate each muscle with contraction prior to inserting the needle no matter how obvious their location, particularly in patients with excess subcutaneous/adipose tissue
– Study the biceps brachii by inserting lateral or just medial of the midline (to avoid the intramuscular septum)
– The anconeus, although oftentimes tender, is a high-yield C7-innervated muscle and useful with radiculopathy work-ups when the triceps is uninvolved
– When assessing cranial-innervated muscles, always study the genioglossus last, and never insert a needle used to assess this muscle (when employing the intraoral/transmucosal approach) into another muscle. This minimizes bacterial translocation and infection risk
Lower limb
– Study the flexor digitorum longus instead of the posterior tibialis or have the patient co-contract both (ask patient to dorsiflex the toes while internally rotating the ankle)
– Save the intrinsic foot muscles, if indicated, for last
– The tensor of fascia lata may be more accessible than gluteus medius in patients with large hips
Either
– Activate the antagonist muscle if necessary to produce transient relaxation
– Support the neck and knees with pillows with slight neck and knee flexion and have the patient gently contract the abdominal/anterior neck muscles (or push the spine backwards) to obtain paraspinal muscle relaxation

between each search to distinguish between normal insertional activity induced by needle movement and abnormally increased insertional activity. The amount of needle searches may be increased or decreased, depending on the level of suspicion for abnormalities and how the patient is tolerating the examination. To assess for MUAP recruitment, the patient is first asked to perform a minimal voluntary contraction with specific directions on how to activate the muscle against resistance. Analyze single MUAPs before requesting full muscle contraction which is usually reserved for the end of the search. With maximal contraction in a normal muscle, the screen should be filled with overlapping MUAPs such that analysis of the firing frequency and configuration of individual MUAPs is difficult, if not impossible (thus, this is referred to as a "full interference pattern").

Ensure that you and the personnel in the EDX laboratory are well-versed on needle EMG safety guidelines. An example of physician safety guidelines is presented in Table 4.5. Growing evidence supports that performing the needle EMG in anticoagulated patients is relatively safe [10, 11]. However, we still leave it to the discretion of individual electrodiagnostic consultants on whether or not they feel comfortable performing extensive needle EMG on multiple limbs or large, deep muscle groups in patients with coagulopathy. Note is also made of the risks of needle EMG in patients with lymphedema. In such scenarios judicious muscle selection is also required to minimize risk of protracted oozing (of serous fluid) and infection.

Table 4.5 Safety guidelines for the needle EMG

Physician safety guidelines
– **Never** recap the needle using both hands
– **Always** recap the needle when moving the patient or performing any task that requires both hands
– The physician should **always** recap and dispose of the needle immediately after the study is complete
– **Always** dispose of the needle after studying the tongue/genioglossus muscle (when employing the intraoral/transmucosal approach) and use a new needle if additional muscles need to be studied
– **Always** use two pairs of gloves when assessing patients with known transmissible infections (including hepatitis, HIV, and any other potential blood-borne pathogens)
– **Remove gloves** when leaving the room and replace with new gloves prior to continuing the needle EMG
– **Always** provide patient pre- and post-needle EMG instructions
– If a contaminated needle stick occurs, ask the patient to remain available for consent for blood draw/potential blood draw as it pertains to ruling out transmissible infections

What Do the Measurements Mean? How Do Different Diseases Affect These Measurements?

MUAP abnormalities correlate with the location of pathology along the peripheral neuro-axis (Table 4.6). Neurogenic changes, e.g., fibrillation potentials and MUAPs of increased amplitude, duration, polyphasia, and reduced recruitment are present with disorders of the AHC, nerve root, plexus, or peripheral nerve. Normal MUAP duration varies with each muscle tested but a general rule of thumb is that duration ranges from ≤10–15 msec and MUAP amplitude ≤2–3 millivolts [3]. With reinnervation, an increased MUAP duration is typically correlated with an increase in phases but not necessarily a proportional increase in amplitude. Moreover, an interpretation of a study being abnormal should not rely on visualization of increased polyphasic MUAPs alone without correlative increases in duration or amplitude or a reduction in MUAP recruitment [8]. Markedly increased MUAP amplitude of 8–10 millivolts or greater invariably represents chronic neurogenic states in which reinnervated has occurred over years, e.g., remote poliomyelitis, late-onset spinal muscular atrophy, or (less typically) chronic radiculopathy.

With disorders of neuromuscular junction (NMJ) transmission, the needle EMG reflects findings that may be similar to myopathic diseases, including MUAPs of short duration, small amplitude, and increased phases or turns. Specifically, the MUAPs seen with NMJ diseases reflect the variability in NMJ transmission as evident by a change in the morphology of individual MUAPs. When assessed using conventional concentric or monopolar needle electrodes, this finding is also referred to as *moment-to-moment amplitude variation (MMAV)* or *jiggle* (Fig. 4.19a, b), in contrast to *jitter* which is seen on single fiber electromyography. The presence of unstable MUAPs is an abnormal but non-specific finding and can be seen with early re-innervation, muscle or NMJ transmission disorders, and segmental demyelinating polyneuropathies [3]. Use of the term "myopathic MUAPs" is discouraged since there are multiple causes for MUAPs of short duration, low amplitude, and increased polyphasia (e.g. nascent units seen in some cases of re-innervation). Thus, a description of the MUAP configuration in the needle EMG results section with a separate statement that the findings are consistent with myopathy

Table 4.6 Patterns of abnormality seen with the needle EMG

Disorder	MUAP duration	Recruitment	Variation/MMAV
Anterior horn cell (ALS)	Decreased/increased	Reduced	Yes/No
Acute radiculopathy	Normal	Variable/reduced	No
Chronic radiculopathy	Increased	Variable/reduced	No
Acute PN – Axon loss – Demyelinating	Normal Normal	Reduced Reduced	No Yes/No
Chronic PN – Axon loss – Demyelinating	Increased Normal	Reduced Increased/Reduced	No Yes/No
Myasthenia gravis	Normal or decreased	Normal	Yes
LEMS	Normal or decreased	Normal	Yes
Botulism	Normal or decreased	Normal	Yes
Early myopathy	Decreased	Normal	No
Late to severe myopathy	Decreased/increased	Early/reduced	No/Yes

MUAP motor unit action potential, *ALS* amyotrophic lateral sclerosis, *PN* polyneuropathy, *LEMS* Lambert-Eaton Myasthenic Syndrome, *MMAV* moment-to-moment amplitude variation
Adapted from [1]

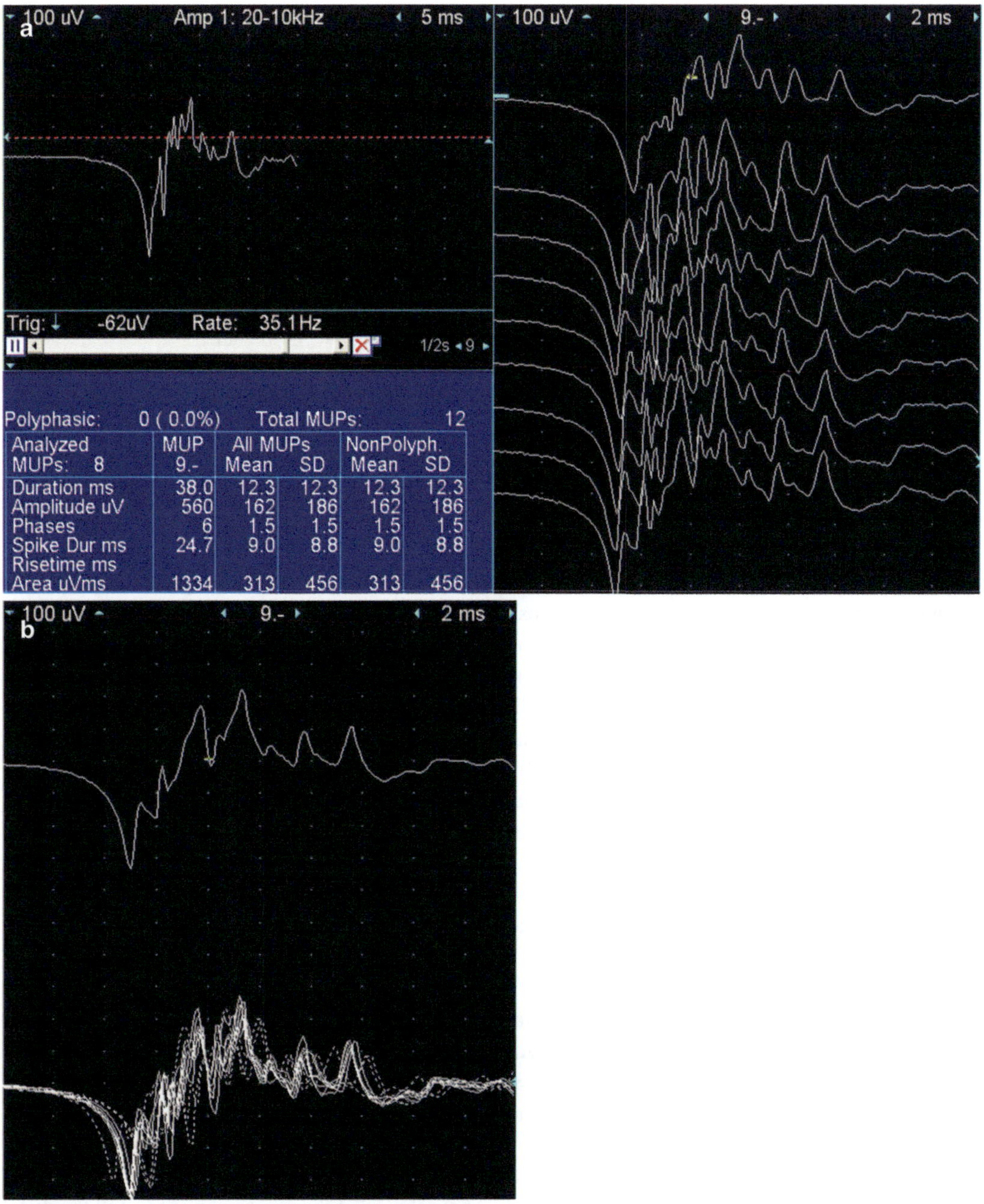

Fig. 4.19 (**a**) Complex MUAP disclosing instability (also referred to as moment-to-moment amplitude variation, MMAV) on the left (5 ms sweep speed), rastered on the right (2 ms sweep speed) displaying the same MUAP from top-to-bottom. Note the variability of the MUAP complexity each time it fires. This is also highlighted in the superimposed tracings of the same MUAP shown in (**b**)

under the interpretation portion of the EDX examination report is more appropriate than simply stating that "myopathic" MUAPs are present.

As with radiculopathy, the electrodiagnostic diagnosis of myopathy primarily relies on the needle EMG. However, the sensitivity of the needle EMG for diagnosing muscle disorders is variable and the specificity is low.

With myopathy, the earliest MUAP change due to muscle fiber loss is a reduction in duration, followed by increased polyphasia or turns and reduced amplitude. *Early or increased recruitment* becomes apparent when there is functional loss of muscle fibers within a motor unit so that more muscle fibers and contraction is required to generate a given force. Although early recruitment is one of the most reliable features of myopathy, it is often only present with moderate to severe disease and, thus, is not an early EDX manifestation [3]. With myopathy, fibrillation potentials indicate there is loss of muscle fiber connectivity to its end plate and supports the presence of inflammation or necrosis of the muscle fiber. However, the presence of fibrillation potentials do not always mean that inflammation will be found on muscle biopsy due to sampling and the patchy nature of some inflammatory myopathies [3]. Similarly, the absence of fibrillation potentials does not indicate that inflammation or necrosis is absent due to needle sampling, the non-uniform nature of inflammatory myopathies, and the fact that inflammatory changes may be obscured by treatment with steroids or other immunomodulating therapy. Myotonic potentials are the next most common spontaneous activity seen with myopathy, yet are non-specific, being compatible with a wide range of myopathies [1].

Certain myopathies may result in a combination of both neurogenic-appearing and myopathic-appearing MUAPs. A classic example is inclusion body myositis, a chronic myopathy in which local inflammation results in denervation and reinnervation of the muscle fibers as well as desychronization and slowing of distal terminal nerve branches [3]. As a result, there are MUAPs of small duration, short amplitude, and increased phases intermixed with MUAPs of increased duration, high amplitude, and increased phases. The MUAP firing pattern may also be comprised of a mixture of early and reduced recruitment.

How Do These Measurements Correlate with Motor NCS?

Both needle EMG and motor NCS assess motor fibers, but the needle EMG is more sensitive in the detection of motor axon loss, i.e., loss of a single motor axon will yield fibrillation potentials if the needle is adjacent to the denervated muscle fibers, whereas it is estimated that approximately 50% of motor axons within a motor unit must be lost before there is an appreciable reduction in compound muscle action potential (CMAP) amplitude. With increasing severity of motor axon loss, there is an increase in fibrillation potentials and reduction of MUAP recruitment. When reinnervation occurs either in the form of collateral sprouting or axonal regeneration (usually after ~3 months have passed), MUAPs with increased duration, amplitude and phases appear. MUAPs with greatly increased amplitude (of >3–4 millivolts) signify a very long-standing process and are typically seen in patients with remote poliomyelitis or other AHC or root level disease.

Whenever focal demyelination is present and the stimulating electrode can be placed proximal and distal to the site of demyelination, the motor NCS can localize the focal conduction defect with a good degree of accuracy. However, if focal demyelination disrupts nerve conduction propagation to a sufficient degree that weakness results and the stimulator can only be placed distal and not proximal to the block, then the distal CMAP will be normal despite clinical deficits. Thus, when NCS are conducted after 5–7 days—the amount of time it typically takes Wallerian degeneration of the distal nerve segment to occur after focal axonal injury—there is weakness of the recorded muscle and the distal CMAP is of normal amplitude, then the likely pathophysiology is demyelinating conduction block proximal to the stimulation site. Assuming there is sufficient demyelinating conduction along the nerve to the weak muscle, the needle EMG in muscles innervated by that nerve segment will demonstrate MUAPs that have normal appearance but are reduced in number in proportion to the number of blocked motor nerve fibers. This combination of a normal CMAP in a weak muscle and reduced MUAP recruitment allows for the EDX medicine consultant to determine indirect evidence of proximal demyelinating conduction block (so-called "inferred" block). This has both diagnostic and treatment implications as incorrectly diagnosing motor axon loss carries a poorer prognosis while persistent proximal demyelinating conduction block can be associated with treatable acquired polyneuropathies (e.g., multifocal motor neuropathy with conduction block).

Another scenario in which the needle EMG is useful is when there is no clinical weakness in a muscle which has a low or reduced CMAP amplitude yet the needle EMG reveals normal MUAP appearance and recruitment. In this instance, the best alternative explanation is that the muscle is receiving its innervation from another nerve which should clue the EDX medicine consultant to perform additional NCS for anomalous innervations.

Finally, when there is chronic motor axon loss followed by adequate reinnervation, the CMAP may be normal in amplitude despite prior loss of motor unit function. When muscle fibers recorded on motor NCS include those re-innervated by surrounding motor units, the amplitude is normal despite varying degrees of reduced MUAP recruitment and large polyphasic MUAPs seen on needle EMG.

Summary

The needle EMG relies on the assessment for spontaneous activity and MUAP recruitment and appearance to evaluate the integrity of the motor unit and together with NCS, can localize and diagnose any number of neuromuscular disorders from the intraspinal canal, nerve roots, plexus, peripheral nerve, neuromuscular junction, and muscle. Recognition of both normal and abnormal spontaneous activity is imperative as is the advanced skill of semi-quantitative assessment of MUAP recruitment and the analysis of MUAP configuration—including duration, amplitude, and phases. The art of performing needle EMG to maximize patient tolerance and diagnostic yield includes using a variety of patient education, sensory/pain distractors, and prioritizing studied muscles. The study can be performed safely in virtually all patients but should be used with caution in patients with lymphedema and anti-coagulation.

References

1. Daube JR. Assessing the motor unit with needle electromyography. In: Clinical neurophysiology. Philadelphia: FA Davis Co; 1996. p. 257–281.
2. Chemali KR, Tsao B. Electrodiagnostic testing of nerves and muscles: when, why, and how to order. Cleveland Clin J Med. 2005;72:37–48.
3. Levin KH. Needle electrode examination. In: Levin KH, Luders HO, editors. Comprehensive clinical neurophysiology. Philadelphia: WB Saunders; 2000. p. 122–39.
4. Dumitru D. Needle electromyography. In: Dumitru D, Amato AA, Zwarts MJ, editors. Electrodiagnostic medicine. 2nd ed. Philadelphia: Hanley & Belfus; 2002. p. 257–91.
5. Preston D, Shapiro B. Basic electromyography: analysis of spontaneous activity. In: Electromyography and neuromuscular disorders. 2nd ed. Boston: Butterworth-Heinemann; 2005. p. 199–213.
6. Rutkove SB. AANEM minimonograph #14: the effects of temperature in neuromuscular electrophysiology. Muscle Nerve. 2001;24:867–82.
7. Preston D, Shapiro B. Basic electromyography: analysis of motor unit action potentials. In: Electromyography and neuromuscular disorders. 2nd ed. Boston: Butterworth-Heinemann; 2005. p. 215–29.
8. Dumitru D. Electrodiagnostic medicine pitfalls. In: Dumitru D, Amato AA, Zwarts MJ, editors. Electrodiagnostic medicine. 2nd ed. Philadelphia: Hanley & Belfus; 2002. p. 541–77.
9. Campbell WW. Needle electrode examination. In: Essentials of electrodiagnostic medicine. Baltimore: Williams & Wilkens; 1999. p. 93–116.
10. Lynch SL, Boon AJ, Smith J, Harper CM Jr, Tanaka EM. Complications of needle electromyography: hematoma risk and correlation with anticoagulation and antiplatelet therapy. Muscle Nerve. 2008;38:1225–30.
11. Boon JA, Bertken JT, Watson JC, Laughlin RS, Strommen JA, Mauermann ML, Sorenson EJ. Hematoma risk after needle electromyography. Muscle Nerve. 2012;45:9–12.

Mononeuropathies

5

Ramon Lugo and Alexandra Soriano

Mononeuropathies, especially those seen with entrapment are among the most common conditions investigated with the use of electrodiagnostic (EDX) studies. These studies not only help to identify the single peripheral nerve involved, but also the site of the lesion, the type of fibers involved (sensory and/or motor), the character of the lesion (axonal vs demyelinating), and the age/chronicity of the lesion. There is also the potential to obtain prognostic information, including features of ongoing reinnervation in axon loss lesions. The most distinctive localizing features occur with focal demyelination (as seen in many entrapment mononeuropathies). These include the presence of conduction block and/or focal conduction slowing, with or without concomitant axon loss features. However, these features may not always be found, and in some cases lesions are not able to be precisely localized with only findings of axonal loss on nerve conduction studies (NCS) and needle electromyography (EMG) in muscles innervated by the affected single nerve. However, knowledge of the anatomy of the course of individual peripheral nerves, and their branches which supply specific muscles allows the electromyographer to at least localize to a particular segment of the nerve in most cases.

In the upper extremity, the most common mononeuropathies include median neuropathy at the wrist (carpal tunnel syndrome), and ulnar neuropathy at the elbow. In the lower extremity, it is peroneal (fibular) neuropathy at the fibular head.

Causes of mononeuropathies include mechanical injury caused by compression or trauma like fractures or joint dislocations, repetitive activities like those seen in typists or carpenters, endocrine disorders like diabetes and hypothyroidism, local tumors like Schwannomas, pregnancy, prolonged limb posture during surgical procedures, among many others.

Most mononeuropathies involve sensory and motor fibers (potentially affecting corresponding sensory and motor responses on NCS), but some are purely motor including the anterior interosseus neuropathy, posterior interosseus neuropathy, long thoracic neuropathy and spinal accessory neuropathy. Others may be purely sensory, like lateral femoral cutaneous neuropathy (meralgia paresthetica), and superficial radial sensory neuropathy (cheiralgia paresthetica).

The EDX study is also very helpful to differentiate between mononeuropathies and other patterns of injury affecting the peripheral nervous system including radiculopathies, plexopathies, and polyneuropathies.

Median Nerve

The sensory fibers of the median nerve come from the cervical root levels 5 and 6 while the motor fibers come from the cervical root levels

R. Lugo (✉)
Cleveland Clinic Florida, Weston, FL, USA
e-mail: lugor@ccf.org

A. Soriano
Braathen Neurological Center, Cleveland Clinic Florida, Weston, FL, USA

Cleveland Clinic Lerner College of Medicine of Case Western Reserve University, Cleveland, OH, USA
e-mail: soriana@ccf.org

N. Galvez-Jimenez et al. (eds.), *Electrodiagnostic Medicine*,
https://doi.org/10.1007/978-3-030-74997-2_5

of C6–T1. This separation of the sensory fibers continue in the brachial plexus with the sensory fibers traveling only through the lateral cord. The motor fibers travel through the lower trunk and medial cord for the C8–T1 components, and follow along with the C6 median sensory fibers through the upper trunk, with the C7 component arising from the middle trunk (these median motor upper and middle trunk components entering into the lateral cord as well). Then, these median lateral and medial cord fibers join to form the median nerve proper. It passes through the upper arm without branching or innervating any muscle. At the antero-cubital area, it is adjacent to the brachial artery. Then it passes in between both heads of the pronator

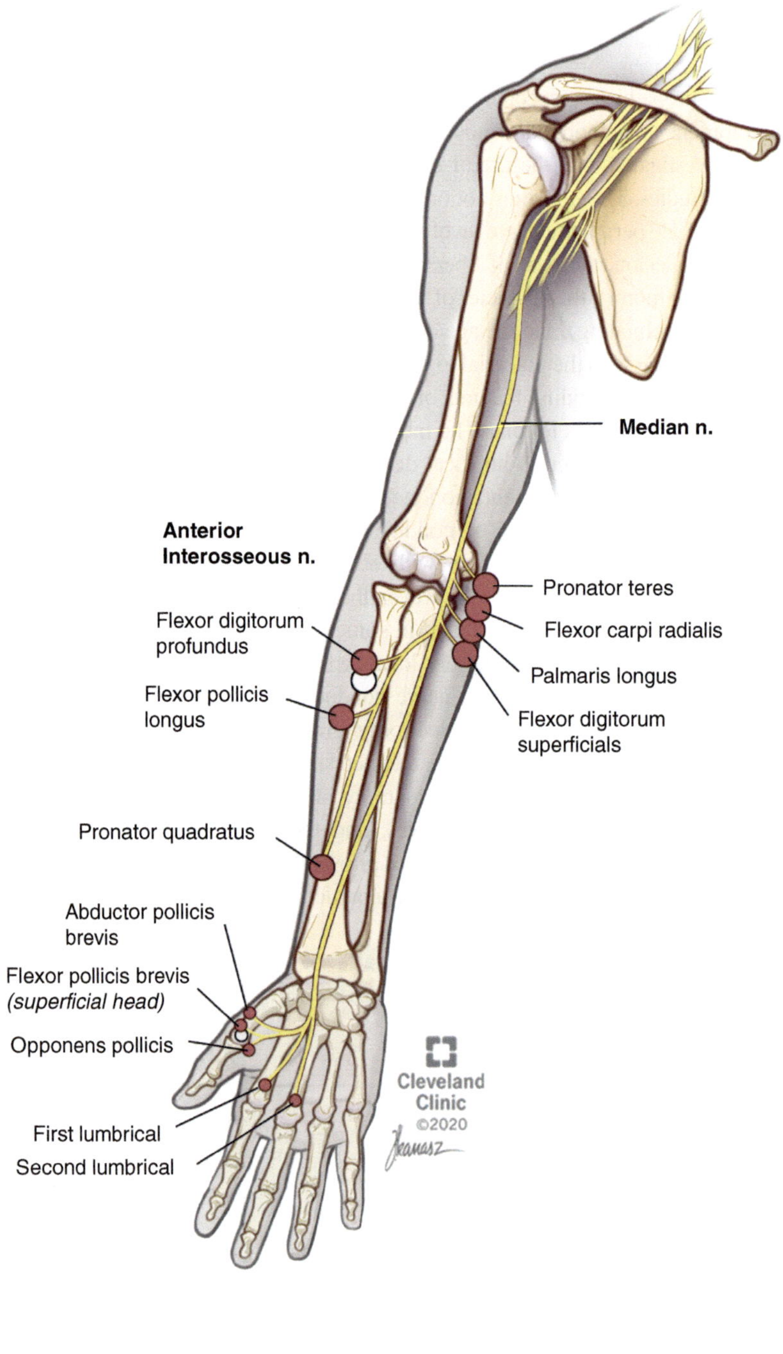

Fig. 5.1 Median nerve: course and branches to key muscles of electrodiagnostic importance

teres to the forearm (see Fig. 5.1). As it pierces the pronator teres it innervates this muscle. Then it branches to innervate several muscles in the anterior portion of the forearm before branching to originate the anterior interosseous nerve (a pure motor branch), which innervates deeper forearm muscles (flexor pollicis longus, pronator quadratus, and the lateral half of flexor digitorum profundus). Before getting in the carpal tunnel it gives the cutaneous palmar branch, that supply cutaneous innervation to the thenar eminence. After passing through the carpal tunnel it gives sensory innervation to the first 3 digits and the lateral half of the fourth finger. The motor branch innervates the first 2 lumbricals and the thenar muscles including the opponens pollicis, abductor pollicis brevis, and superficial part of flexor pollicis brevis (muscles supplied by the recurrent branch of the median nerve).

The most common sites of entrapment are at the carpal tunnel (wrist) [1–4] and while piercing the pronator teres muscle (pronator teres syndrome).

Median Neuropathy at the Wrist (Carpal Tunnel Syndrome)

It affects around 3–5% of Americans [1, 2, 5–7], with a peak incidence between 40 and 60 years old, and more frequent in females than male (3:1). Dominant hand tends to be affected first and more severely. The clinical syndrome is known as carpal tunnel syndrome and may include symptoms of pain or paresthesia located in the wrist, hand, fingers, at times in forearm (and even as proximal as the shoulder), this pain is usually worst with repetitive hand use, and at night, often awaking patients. Paresthesia and sensory loss features are appreciated especially in the first three digits, and sometimes the lateral half of the fourth finger. Weakness of the hand can also develop, particularly involving the median-innervated muscles of the thenar eminence, with atrophy of these muscles seen in more severe cases.

Common risk factors for median neuropathy at the wrist include diabetes mellitus, hypothyroidism, obesity, wrist trauma, pregnancy, and repetitive mechanical wrist movement/hand use [1, 8–12]. Other causes include congenital small caliber of carpal tunnel, use of vibrating tools, renal failure, amyloidosis, and arthritis.

Electrodiagnostic studies can help confirm the diagnosis and assess the severity of the median neuropathy. The nerve conduction study findings include:

1. Focal slowing across the carpal tunnel, manifested by a prolonged peak latency of the sensory nerve action potential first, and then decreased amplitude of the sensory response. The motor responses abnormalities include first prolonged onset distal latency of the compound motor action potential across the wrist, and later on decrease amplitude of the motor response. Marked decreased amplitude may suggest a poorer prognosis.

The routine electrodiagnostic studies for a median neuropathy at the wrist should include:

1. Motor nerve conduction of the median nerve at the wrist and at the elbow while recording at the abductor pollicis brevis.
2. Ulnar motor studies with stimulation at the wrist, below the elbow and above the elbow while recording at the abductor digiti minimi.
3. Sensory nerve studies of the median and ulnar nerves must be done. Sometimes, in milder cases, comparison studies are necessary, including comparison of latency between the median palmar and ulnar palmar mixed nerve response, among others.
4. Needle electromyography must include at least 2 C6–C7 innervated muscles, abductor pollicis brevis, and 2 median-innervated muscles proximal to the wrist and 2 C8–T1 non-median-innervated muscles.

Anterior Interosseous Nerve (AIN) Syndrome

This is a predominantly motor syndrome, with presence of weakness of the thumb and index finger with difficulty pinching items between these two fingers due to weakness of the lateral half of flexor digitorum profundus and flexor pollicis longus muscles (patient unable to make the "OK sign" with fingers). Pain can be present, but sensory loss should not. The place of entrapment of this nerve is variable, but mostly at the forearm.

Nerve conduction studies may be normal, or show reduced amplitudes of median motor responses. EMG will show denervation changes in the flexor pollicis longus, flexor digitorum profundus to second and third digits, and/or pronator quadratus.

Median Mononeuropathy at the Proximal Medial Forearm (Pronator Teres Syndrome)

When the median nerve passes in between the two heads of the pronator teres muscle it can be compressed at this level due to various reasons including, hypertrophied pronator teres muscle, repetitive pronation/supination motion, acute forceful pronation, anomalous arteries, postoperative scarring, and compression on the proximal forearm by heavy bag with narrow handles (grocery-bag neuropathy). Compression of the median nerve in the proximal forearm can also occur at the edge of the flexor digitorum sublimis (flexor digitorum superficialis) arch.

The clinical symptoms with entrapment of the median nerve at these proximal forearm sites are like those of carpal tunnel syndrome with paresthesias mostly in the second and third digits, but lack of nocturnal worsening of the symptoms, with also dull ache around the forearm that is exacerbated with forced arm pronation. Physical exam findings may include tenderness on palpation of the pronator teres, increased pain and paresthesias with pronation of the arm, weakness and atrophy of forearms flexors (typically sparing pronator teres). Nerve conduction studies can show:

1. Median motor and sensory responses which are either reduced or absent. A normal median peak/distal latency or conduction velocity at the wrist segment can help distinguish this from carpal tunnel syndrome.
2. On needle examination, there may be features of denervation of all the median-innervated muscles distal to the pronator teres, with relative sparing of the pronator teres.

Ulnar Nerve

The sensory and the motor fibers of the ulnar nerve originate at the level of C8 and T1 nerve roots, then traveling through the inferior/lower trunk and in the medial cord before forming the ulnar nerve proper (see Fig. 5.2). In the arm (above elbow) it does not provide any innervation and travels together with the brachial artery, vein and the median nerve. Then passing through the ulnar groove at the elbow between the medial epicondyle of the humerus and the olecranon process of the ulna. It enters the forearm through the aponeurotic arcade known as the cubital tunnel. There it provides innervation to the flexor carpi ulnaris muscle, and travels in its belly, exiting later to innervate the flexor digitorum profundus to the ring and little fingers. At about the mid-forearm it gives the dorsal cutaneous branch to the dorsal surface of the medial one and a half fingers, and the associated dorsal hand area, separate from the palmar cutaneous branch to the medial aspect of the palm including the proximal aspect of the ring and little fingers. The final sensory component is the superficial branch which arises in the hand itself and innervates the palmar surface of the medial one and a half fingers. There is no consistent sensory innervation from the ulnar nerve to the forearm itself. When the ulnar nerve reaches the wrist, it passes through the Guyon's canal, formed by the pisiform medially and the hook of the hamate laterally. There it divides in to superficial and deep branches to intrinsic hand muscles.

The most common sites of compression of the ulnar nerve are at the elbow (retrocondylar groove and/or ulnar groove and cubital tunnel), and at the wrist (Guyon's canal) [13–15].

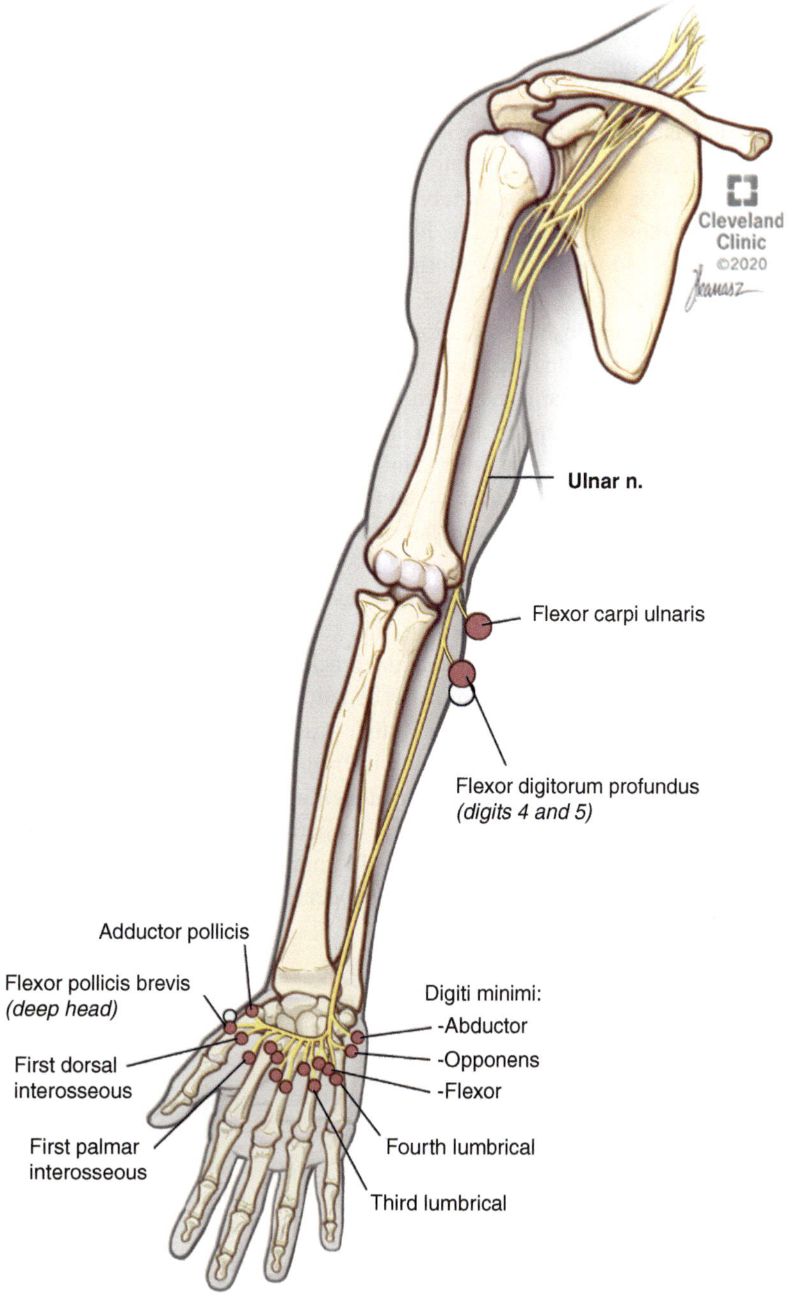

Fig. 5.2 Ulnar nerve: course and branches to key muscles of electrodiagnostic importance

Ulnar Neuropathy at the Elbow

Compression of ulnar nerve at the elbow can occur either at the retrocondylar grove and/or ulnar groove (between the medial epicondyle and the olecranon, especially with nerve subluxation or dislocation) or 1–2 cm distally at the cubital tunnel. At the retrocondylar grove this can be caused by repeated trauma such as leaning on the elbow, sustained hyperflexion of the elbow, distal humerus fractures or elbow dislocation, degenerative joint disease, immobilization during surgery.

Patients may present with sensory symptoms and pain in the sensory distribution at the hand, including dorsum of the hand, with pain or tenderness at the elbow, and when motor symptoms present: weakness and muscle wasting of the first dorsal interosseous (FDI), abductor digiti minimi (ADM) and/or other ulnar innervated muscles (including those in the forearm like the flexor carpi ulnaris and the flexor digitorum profundus to digits 4&5).

The electrodiagnostic evaluation of an ulnar neuropathy must include motor nerve conduction studies of the ulnar nerve when recording at the abductor digiti minimi and, if needed, the first dorsal interosseus and with stimulations at the wrist, below and above the elbow (with the elbow flexed at 90 degrees). Median nerve conduction studies should be done as well. Median and ulnar F-waves should be evaluated as well sensory responses of the median and ulnar nerves. Dorsal ulnar and medial antebrachial cutaneous sensory responses may be beneficial as well, depending on the need for further lesion localization refinement. The needle electromyography should include ulnar-innervated muscles distal to the wrist, the forearm ulnar-innervated muscles, other C8–T1 non-ulnar innervated muscles, and C8–T1 (low cervical) paraspinals.

Electrodiagnostic findings may show:

1. Slowing of conduction velocity or conduction block at the culprit segment (typically between the above-elbow and below-elbow stimulation sites).
2. Absent or reduced superficial sensory +/− dorsal ulnar cutaneous responses (both usually affected when ulnar lesion is at the elbow, but fascicular sparing may occur).
3. EMG abnormalities may be found in the FDI, ADM, as well as the flexor carpi ulnaris and flexor digitorum profundus (to digits 4&5)—ulnar-innervated intrinsic hand and forearm muscles usually affected when ulnar lesion is at the elbow, but fascicular sparing may occur).

Ulnar neuropathy at the wrist (Guyon's canal).

Entrapment at the wrist can be associated with mass lesions such as ganglion cyst, lipomas, or chronic mechanical compression due to use of crutches, compression in bicycle bars, etc.

Compression at and around this site may involve specific branches of the nerve and produce various patterns as follows:

- Type 1 (only subtype where lesion is actually in Guyon's canal) involves compression of both the deep and superficial branches of the ulnar nerve. There is weakness in the intrinsic hand muscles and sensory loss in digits 4&5, though there is sparing in the distributions of the palmar and dorsal ulnar cutaneous branches.
- Type 2 is manifested by exclusive involvement of the deep branch, affecting the distal components of both the hypothenar branch and the terminal branch (to the interossei and lumbricals). Accordingly, sensory deficits are absent. Compression in this scenario occurs distal to Guyon's canal but proximal to the hypothenar branch.
- Type 3 occurs when there is compression of the deep branch distal to the hypothenar branch, thereby sparing the hypothenar muscles (the interossei and third and fourth lumbricals are affected). Sensory function is not affected.
- Type 4 is rare and comprises compression distal to Guyon's canal involving the superficial branch exclusively, so motor function is spared (exception being the palmaris brevis muscle).

The role of electrodiagnostic studies is essentially to rule out more common ulnar nerve lesions, such as at the elbow. If there is an abnormality of the dorsal ulnar sensory response, this may suggest a process/lesion proximal to the wrist. If the ulnar sensory response, when recorded at the fifth finger is affected and there is a normal dorsal ulnar sensory response, this favors an ulnar lesion distal to the mid-forearm and most likely at the wrist. Sometimes to further assess the possibility of a palmar process affecting the ulnar nerve, comparing the onset latencies of the ulnar motor response when recorded at the abductor digiti minimi versus the first dorsal interoseous with wrist stimulation may be performed. More than

2 milliseconds in difference may be a discriminating feature. On needle electromyography, there may be signs of denervation in ulnar-innervated hand muscles with sparing of ulnar-innervated forearm muscles. However, sometimes this pattern may also be seen in ulnar neuropathy at the elbow with fascicular sparing and close analysis of the nerve conduction studies will usually help with distinguishing localization.

Radial Nerve

The radial nerve receives fibers from C5 to C8. These fibers arise from the posterior cord where the terminal branch becomes the radial nerve (remaining fibers after the axillary nerve branches off)—see Fig. 5.3. It travels posterior to the axillary artery and goes across the back of the humerus through the spiral grove. In the arm it gives innervation to the triceps, anconeous

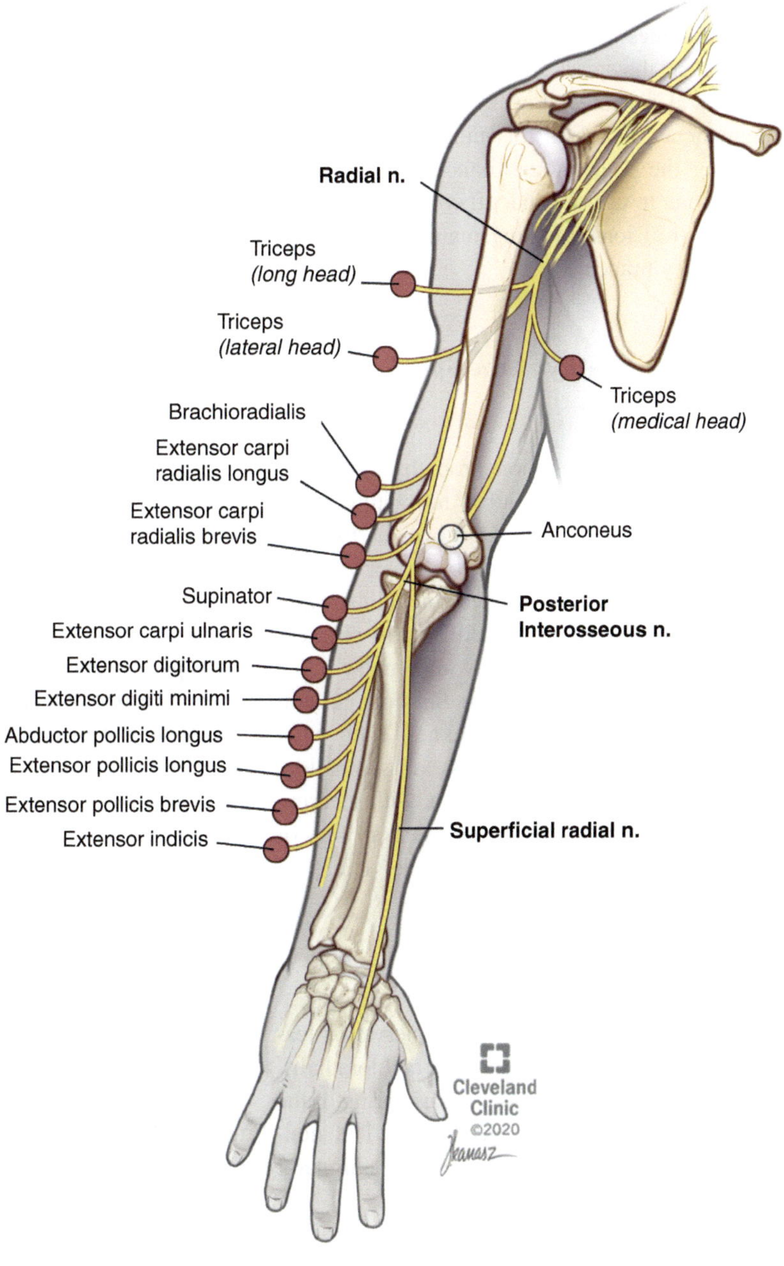

Fig. 5.3 Radial nerve: course and branches to key muscles of electrodiagnostic importance

and brachioradialis. There it come across the elbow and divides into the superficial and deep branch of the radial nerve. The superficial branch is purely sensory to the dorsum of the hand lateral to the ring finger. The deep motor branch/posterior interosseous nerve (PIN) supplies multiple muscles including the supinator, extensor carpi ulnaris, extensor digitorum (communis), extensor digiti minimi, abductor pollicis longus, extensor pollicis longus and brevis and extensor indicis.

The radial nerve can be injured at multiple levels, including the brachio-axillary angle due to use of crutches or proximal humeral fractures; at the level of the spiral grove due to compression or humeral fractures as well; at the level of the supinator as it crosses this muscle, specifically affecting the deep motor branch/PIN; or more distally due to use of handcuffs or complications from IV infusions affecting mainly the superficial sensory branch.

Radial Neuropathy at the Spiral Groove

Radial compression mononeuropathy at the spiral grove can happen secondary to fracture of the humeral shaft at the spiral groove, or by prolonged external compression of the nerve when the arm is over a chair or bed, including while sleeping, this classically occurring in sedated/intoxicated patients ("Saturday night palsy").

The clinical features of a radial compression at this level may include, weakness with wrist and finger extension, weakness of supination, mild weakness with elbow flexion, with spearing of elbow extension (triceps) and sensory loss of the dorsum of the hand mostly in the vicinity of the first web space.

Electromyography findings include:

1. Reduced or absent radial sensory responses.
2. On needle electromyography denervation features may be found in the brachioradialis, wrist and finger extensors, with sparing of the triceps and anconeus. Needle EMG of non-radial-innervated C7 muscles (e.g. pronator teres, and flexor carpi radialis) is needed to exclude a C7 radiculopathy.

Radial Neuropathy at the Elbow

Compression of the radial nerve at the elbow happens when the posterior interosseus branch of the radial nerve pass in between the two heads of the supinator muscle in the arcade of Frohse. This may be due to repetitive supinator use with muscle hypertrophy, fracture of the proximal radius, nearby lipomas or other mass lesions. The symptoms are purely motor, affecting mostly finger extension and sparing supination (with partial sparing of wrist extension).

Electromyography studies will show:

1. Normal radial sensory response.
2. Abnormal radial motor nerve responses, with possible reduction in conduction velocity with motor amplitude.
3. Needle EMG with evidence of denervation in all muscles supplied by the PIN, with normal triceps, anconeous, brachioradialis, extensor carpi radialis which are supplied by the (more proximal) radial nerve.

Radial Neuropathy at the Wrist

When compressed at the wrist, the radial neuropathy is purely sensory (cheiralgia paresthetica), this typically caused by use of handcuffs, tight watches or bracelets. Patients present with sensory changes in the radial dorsum of the hand (mostly around first web space), with no motor involvement.

The electrodiagnostic studies typically disclose a reduced or absent superficial radial sensory response, with normal radial motor studies and normal needle EMG findings.

Peroneal (Fibular) Nerve

The peroneal (fibular) nerve derives mostly from the L5 and (to a lesser extent) S1 spinal nerve roots. Parent fibers travel through the lumbosacral plexus and becomes part of the sciatic nerve. While passing through the thigh it supplies what may be considered the only peroneal (fibular)-innervated muscle proximal to the fibular head, the short head of bicep femoris (alternatively considered to be innervated by the peroneal (fibular) division of the sciatic nerve). The sciatic nerve divides into the common peroneal (fibular) and the tibial nerves behind the knee, above the popliteal fossa. It gives out the lateral cutaneous nerve of the knee just before passing through the fibular tunnel. It passes through the fibular tunnel and then branch into the superficial peroneal (fibular) and deep peroneal (fibular) branches (see Fig. 5.4). The deep peroneal (fibular) nerve innervates mainly the foot dorsiflexors while the superficial peroneal (fibular) nerve innervates mainly the foot evertors, also supplying sensation to the lateral calf and the dorsum of the foot.

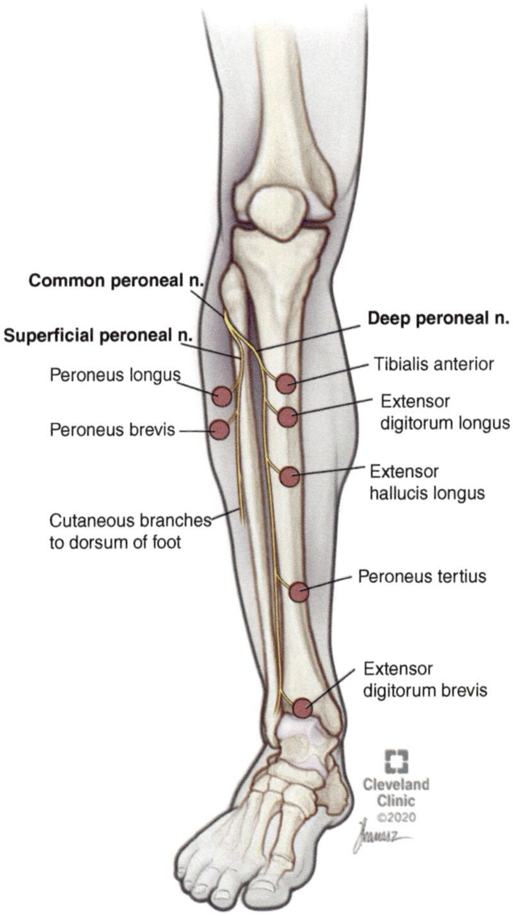

Fig. 5.4 Peroneal (fibular) nerve: course and branches to key muscles of electrodiagnostic importance

The most common site of peroneal (fibular) compression neuropathy is at the knee, right at the fibular neck [16, 17]. At this location, both the deep and superficial peroneal (fibular) nerves are involved, and patients present with weakness in toes and foot dorsiflexion, resulting in foot drop, and weakness in foot eversion. There are also sensory symptoms in the lateral aspect of the calf, and in the dorsum of the foot including the first web space.

Peroneal (fibular) neuropathy at the fibular neck occurs secondary to direct trauma, stretch injuries, or prolonged inadvertent compression in patients following heavy sedation or anesthesia. Ganglion cyst (intraneural) or a nerve sheet tumor, repetitive leg crossing or repetitive squatting can also be a cause/contributor.

Electrodiagnostic findings include:

1. In peroneal (fibular) motor studies there can be focal slowing or conduction block across the fibular neck. Any slowing 10 m/s or more, or a reduction in amplitude of 20% or more (with proximal/above fibular neck site stimulation) may be considered significant.
2. Reduction of motor amplitudes are present when axonal loss occurs, typically in conjunction with reduction in the amplitude of the superficial peroneal (fibular) sensory nerve action potential.
3. Focal slowing or conduction block in peroneal (fibular) motor studies recording at the tibialis anterior (TA) muscle, if this is not present when doing motor studies at the extensor digitorum brevis (EDB).
4. Needle electrode evidence of denervation in muscles supplied by the deep and superficial peroneal (fibular) nerves. Other non-peroneal (fibular) innervated muscles supplied by the L5–S1 roots should be examined to rule out the possibility of a more proximal sciatic neuropathy, lumbosacral plexopathy or L5–S1 lumbar radiculopathy. As part of this approach, pertinent muscles above the fibular neck (in particular, the short head of biceps femoris) should be tested to exclude a sciatic neuropathy.

5. Prolonged or absent peroneal (fibular) Fwave response may be seen.

Tibial Nerve

Most of the fibers from the tibial nerve come from the L5, S1 and some S2 roots. They travel through the lumbosacral plexus and become the tibial division of the sciatic nerve. Behind the knee, the sciatic nerve gives rise to the tibial nerve after the peroneal (fibular) division branches off (see Fig. 5.5). The tibial nerve travel behind the calf innervating the plantar flexors and foot invertor muscles before passing through the tarsal tunnel. It runs distal to the medial malleolus beneath the flexor retinaculum on the medial side of the ankle. In the tarsal tunnel, the tibial nerve travels with the tibial artery, tendon of the flexor hallucis longus, tibialis posterior and flexor digitorum longus. Then the tibial nerve divides in to the medial and lateral calcaneal sensory nerves, providing sensation to the heel of the sole, and the medial and lateral plantar mixed nerves providing innervation to medial and lateral sole of the foot. These plantar mixed nerves innervate muscles of the foot that can be tested during EMG, such as the abductor hallucis (AH), flexor digitorum brevis (FDB), abductor digiti quinti pedis (ADQP) muscles.

Compression of the tibial nerve under the flexor retinaculum at the medial ankle, potentially results in tarsal tunnel syndrome, which can follow trauma (sprains or fractures), but has also been attributed to inflammation or tumors [18, 19].

The clinical picture in tarsal tunnel syndrome is perimalleolar pain, ankle and sole burning pain that is worse with weight bearing, especially at night. Ankle jerk is spared as well as sensationin the dorsum and lateral aspect of the foot.

The electrodiagnostic findings include:

1. Reduction in the tibial compound motor action potentials when recording the abductor hallucis and abductor digiti quinti pedis muscles. Contralateral examination is strongly recommended in these cases to demonstrate significant asymmetry of findings (when the lesion is unilateral).
2. Needle EMG may show motor axon loss changes in the tibial/plantar-innervated intrinsic foot muscles, with sparing of the calf muscles and the peroneal (fibular)-innervated intrinsic foot muscles (like the extensor digitorum brevis). Needle EMG of foot muscles can be difficult to be tolerated by the patient, but again, contralateral studies are strongly recommended in order to increase diagnostic certainty (including the assurance that there are motor axon loss features on the affected side beyond chronic denervation changes often seen in intrinsic foot muscles secondary to chronic local trauma, as attributable to footwear).

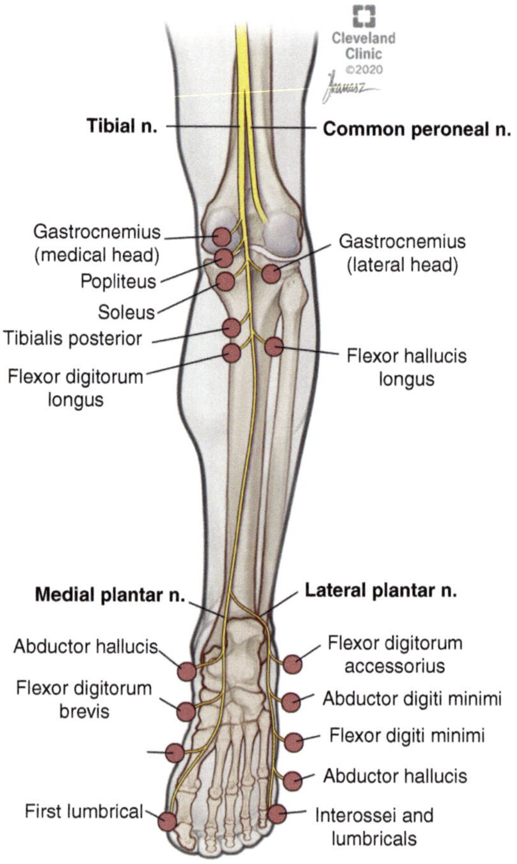

Fig. 5.5 Tibial nerve: course and branches to key muscles of electrodiagnostic importance

Sciatic Nerve

The sciatic nerve is derived from the L4–S2 nerve roots. It is essentially composed of compartmentalized common peroneal (fibular) and tibial parent nerve fibers along its course, comprising the lateral and medial divisions, respectively. After exiting the pelvis at the sciatic notch, the nerve passes under the piriformis muscle (see Fig. 5.6). As the sciatic nerve courses through the posterior thigh, the tibial nerve component fibers innervate several hamstring muscles (semimembranosus, semitendinosus, and the long head of biceps femoris). The short head of bicep femoris is considered the only hamstring muscle innervated by the common peroneal (fibular) nerve. The adductor magnus (hamstring portion) is also innervated by the tibial component of the sciatic nerve (the adductor portion of this muscle is supplied by the obturator nerve). Of note, most lesions of the proximal sciatic nerve (for example at the upper thigh and hip) tend to affect the lateral division/common peroneal (fibular) nerve fibers.

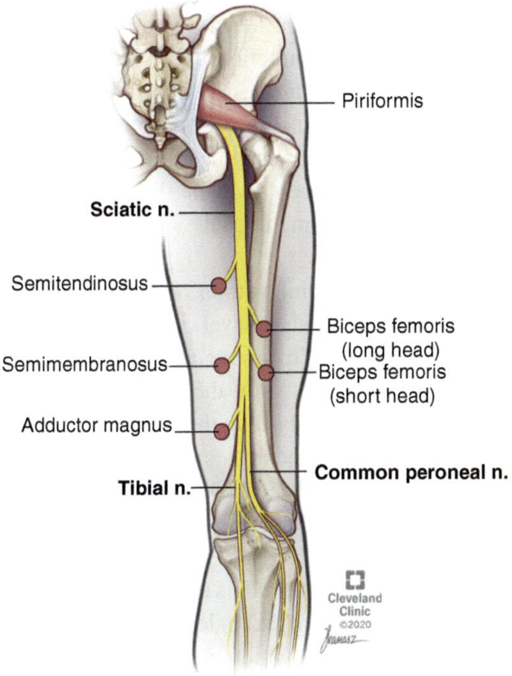

Fig. 5.6 Sciatic nerve: course and branches to key muscles of electrodiagnostic importance

Accordingly, the clinical and electrodiagnostic characteristics of sciatic mononeuropathies represent a combination of the individual features seen with common peroneal (fibular) and tibial mononeuropathies, with additional hamstring muscle involvement (muscles innervated by the superior and inferior gluteal nerves, as well as the femoral and obturator nerves spared).

Femoral Nerve

The femoral nerve comes from the lumbar plexus and receives branches from L2, L3 and L4 nerve roots. Parent nerve fibers cross the pelvis behind the psoas muscle, deep and above the iliacus muscle, which it also supplies (see Fig. 5.7). It enters the thigh together with the femoral artery and vein. It divides into the anterior division which gives the medial and intermediate cutaneous nerves of the thigh, and motor branches to sartorius and pectineus muscles; the posterior division innervates the quadriceps femoris muscle, continuing then as the saphenous (sensory) nerve.

Causes of femoral neuropathy include prolonged compression during pelvic or abdominal surgeries, or during labor or delivery. Trauma to the nerve may also occur in total hip replacement surgeries. Retroperitoneal hemorrhages or hematomas of the inguinal region may also injure the femoral nerve.

Patients typically present with symptoms of sensory changes in the anterior/medial thigh, and medial calf, with weakness of the quadriceps and iliopsoas muscles, usually manifesting with knee buckling/weakness of knee extension and weakness of hip flexion.

Electrodiagnostic findings include:

1. Reduced femoral nerve motor amplitude (in cases of axonal loss) recording at the quadriceps muscle (rectus femoris or vastus lateralis). Side to side comparison is strongly recommended to demonstrate significant asymmetry and increase diagnostic certainty.
2. Reduced saphenous sensory nerve amplitudes. Similarly, side-to-side comparison studies are needed in these cases, with iso-

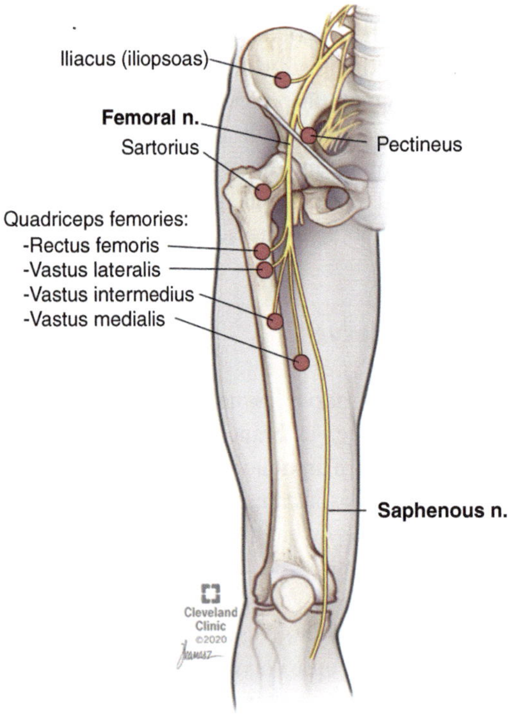

Fig. 5.7 Femoral nerve: course and branches to key muscles of electrodiagnostic importance

lated bilaterally absent saphenous responses considered insufficient for diagnostic purposes (often technically difficult to obtain, especially in overweight or obese patients).

3. Needle EMG of the iliacus (for lesions above the inguinal ligament) and two heads of the quadriceps muscle (usually rectus femoris and vastus lateralis) typically shows motor axon loss changes. Other L2–L4-innervated muscles must be sampled to exclude the presence of a lumbar plexopathy, or L2–L4 motor radiculopathy.

Facial Nerve

The facial nerve (cranial nerve VII) originates from the union of the axons coming from the facial motor nucleus (primarily motor fibers for facial expression muscles) and the *nervus intermedius* (giving parasympathetic, taste, and non-taste sensory fibers). It exits the brainstem at the cerebellopontine angle, next to cranial nerve VIII and both nerves enter the internal auditory meatus. Then the facial nerve (sensory component) fibers pass through the geniculate ganglion before getting into the facial nerve canal. Some of the parasympathetic fibers branches out to the greater and lesser petrosal nerves to get to the pterygopalatine and otic ganglia. The next fibers to branch out are the motor fibers which innervate the stapedius muscle in the ear. Next, the chorda tympani carry special sensory fibers for taste supplying the anterior 2/3 of the tongue, and parasympathetic fibers to the submandibular and sublingual glands. The facial nerve then exits the cranium through the stylomastoid foramen. After exiting, it innervates the posterior belly of the digastric and the stylohyoid muscles. It then gives the posterior auricular branch. At this point, the facial nerve continues towards the face to branch out into the five main branches (temporal, zygomatic, buccal, mandibular and cervical).

The most common facial neuropathy is idiopathic Bell's palsy. The etiology is still unclear, although it is believed to be a neuritis caused by a viral infection, possibly herpes viruses. Other possible etiologies for facial neuropathy include tumor, trauma or infectious [20, 21]. Bilateral facial neuropathies are less common but may be seen with, Guillain-Barré syndrome or other inflammatory/infectious processes affecting the base of the brain such as Lyme disease, sarcoidosis, or leptomeningeal lymphomatosis/carcinomatosis.

The clinical manifestation of facial neuropathy depends on what level is the pathology. Processes affecting the nerve as it exits the brain stem may affect not only the muscles of facial expression, but also taste in the anterior 2/3 if the tongue, hearing (hyperacusis) and tearing (lacrimation) ipsilaterally. Processes affecting the nerve distal to the chorda tympani will affect only the motor fibers.

Electrodiagnostic studies can be used to determine the amount of axon loss associated with facial nerve lesions, which may help in prognostication. These studies typically employed are facial nerve conduction studies with needle electromyography and blink reflexes.

The muscle typically recorded for facial motor nerve conduction studies is the nasalis. This muscle may also be examined by needle electrode, together with the frontalis, orbicularis oculus, orbicularis oris, and the mentalis muscles.

The nerve conduction studies should be done at least 10 days after the onset of the neuropathy to allow for Wallerian degeneration to take place (to reduce the likelihood of false negative/confounding results). The blink reflexes may help to assess the portion of the facial nerve proximal to the stylomastoid foramen. The reader is referred to Chap. 1 for further details about blink reflex testing.

Less Common Mononeuropathies

Suprascapular Neuropathy

The suprascapular nerve fibers arise from the C5–C6 anterior horn cells and its spinal nerve roots/segments passing through the upper trunk of the brachial plexus. The nerve itself passes posterior to the trapezius muscle, then through the suprascapular notch of the scapula (space located in the superior border of the scapula covered by the superior transverse scapular ligament. The nerve first supplies the supraspinatus muscle, then traverses the spinoglenoid notch to innervate the infraspinatus muscle.

Entrapment is more common at the suprascapular notch, and less common at the spinoglenoid notch. Some causes for entrapment include repetitive movement of the shoulder and scapula, commonly observed in weight lifters, prolonged positioning during surgical procedures, volleyball players, baseball pitchers and dancers. The nerve can also be involved in cases of neuralgic amyotrophy. Some masses such as ganglion cysts, sarcomas or metastatic carcinomas may cause entrapment of this nerve; rotator cuff tear can potentially cause nerve compression due to medial retraction of the tendons of the supraspinatus and infraspinatus muscles.

Patients may present with various symptoms and exam findings, depending on the site of entrapment. If entrapment occurs at the suprascapular notch, patients may develop shoulder pain that may worsen with shoulder movement, weakness with shoulder abduction and external rotation. Atrophy may be noted in the supraspinatus and infraspinatus muscles. If entrapment occurs distally at the spinoglenoid notch, patients may develop relatively painless weakness and atrophy of the infraspinatus muscle alone.

Differential diagnosis of suprascapular neuropathy includes cervical (C5–C6) radiculopathy, upper brachial plexopathy including neuralgic amyotrophy, rotator cuff tear and other musculoskeletal shoulder injuries.

Electrodiagnostic studies may help confirm the diagnosis and assess the severity of the mononeuropathy. In these studies, needle EMG may be useful in confirming and localizing the lesion, and excluding a cervical radiculopathy. Nerve conduction studies are particularly useful in excluding a brachial plexopathy (for e.g. by demonstrating an intact lateral antebrachial cutaneous sensory response).

Studies of nerves that pass through the upper trunk of the brachial plexus should be done including the lateral antebrachial cutaneous nerve, as well as the median and radial sensory nerves recording from the thumb. Other than "routine" motor nerve conduction studies of the upper extremity, motor nerve conduction studies of the supraspinatus and infraspinatus can be done using a monopolar needle electrode in either muscle for recording, and stimulating at the Erb's point.

Needle EMG of the upper extremity including the supraspinatus and infraspinatus should be done. Motor axon loss needle EMG abnormalities will typically be found in both the supraspinatus and infraspinatus muscles if the nerve is entrapped at the suprascapular notch. However, these abnormalities will only be found in the infraspinatus muscle if the lesion is at the spinoglenoid notch. Other C5–C6 innervated muscles and the cervical paraspinals, should be sampled to rule out a cervical motor radiculopathy and/or other intraspinal processes.

Axillary Neuropathy

The posterior cord of the brachial plexus gives rise to the axillary nerve, with fibers coming from the C5–C6 anterior horn cells and spinal nerve roots/segments, passing through the upper trunk. The axillary nerve then exits the axilla though a space delineated by the humerus, teres minor, teres major and long head of the triceps muscles, called the *quadrilateral space*. Then it divides into two trunks, the posterior trunk supplying the teres minor muscle as well as the posterior head of the deltoid muscle, terminating in the lateral brachial cutaneous nerve conveying sensation over the lateral shoulder. The anterior trunk supply the middle and anterior heads of the deltoid muscle and gives deep sensory branches to the shoulder joint.

Common causes of axillary neuropathy include direct trauma, shoulder dislocations or humeral fractures. Symptoms include numbness over the lateral shoulder and weakness of shoulder abduction and external rotation. The extent of clinical deficits may be quite variable across cases. Additionally, brachial plexopathy can present with axon loss features predominantly in the axillary nerve distribution.

Electrodiagnostic studies should include sensory nerves that run through the posterior cord and upper trunk of the brachial plexus, including radial and lateral antebrachial cutaneous sensory nerves, and the median nerve recording at the thumb. Motor studies of the axillary nerve are done by stimulating at the Erb's point and recording with a surface electrode over the deltoid muscle. Reduction in the CMAP can be found, and side-to-side comparison should be done. A drop of more than 50% in CMAP amplitude (compared to the contralateral/normal side) is considered abnormal.

Needle EMG should be performed in the teres minor and deltoid muscles, as well as other muscles innervated by the upper trunk and posterior cord of the brachial plexus (e.g. supraspinatus, infraspinatus, biceps, triceps, brachioradialis, cervical paraspinals) to exclude a more widespread lesion like a brachial plexopathy or a C5–C6 cervical motor radiculopathy.

Musculocutaneous Neuropathy

From the lateral cord of the brachial plexus, with fibers coming from the C5–C6(+/-C7) anterior horn cells and spinal nerve roots/segments, passing through the upper trunk, the musculocutaneous nerve innervates the brachialis, coracobrachialis and biceps brachii muscles. Coursing below the elbow it ends as the lateral antebrachial cutaneous sensory nerve.

Mononeuropathies of this nerve are uncommon and can occur in cases of direct trauma, surgery, compression (e.g. prolonged resting head during sleep), or stretch injury (lifting a particularly heavy weight). The lesion of this nerve can cause symptoms of paresthesia in the lateral forearm, and weakness of elbow flexion. Rarely, the lateral antebrachial cutaneous sensory nerve may be entrapped at the elbow between the biceps tendon and the brachialis muscle, this leading to increased pain or paresthesia in lateral forearm with pronation and arm extension.

Electrodiagnostic studies are used to exclude or isolate a mononeuropathy of this nerve, differentiating from a more widespread lesion like a brachial plexopathy, or cervical radiculopathy. For this, motor neve conduction studies can be done by stimulating the musculocutaneous nerve at the axilla and Erb's point while recording at the biceps muscle. For sensory studies, testing the lateral antebrachial cutaneous response is essential. Side-to-side comparisons of these motor and sensory responses is highly recommended.

In proximal lesions of the musculocutaneous nerve, needle EMG would typically show motor axon loss changes in the biceps muscle. Other muscles innervated by the upper trunk and lateral cord (e.g. pronator teres, flexor carpi radialis, deltoid, brachioradialis, supraspinatus and infraspinatus, and cervical paraspinals) should be tested as well to exclude a more widespread lesion e.g. brachial plexopathy, or C5–C6 cervical motor radiculopathy.

Long Thoracic Neuropathy

This nerve arises directly from the cervical spinal nerve roots C5–C6–C7 and strictly speaking, does not enter the brachial plexus. It innervates the serratus anterior muscle only. This muscle produces scapular protraction and stabilization, together with augmenting upward rotation of the scapula. Damage to this nerve alone is relatively uncommon, but has been described in cases of trauma to the cervical spine and chest wall, or stretch injuries as may occur in a variety of sports and recreational activities, or even during surgical procedures/positioning. In some cases of neuralgic amyotrophy, it may also be the only nerve involved.

Symptoms may include pain around the shoulder and weakness around the shoulder, particularly affecting scapular stabilization and producing scapular winging. This is best seen when the arm is placed (flexed) in front of the body and the hand is pushed firmly against a wall, producing medial winging of the scapula.

Needle EMG is most helpful when studying this nerve, as there is no specific or reliable way to stimulate this nerve exclusively. Abnormalities should only be found in the serratus anterior muscle with isolated lesions, always using abundant caution when inserting the needle to prevent iatrogenic pneumothorax with pleural puncture (recommended to insert over the rib and not in the interspace). One should always sample other C5–C6 and C7 muscles, as well as paraspinal muscles to exclude a cervical motor radiculopathy or a brachial plexopathy. Nerve conduction studies should be aimed at ruling out a more widespread process involving the brachial plexus, especially studying nerves that travel though the upper and middle brachial plexus and are derived from the same roots [i.e. lateral antebrachial cutaneous, median (recording at the thumb) and radial sensory nerves].

Spinal Accessory Neuropathy

This pure motor nerve comes from the C1 to C4 cervical roots and does not enter the brachial plexus. It passes through the foramen magnum and then though the jugular foramen supplying the sternocleidomastoid muscle, and finally through the posterior cervical triangle to innervate the trapezius muscle.

Lesion to this nerve occurs most commonly at the posterior cervical triangle, due to external compression, stretch or following local surgery such as cervical lymph node biopsy. This causes weakness of the trapezius muscle resulting in shoulder drop by affecting shoulder abduction. A shoulder drop may result in traction of the brachial plexus leading to shoulder pain and paresthesia, which may lead to the clinical suspicion of brachial plexopathy. If the lesion is more proximal, then weakness of the sternocleidomastoid muscle is seen with difficulty turning head and neck to contralateral side (as well as having some weakness in neck flexion).

The electrodiagnostic studies of this nerve can be performed by stimulating posterior to the middle of the sternocleidomastoid, recording over the upper trapezius. Comparison to the contralateral side is recommended. Sensory nerves traveling through the upper trunk of brachial plexus [i.e. lateral antebrachial cutaneous, median (recording at the thumb) and radial sensory] should be studied to exclude a more widespread process.

The EMG portion is useful in studying the trapezius and sternocleidomastoid muscles. When studying the trapezius, caution should be taken not to insert the needle too deep and sample underlying muscles, such as rhomboids or supraspinatus. Other muscles (especially those innervated by C5–C6 spinal nerve roots/segments) should be tested including deltoid, infraspinatus, supraspinatus and rhomboids and cervical paraspinals, to rule out a more widespread process.

Sample Cases

Median Neuropathy (at the Wrist)

History of Presentation and Exam Findings

A 72-year-old man presented with right hand and finger numbness of 1 year duration. Symptoms are intermittent and made worse by hand use, such as holding a book to read, using mechanical tools or driving. At times, he has been awakened during sleep with pain and numbness of the entire right hand, finding relief by changing arm position and flicking his wrist. On exam he had reduced sensation to light touch and pinprick in the distal index finger and thumb. There is no upper limb muscle weakness or atrophy, except for some noted in the right abductor pollicis brevis (which was also moderately weak).

Electrodiagnostic studies were done (see Table 5.1) primarily to evaluate for a neuropathy of the right median nerve, either at/distal or proximal to the wrist, or a C6–C7 radiculopathy.

There was an absent right median sensory response. Markedly prolonged right median motor distal latency with reduced amplitude were demonstrated. The median minimal F-wave latency was prolonged. Ulnar motor and sensory studies were normal, as was the radial sensory study.

The needle EMG findings included moderately reduced recruitment of motor unit action potentials (MUAPs) in the right abductor pollicis brevis muscle, with increased MUAP amplitude, duration and the presence of polyphasic MUAP's. No active/ongoing denervation features were detected. The absence of abnormal findings in more proximal median-innervated muscles such as the flexor pollicis longus and flexor carpi radialis excludes a proximal median neuropathy like that at the forearm, and the normal studies of other C8–T1 muscles do not favor a cervical motor radiculopathy at these levels.

In this case, *the electrodiagnostic findings are consistent with a severe and chronic right median neuropathy at or distal to the wrist, corresponding to the clinical diagnosis of carpal tunnel syndrome. This is supported by the prolongation of the right median motor distal latency with stimulation at the wrist, as well as reduced right median motor amplitude, and prolongation of the right median F-wave latency in the context of an absent right median sensory response.*

Ulnar Neuropathy (at the Elbow)

History of Presentation and Exam Findings

A 54-year-old man had symptoms of left-hand numbness mainly in the fifth digit for 6 months. He had also noticed loss of muscle bulk of the left-hand muscles, with pain in the elbow and intermittent neck pain. On exam, there was moderate intrinsic left hand muscle atrophy involving ulnar-innervated muscles, and significant reduced sensations to light touch and pin prick in the fifth digit only.

Electrodiagnostic study (see Table 5.2) was done to work up the differential diagnoses of a left ulnar neuropathy at the elbow or at the wrist, a lower brachial plexopathy or a radiculopathy involving C8–T1 nerve roots.

Findings included an absent left ulnar sensory response recording the fifth digit, with a reduced amplitude of the left ulnar sensory response recording the dorsal hand. Ulnar motor responses recording at the abductor digiti minimi (ADM) showed normal distal latencies with reduced amplitude and markedly reduced conduction velocity between the above-elbow and below-elbow stimulation sites (i.e. the elbow segment). A complete left ulnar motor conduction block (amplitude drop >50%) was demonstrated between these two stimulation sites as well. Additionally, ulnar motor responses recording at the first dorsal interosseous (FDI) muscle showed normal distal latency and reduced amplitude, with reduced conduction velocity at the elbow segment. However, no definite conduction blocks were demonstrated in this or other segments studied. The ulnar F-wave latency was significantly prolonged. Median sensory and motor nerve conduction studies were within normal limits.

The findings on needle EMG included fibrillation potentials in the FDI and ADM muscles, few fasciculation potentials seen in the FDI, with reduced recruitment of the motor unit action potentials (MUAPs) firing at a rapid rate in both these muscles, as well as the flexor digitorum profundus (to digits 4&5) and the flexor carpi ulnaris muscles. The MUAPs in these four muscles were also increased in amplitude and duration, with some polyphasia. Other C8–T1 innervated muscles as well as lower cervical paraspinal muscles were normal on needle EMG.

In this case, *the electrodiagnostic findings are consistent with a subacute on chronic left ulnar mononeuropathy localizable at the elbow. This lesion which is severe in degree electrically exhibits focal demyelinating (at the elbow segment) as well as marked axon loss characteristics.*

Table 5.1 Case electrodiagnostic data

Sensory nerve conduction studies

Nerve	Stimulus	Recording	B-P Amp (µV) L	B-P Amp (µV) R	LatNPk (ms) L	LatNPk (ms) R	CV (m/s) L	CV (m/s) R	Dist (mm) L	Dist (mm) R	Norm B-P Amp (µV)	Norm LatNPk (ms)	Norm CV (m/s)	Temp (°C) L	Temp (°C) R
Median	Wrist	Index finger		**Absent**		**Absent**		**Absent**		130	>10	<3.6	>50		33.1
Ulnar	Wrist	Digit 5		23.9		3.1		55		110	>10	<3.2	>50		33.3
Radial	Forearm	Thumb		21.2		2.4		57		100	>14	<2.7	>50		33.1

Motor nerve conduction studies

Nerve	Recording	Stimulus	B-P Amp (mV) L	B-P Amp (mV) R	LatOn (ms) L	LatOn (ms) R	CV (m/s) L	CV (m/s) R	Dist (mm) L	Dist (mm) R	Norm B-P Amp (mV)	Norm LatON (ms)	Norm CV (m/s)	Temp (°C) L	Temp (°C) R
Median	Abductor pollicis brevis	Wrist		**1.8**		**12.5**				50	>6	<4	>50		33.2
		Elbow		**1.5**		18.2		**40.0**		230					
Ulnar	Abductor digiti minimi	Wrist		12.2		1.8				50	>7	<3.1	>50		33.2
		Below elbow		12.1		5.1		58.5		190					
		Above elbow		11.7		6.8		58.0		290					

F-wave studies

Nerve	Stimulus	Recording	F-waves Lat (ms) L	F-waves Lat (ms) R
Median	Wrist	Abductor pollicis brevis		**35.3** (NL 22–31)
Ulnar	Wrist	Abductor digiti minimi		28.9 (NL 21–32)

Needle EMG summary

Side	Muscle	Ins Act	Fib	PW	Fasc	Other	Number	Recruit	Dur	Dur	Amp	Amp	Poly	Poly	Descript
R	Deltoid	Norm	0	0	0		Norm	Full		Norm		Norm		Norm	NC
R	Flexor carpi radialis	Norm	0	0	0		Norm	Full		Norm		Norm		Norm	NC
R	Abductor pollicis brevis	Norm	0	0	0		−2	Rapid	Many	1+	Many	1+	Many	1+	NC
R	Flexor pollicis longus	Norm	0	0	0		Norm	Full		Norm		Norm		Norm	NC
R	First dorsal interosseous	Norm	0	0	0		Norm	Full		Norm		Norm		Norm	NC
R	Biceps brachii	Norm	0	0	0		Norm	Full		Norm		Norm		Norm	NC
R	Triceps	Norm	0	0	0		Norm	Full		Norm		Norm		Norm	NC

Table 5.2 Case electrodiagnostic data

Sensory nerve conduction studies

Nerve	Stimulus	Recording	B-P Amp (μV)		LatNPk (ms)		CV (m/s)		Dist (mm)		Norm B-P Amp (μV)	Norm LatNPk (ms)	Norm CV (m/s)	Temp (°C)	
			L	R	L	R	L	R	L	R				L	R
Median	Wrist	Index finger	18.7		3.4		60.1		130		>15	<3.6	>50	33.2	
Ulnar	Wrist	Digit V	**Absent**		**Absent**		**Absent**		110		>10	<3.1	>50	33.0	
Ulnar	Wrist	Dorsum of hand	**5.1**		2.9		51.5		100		>10	<3.1	>50	33.1	

Motor nerve conduction studies

Nerve	Recording	Stimulus	B-P Amp (mV)		LatOn (ms)		CV (m/s)		Dist (mm)		Norm B-P Amp (mV)	Norm LatON (ms)	Norm CV (m/s)	Temp (°C)	
			L	R	L	R	L	R	L	R				L	R
Median	Abductor pollicis brevis (APB)	Wrist	9.9		3.9				50		>6	<4	>50	33.2	
		Elbow	8.2		10.9		51.2		320						
Ulnar	Abductor digiti minimi (ADM)	Wrist	**3.7**		3.0				50		>7	<3.1	>50	33.1	
		Below elbow	**3.0**		7.5		53.3		240						
		Above elbow	**1.4**		17.1		**24.1**		340						
Ulnar	First dorsal interosseous	Wrist	**5.4**		4.4				50		>7	<4.5	>50	33.1	
		Below elbow	**4.4**		8.5		58.5		240						
		Above elbow	**3.7**		18		**25.0**		340						

F-wave studies

Nerve	Stimulus	Recording	F-waves Lat(ms) L	F-waves Lat(ms) R
Median/APB	Wrist	Abductor pollicis brevis	29.9 (NL 22–31)	
Ulnar/ADM	Wrist	Abductor digiti minimi	**45.5** (NL 21–32)	

Needle EMG summary

Side	Muscle	Ins Act	Fib	PW	Fasc	Other	Number	Recruit	Dur	Dur	Amp	Amp	Poly	Poly	Descript
Left	First dorsal interosseous	1+	1+	1+	1+		2–	Rapid	Many	1+	Some	1+	Few	1+	NC
Left	Abductor digiti minimi	1+	1+	1+	0		2–	Rapid	Many	1+	Some	1+	Some	2+	NC
Left	Flexor digitorum profundus to digits 5 and 4	0	0	0	0		2–	Rapid	Some	1+	Some	1+	Few	1+	NC
Left	Flexor carpi ulnaris	0	0	0	0		2–	Rapid	Many	1+	Some	1+	Some	1+	NC
Left	Pronator teres	0	0	0	0			Full		Norm		Norm		Norm	NC
Left	Biceps brachii	0	0	0	0			Full		Norm		Norm		Norm	NC
Left	Triceps	0	0	0	0			Full		Norm		Norm		Norm	NC
Left	Low cervical paraspinals	0	0	0	0			Full		Norm		Norm		Norm	NC

This is supported by the findings of active/ongoing and chronic denervation features in the ulnar-innervated hand and forearm muscles, and normal findings in other C8–T1 innervated muscles, with abnormal ulnar sensory (recording fifth digit & dorsal hand) and abnormal ulnar motor responses recording the ADM and FDI muscles. Localization of the lesion at the elbow is based on the demonstration of conduction velocity reduction/slowing and conduction block in this segment.

Radial Neuropathy

History of Presentation and Exam Findings

A 44-year-old woman presented with a 4 month history of a left wrist and finger drop, initially noticed after awakening from a prolonged and deep sleep, in the context of heavy alcohol use before falling asleep on a couch "in an awkward position". She also noticed numbness in the dorsum of her left hand, mostly around the first web space. There was no significant pain, nor history of known trauma. On exam she had a left wrist and finger drop with significant weakness graded as 2/5 on the Medical Research Council (MRC) scale. There was modest weakness in hand grip, but finger flexion was normal, as well as strength in the rest of the left upper limb. On sensory exam there was reduced sensation to light touch and pinprick in the dorsum of the left hand between the thumb and index fingers only. Deep tendon reflexes were normal throughout.

Electrodiagnostic studies (see Table 5.3) were done to work up a differential diagnosis of a left radial neuropathy at the spiral grove versus at other level, a left brachial plexopathy (especially one involving the posterior cord), or a radiculopathy involving the C7 nerve root.

Left radial motor nerve conduction studies recording both the extensor indicis (proprius) and the extensor digitorum (communis) muscles showed a normal motor amplitude and latency when stimulating at the elbow and distal spiral groove site, but the amplitude significantly reduced by >50% when stimulating at the proximal spiral groove site, which indicates presence of a conduction block at the spiral groove segment (in which there is also conduction slowing/velocity reduction). Right radial motor studies were done for comparison, and the responses were normal. The left median and ulnar motor studies were also normal.

The left radial sensory response was markedly reduced in amplitude with normal peak latency, and the right radial sensory response showed normal amplitude and peak latency. The left median and ulnar sensory studies were normal.

The needle EMG demonstrated fibrillation and positive sharp wave potentials in the left brachioradialis, extensor digitorum (communis) and extensor indicis (proprius) muscles. On needle EMG, these three muscles showed markedly reduced recruitment with at least a few to some motor unit action potentials (MUAPs) displaying large amplitudes, increased duration and polyphasia.

In this case, *the electrodiagnostic findings are consistent with a subacute to early chronic left radial neuropathy, localizable at the spiral groove. The lesion is at least moderate in degree electrically and exhibits focal demyelinating (at the spiral groove segment) as well as marked axon loss characteristics. This is supported by the presence of a conduction block (with slowing/velocity reduction) at the spiral groove, with preserved distal radial motor amplitudes, but significant (>50%) amplitude drop when stimulating at the proximal spiral groove site, together with the presence of fibrillation and positive sharp wave potentials, and reduced recruitment with some large-sized MUAPs (with polyphasia) in all radial-innervated muscles examined below the spiral groove [i.e. brachioradialis, extensor indicis (proprius) and extensor digitorum (communis)].*

Suprascapular Neuropathy

History of Presentation and Exam Findings

A 52-year-old patient presented to the clinic with a 2-month history of right arm weakness with external rotation and somewhat with elevating the arm above the shoulder. She had posterior shoulder pain, but this was not a prominent symptom. She denies trauma to the neck and shoulder

Table 5.3 Case electrodiagnostic data

Sensory nerve conduction

Nerve	Stimulus	Recording	B-P Amp (μV)		LatNPk (ms)		Dist (mm)		Norm B-P Amp	Norm LatNPk	Temp (°C)	
			L	R	L	R	L	R			L	R
Median	Wrist	Index	49.20		2.70		130		>20 μV	<3.4 ms	33.2	
Ulnar	Wrist	5th dig	42.70		2.60		110		>12 μV	<3.1 ms	33.2	
Radial	Forearm	Thumb	**10.50**	47.50	2.20	2.10	100	100	>18 μV	<2.7 ms	32.5	32.8

Motor nerve conduction

Nerve	Recording	Stimulus	B-P Amp (mV)		LatOn (ms)		CV (m/s)		Dist (mm)		Norm B-P Amp	Norm LatOn	Norm CV	Temp (°C)	
			L	R	L	R	L	R	L	R				L	R
Median	APB	Wrist	10.50		2.60		n/a		50		>6 mV	<3.9 ms	>50 m/s	32.3	
		Elbow	10.00		6.50		65.4		255					32.2	
Ulnar/ ADM	ADM	Wrist	11.10		2.00		n/a		50		>7 mV	<3.1 ms	>50 m/s	32.9	
		Below Elbow	10.80		5.30		59.1		195					32.9	
		Above Elbow	10.30		7.40		54.0		295					32.0	
Radial/ EDC	EDC	Elbow	6.70	7.10	1.30	1.00	n/a	n/a			>6 mV	<3.1 ms	>50 m/s	32.0	32.1
		Dist. Spir. Groove	6.10	7.00	2.60	2.60	81.5	68.8	110	110				32.7	32.0
		Prox. Spir. Groove	**1.30**		7.70		31.3		200					32.7	
Radial/ EIP	EIP	Elbow	7.80	7.70	2.20	2.20	n/a	n/a			>6 mV	<3.1 ms	>50 m/s	32.6	32.7
		Dist. Spir. Groove	6.10	6.70	4.20	3.70	60.0	80.0	120	120				32.5	32.6
		Prox. Spir. Groove	**1.42**		6.40		**40.5**		170					32.5	

F-wave side-to-side comparison table

Nerve	Stimulus	Recording	F-Waves	
			Lat (ms)	
			L	R
Ulnar/ADM	Wrist	ADM	25.80	

Needle EMG summary

Side	Muscle	Ins Act.	Fib	PW	Fasc	Other	Number	Recruit	Dur	Dur	Amp	Amp	Poly	Poly	Descript	Descript	Descript
L	1st Dorsal Interosseous	Norm	0	0	0		2–	Mod		Norm		Norm		Norm	NC		
	Flex.Pollicis Longus	Norm	0	0	0		2–	Mod		Norm		Norm		Norm	NC		
	EIP	Norm	2+	1+	0		3–	Rapid	Some	1+	Some	1+	Few	1+	NC		
	Pronator Teres	Norm	0	0	0		1–	Mod-V		Norm		Norm		Norm	NC		
	EDC	Norm	2+	0+	0		3–	Rapid	Many	1+	Some	1+	Many	1+	NC		
	Brachioradial	Norm	1+	2+	0		3–	Rapid	Some	1+	Few	1+	Few	1+	NC		
	Anconeus	Norm	0	0	0		2–	Mod		Norm		Norm		Norm	NC		
	Biceps Brachii	Norm	0	0	0		1–	Mod		Norm		Norm		Norm	NC		
	Triceps—Lateral head	Norm	0	0	0		1–	Mod-V		Norm		Norm		Norm	NC		
	Deltoid–Middle head	Norm	0	0	0		1–	Mod		Norm		Norm		Norm	NC		

APB Abductor pollicis brevis, *ADM* Abductor digiti minimi, *EDC* Extensor digitorum communis, *EIP* Extensor indicis proprius area, and there is no definite numbness or paresthesia. The patient states that she carries a heavy handbag frequently over her right shoulder.

Examination revealed weakness of external shoulder rotation on the right, with normal strength in the rest of the muscle groups. There was no appreciable muscle atrophy, and there were intact deep tendon reflexes and a normal sensory exam.

Electrodiagnostic studies of the upper extremity (see Table 5.4) were performed to work up the differential diagnoses which included a cervical radiculopathy, a brachial plexopathy or a proximal upper limb mononeuropathy.

All motor responses, including axillary, musculocutaneous, ulnar and median had normal amplitudes, distal latencies and conduction velocities. Sensory nerve conduction studies, including the median nerve recording at digits 1, 2 and 3, the ulnar, radial, as well as the lateral and medial antebrachial cutaneous responses were also with normal peak latencies and amplitudes. These normal responses essentially ruled out a right brachial plexopathy.

Needle EMG showed the presence of fibrillation potentials with reduced recruitment and rapid firing pattern (of normal-sized motor unit potentials) in the infraspinatus muscle only. The supraspinatus and other muscles in the C5–C6 myotomes were normal, effectively excluding the presence of a C5–C6 cervical motor radiculopathy.

In this case, *the electrodiagnostic findings are consistent with a subacute axon loss lesion of the distal right suprascapular nerve, favoring localization at the spinoglenoid notch, moderate in degree electrically, with evidence of active/ongoing motor axon loss. This is supported by the needle EMG findings of active/ongoing denervation features and reduced recruitment of normal-sized motor unit action potentials (too early for remodeling and enlargement) in the infraspinatus muscle, sparing the supraspinatus muscle.*

The finding of denervation features in the infraspinatus muscle only supports the diagnosis of suprascapular neuropathy localizable at the spinoglenoid notch, with little pain mainly due to sparing of the deep sensory branches that supply the glenoacromial and acromioclavicular joints.

Axillary Neuropathy

History of Presentation and Exam Findings

A 72-year-old man was evaluated 3 months after right shoulder dislocation in the context of a fall which was treated conservatively in the emergency department. Now, he presents with persistent numbness in the lateral aspect of his right shoulder, with loss of muscle bulk around the point of the shoulder and weakness with significant difficulty raising the arm above the shoulder level. This had not improved following months of physical therapy.

On exam, there was atrophy of the right deltoid, moderate weakness with right shoulder abduction and (to a lesser degree) with arm/shoulder flexion and extension as well. However, there was no scapular winging, and the rest of the right arm muscles demonstrated normal strength; deep tendon reflexes were normal. There were no sensory deficits, except for reduced sensation to light touch and pinprick in small area of the right lateral shoulder.

Electrodiagnostic studies of the upper extremities (see Table 5.5) were performed to work up the differential diagnoses including a right cervical radiculopathy at C5–C6, a brachial plexopathy (especially one involving the upper trunk), or a proximal upper limb mononeuropathy.

The right axillary motor response recording the deltoid muscle was absent. All other motor responses (including the right median, right ulnar, left axillary and bilateral musculocutaneous) were with normal amplitudes, distal latencies, and conduction velocities. Sensory nerve conduction studies, including the right median nerve recording at digits 1, 2 and 3, the right ulnar, radial, as well as the lateral and medial antebrachial cutaneous responses were also with normal peak latencies and amplitudes. These other normal motor responses and sensory responses essentially ruled out a right brachial plexopathy.

Table 5.4 Case electrodiagnostic data

Sensory nerve conduction studies

Nerve	Stimulus	Recording	B-P Amp (μV) L	B-P Amp (μV) R	LatNPk (ms) L	LatNPk (ms) R	CV (m/s) L	CV (m/s) R	Dist (mm) L	Dist (mm) R	Norm B-P Amp (μV)	Norm LatNPk (ms)	Norm CV (m/s)	Temp (°C) L	Temp (°C) R
Median	Wrist	Index (D2) Middle (D3) Thumb (D1)		58.9 52.5 40.8		2.8 2.8 2.4		63		130	>10	<3.6	>50		33.4
Ulnar	Wrist	Digit 5		56.9		2.5		55		110	>10	<3.1	>50		33.2
Radial	Forearm	Thumb (D1)		50.4		2.2		57		100	>14	<2.7	>50		33.0
Medial antebrachial cutaneous	Medial elbow	Medial forearm		19.3		2.4		63		120	>8	<2.9	>55		33.0
Lateral antebrachial cutaneous	Antecubital fossa	Lateral forearm		19.4		2.2		60		120	>10	<2.9			33.0

Motor nerve conduction studies

Nerve	Recording	Stimulus	B-P Amp (mV) L	B-P Amp (mV) R	LatOn (ms) L	LatOn (ms) R	CV (m/s) L	CV (m/s) R	Dist (mm) L	Dist (mm) R	Norm B-P Amp (mV)	Norm LatON (ms)	Norm CV (m/s)	Temp (°C) L	Temp (°C) R
Median	Abductor pollicis brevis	Wrist		10.4		2.9				50	>6	<4	>50		33.2
		Elbow		10.2		7.4		57.8		260					
Ulnar	Abductor digiti minimi	Wrist		8.9		2.1				50	>7	<3.1	>50		33.1
		Below elbow		8.8		4.8		69.1		190					
		Above elbow		8.7		6.8		61.7		290					
Musculocutaneous	Biceps	Axilla		5.3		3.4					>4	<3.5			33.5
Axillary	Deltoid	Erb's point		10.7		3.1					>4	<4.9			33.5

F-wave studies

Nerve	Stimulus	Recording	F-waves Lat (ms) L	F-waves Lat (ms) R
Median	Wrist	Abductor pollicis brevis		24.6 (NL 22–31)
Ulnar	Wrist	Abductor digiti minimi		23.3 (NL 21–32)

(continued)

Table 5.4 (continued)

Needle EMG summary											
Side	Muscle	Insertional activity	Positive Sharp Wave	Fibrillation	Fasciculation	Recruitment	Firing pattern	Amp	Duration	Polyphasia	Descript
R	Infraspinatus	1+	None	2+	0	2-	Rapid	Normal	Normal	Normal	NC
R	Supraspinatus	Normal	0	0	0	Normal	Normal	Normal	Normal	Normal	NC
R	Rhomboid major	Normal	0	0	0	Normal	Normal	Normal	Normal	Normal	NC
R	Deltoid	Normal	0	0	0	Normal	Normal	Normal	Normal	Normal	NC
R	Pronator teres	Normal	0	0	0	Normal	Normal	Normal	Normal	Normal	NC
R	Biceps brachii	Normal	0	0	0	Normal	Normal	Normal	Normal	Normal	NC
R	Triceps	Normal	0	0	0	Normal	Normal	Normal	Normal	Normal	NC
R	1st dorsal interosseous	Normal	0	0	0	Normal	Normal	Normal	Normal	Normal	NC
R	Cervical paraspinals (mid)	Normal	0	0	0	Normal	Normal	Normal	Normal	Normal	NC

Table 5.5 Case electrodiagnostic data

Sensory nerve conduction studies

Nerve	Stimulus	Recording	B-P Amp (μV) L	B-P Amp (μV) R	LatNPk (ms) L	LatNPk (ms) R	CV (m/s) L	CV (m/s) R	Dist (mm) L	Dist (mm) R	Norm B-P Amp (μV)	Norm LatNPk (ms)	Norm CV (m/s)	Temp (°C) L	Temp (°C) R
Median	Wrist	Index (D2)		28.1		3.5		54		130	>10	<3.6	>50		33.2
		Middle (D3)		17.7		3.5				130					33.2
		Thumb (D1)		17.7		3.4				130					33.2
Ulnar	Wrist	Digit 5		11.0		2.5		51		110	>10	<3.2	>50		33.5
Radial	Forearm	Thumb		14.8		2.3		50		100	>14	<2.7	>50		33.5
Medial antebrachial cutaneous	Medial elbow	Medial forearm		10.8		2.6		56		120	>8	<2.9	>55		33.2
Lateral antebrachial cutaneous	Antecubital fossa	Lateral forearm		12.3		2.8		55		120	>10	<2.9			33.2

Motor nerve conduction studies

Nerve	Recording	Stimulus	B-P Amp (mV) L	B-P Amp (mV) R	LatOn (ms) L	LatOn (ms) R	CV (m/s) L	CV (m/s) R	Dist (mm) L	Dist (mm) R	Norm B-P Amp (mV)	Norm LatON (ms)	Norm CV (m/s)	Temp (°C) L	Temp (°C) R
Median	Abductor pollicis brevis	Wrist		8.7		3.9				50	>6	<4	>50		33.5
		Elbow		8.6		9.5		58.9		330					
Ulnar	Abductor digiti minimi	Wrist		8.0		2.8				50	>7	<3.1	>50		33.5
		Below elbow		7.2		6.9		55.4		230					
		Above Elbow		7.1		8.9		54.1		330					
Musculocutaneous	Biceps	Axilla	8.5	7.9	2.9	3.0					>4	<3.1		33.5	33.2
Axillary	Deltoid	Erb's point	4.3	**0**	4.3	**0**					>4	<4.9		33.2	33.2

F-wave studies

Nerve	Stimulus	Recording	F-waves Lat (ms) L	F-waves Lat (ms) R
Median	Wrist	Abductor pollicis brevis		29.3 (NL 22–31)
Ulnar	Wrist	Abductor digiti minimi		28.2 (NL 21–32)

(continued)

Table 5.5 (continued)

							Needle EMG Summary								
Side	Muscle	Ins Act	Fib	PW	Fasc	Other	Number	Recruit	Dur	Dur	Amp	Amp	Poly	Poly	Descript
R	Infraspinatus	0	0	0	0		Norm	Full		Norm		Norm		Norm	NC
R	Supraspinatus	0	0	0	0		Norm	Full		Norm		Norm		Norm	NC
R	Deltoid, middle head	1+	1+	1+	0		3–	Rapid	Many	1+	Many	1+	Many	1+	NC
R	Extensor indicis proprius	0	0	0	0		Norm	Full		Norm		Norm		Norm	NC
R	Pronator teres	0	0	0	0		Norm	Full		Norm		Norm		Norm	NC
R	First dorsal interosseous	0	0	0	0		Norm	Full		Norm		Norm		Norm	NC
R	Biceps Brachii	0	0	0	0		Norm	Full		Norm		Norm		Norm	NC
R	Teres minor	1+	3+	1+	0		3–	Rapid	Most	1+	Many	1+	Some	2+	NC
R	Triceps	0	0	0	0		Norm	Full		Norm		Norm		Norm	NC
R	Mid cervical paraspinals	0	0	0	0		Norm	Full		Norm		Norm		Norm	NC

The needle EMG showed fibrillation potentials and positive sharp waves in the middle head of the deltoid muscle and the teres minor muscle, with motor unit action potentials demonstrating severely reduced recruitment, rapid firing pattern, increase in amplitude, duration and polyphasia. All other muscles in the C5–C6 myotomes, as well as paraspinal muscles were normal, essentially ruling out a cervical motor radiculopathy.

In this case, *the electrodiagnostic findings are consistent with a subacute on early chronic axon loss lesion of the right axillary nerve, severe in degree electrically. This is supported by an absent right axillary motor response, and active/ongoing denervation features with severe motor unit dropout demonstrated by needle EMG in the right deltoid and teres minor muscles.*

As in this case of a shoulder dislocation following a fall, isolated axillary neuropathies are usually secondary to trauma. The typical findings of weakness of shoulder abduction > arm/shoulder flexion and extension, as well as sensory loss over proximal lateral shoulder, and the EMG findings of motor axon loss changes in the axillary nerve distribution (including in the deltoid and teres minor muscles) are all strong supportive evidence of an axillary neuropathy.

Anterior Interosseous Neuropathy

History of Presentation and Exam Findings

A 44-year-old man presented with left forearm pain over the past 5 weeks, noticed soon after surgery for left thumb carpometacarpal joint arthrodesis with bone graft. He had been in a left arm cast for about 4 weeks postoperatively (recently removed), but was still having pain in the forearm, as well as weakness with thumb and index finger flexion, often dropping keys and other items requiring a secure pincer grasp.

Examination of the left upper limb revealed severe weakness of flexion of the distal phalanx of the thumb and the index, and mild weakness of pronation with the elbow flexed. The patient was unable to make the "OK" sign with left hand, had some tenderness to touch in distal left forearm, but no definite sensory deficits.

Electrodiagnostic studies (see Table 5.6) were done to work up the differential diagnoses which included an anterior interosseous neuropathy versus a more proximal median neuropathy, a lower brachial plexopathy or a radiculopathy involving predominantly C8–T1 nerve roots.

Nerve conduction studies demonstrated normal left median and ulnar motor responses, as well as normal left median, ulnar and radial sensory responses. Corresponding left median and ulnar F-wave latencies were also within normal limits.

Needle EMG disclosed abundant fibrillation potentials and positive sharp waves in the left flexor pollicis longus (FPL) and pronator quadratus (PQ) muscles. No motor unit action potential (MUAP) recruitment was found in these two muscles (suggesting loss of nerve continuity to these muscles). Needle EMG of the left flexor digitorum profundus to digits 2&3 (FDP-2&3) disclosed fibrillation potentials as well, but also markedly reduced recruitment with a few residual MUAPs of normal size and morphology, firing moderately fast to rapidly. All other muscles examined were normal, including the remaining median-innervated muscles (the left flexor carpi radialis, pronator teres, and abductor pollicis brevis), the left first dorsal interosseous, biceps brachii, deltoid and triceps.

In this case, *the electrodiagnostic findings are consistent with a subacute left anterior interosseous neuropathy, very severe in degree electrically, with evidence of active/ongoing motor axon loss. This is supported by findings on needle EMG, particularly abundant fibrillation and/or positive sharp potentials without chronic denervation MUAP changes (actually nerve discontinuity suggested by lack of MUAPs in the left FPL and PQ), exclusively in the left anterior interosseous nerve (AION) distribution (FPL, PQ, FDP-2&3). The normal left median sensory and motor nerve conduction studies are also compatible*

Table 5.6 Case electrodiagnostic data

Sensory nerve conduction studies

Nerve	Stimulus	Recording	B-P Amp (μV) L	B-P Amp (μV) R	LatNPk (ms) L	LatNPk (ms) R	CV (m/s) L	CV (m/s) R	Dist (mm) L	Dist (mm) R	Norm B-P Amp (μV)	Norm LatNPk (ms)	Norm CV (m/s)	Temp (°C) L	Temp (°C) R
Median	Wrist	Index finger	44.5		3.0		60.1		130		>20	<3.4	>50	33.2	
Ulnar	Wrist	Digit V	24.6		2.6		58		110		>12	<3.1	>50	33.0	
Radial	Forearm	Thumb	24.7		2.1		52		100		>18	<2.7	>50	30.8	

Motor nerve conduction studies

Nerve	Recording	Stimulus	B-P Amp (mV) L	B-P Amp (mV) R	LatOn (ms) L	LatOn (ms) R	CV (m/s) L	CV (m/s) R	Dist (mm) L	Dist (mm) R	Norm B-P Amp (mV)	Norm LatON (ms)	Norm CV (m/s)	Temp (°C) L	Temp (°C) R
Median	Abductor pollicis brevis	Wrist	6.8		2.9				50		>6	<4	>50	33.2	
		Elbow	6.5		7.3		54.5		240						
Ulnar	First dorsal interosseous	Wrist	10.1		2.2				50		>7	<4.5	>50	33.1	
		Below elbow	8.1		6.2		52.0		210						
		Above elbow	7.9		8.3		51.2		310						

F-wave studies

Nerve	Stimulus	Recording	F-waves Lat (ms) L	F-waves Lat (ms) R
Median	Wrist	Abductor pollicis brevis	28.2 (NL 22–31)	
Ulnar	Wrist	Abductor digiti minimi	28.6 (NL 21–32)	

Needle EMG Summary

Side	Muscle	Ins act	Fib	PW	Fasc	Other	Number	Recruit	Dur	Dur	AMP	Amp	Poly	Poly	Descript
Left	First dorsal interosseous	0	0	0	0			Full		Norm		Norm		Norm	NC
Left	Flexor pollicis longus	1+	2+	1+	0			None							NC
Left	Abductor pollicis brevis	0	0	0	0			Full		Norm		Norm		Norm	NC
Left	Pronator quadratus	1+	2+	2+	0			None							NC
Left	Pronator teres	0	0	0	0			Full		Norm		Norm		Norm	NC
Left	Flexor carpi radialis	0	0	0	0			Full		Norm		Norm		Norm	NC
Left	Flexor digitorum profundus (to D2&3)	1+	1+	0	0		3–	Mod-R		Norm		Norm		Norm	NC
Left	Biceps	0	0	0	0			Full		Norm		Norm		Norm	NC
Left	Triceps	0	0	0	0			Full		Norm		Norm		Norm	NC
Left	Deltoid	0	0	0	0			Full		Norm		Norm		Norm	NC

with this diagnosis, ruling out a median neuropathy at or distal to the wrist (as seen with carpal tunnel syndrome), or one more proximal to the branchpoint of the AION.

Sciatic Neuropathy

History of Presentation and Exam Findings

A 64-year-old woman presented with persistent left leg weakness and pain that was worst at the end of the day. Pain would radiate from posterior left hip to the dorsum of the foot, with stabbing and electrical-like sensations. Symptoms began immediately after a left hip replacement surgery 6 months ago. Her exam revealed moderate atrophy of left leg muscles, particularly those below the knee, with marked weakness of knee flexors, and also severe weakness with ankle dorsiflexion, plantarflexion, inversion and eversion. The left ankle deep tendon reflex was absent, and sensory exam showed absent perception to light touch and pin prick in the dorsal and lateral left foot and calf. To walk she required the help of a walker and had a pronounced foot drop.

Electrodiagnostic studies (see Table 5.7) were done to work up the differential diagnoses including a left sciatic mononeuropathy, peroneal (fibular) mononeuropathy, lumbosacral plexopathy or a (mostly L5) radiculopathy.

Findings were notable for an absent left tibial (recording abductor hallucis) and peroneal [fibular] (recording both extensor digitorum brevis and tibialis anterior) motor nerve responses, as well as absent left sural and superficial peroneal [fibular] sensory responses. The tibial H-reflex was absent on the left as well. Contralateral responses obtained were normal.

The needle EMG showed abundant fibrillation and/or positive sharp wave potentials in the left abductor hallucis (AH), extensor digitorum brevis (EDB), medial gastrocnemius, tibialis anterior, tibialis posterior (TP), and the short head of the biceps femoris muscle. On needle EMG, recruitment was absent (no residual motor units detected) in the left AH, EDB and TP, with the other aforementioned muscles (plus the left semitendinosus) displaying electrically moderate-to-severe chronic denervation changes, including reduced recruitment with rapidly-firing large MUAPs.

Other left non-sciatic L5 and S1-innervated muscles tested, including gluteus medius as well as the left low lumbar paraspinal muscles showed no definite evidence of motor axon loss. This helped exclude a left L5–S1 lumbar radiculopathy or a left lumbosacral plexopathy (noting needle EMG of the left rectus femoris was also normal).

In this case, *the electrodiagnostic findings are consistent with a subacute to chronic left sciatic mononeuropathy, axon loss in character and severe in degree electrically. This impression is supported by the absent motor responses of the left tibial and peroneal [fibular] nerves (derivatives of the sciatic nerve), an absent left tibial H-reflex, as well as absent left sural and superficial peroneal [fibular] sensory responses, with needle EMG findings of active/ongoing and chronic denervation changes in left peroneal [fibular] and tibial nerve supplied muscles below the knee as well as direct sciatic-innervated hamstring muscles, with sparing of the more proximal (non-sciatic supplied) L5 and S1 innervated muscles, including the gluteal and lumbosacral paraspinal muscles.*

Peroneal (Fibular) Neuropathy

History of Presentation and Exam Findings

A 56-year-old woman presented with 5 weeks of burning pain and numbness in the right anterior leg below the knee and on the dorsum of the foot. Upon further questioning she mentioned frequently tripping over her "floppy" right foot, but no falls. Just prior to symptom onset, she had resumed frequent leg-crossing after losing 100 pounds over 9 months in the wake of bariatric surgery.

Table 5.7 Case electrodiagnostic data

Sensory nerve conduction

Nerve	Stimulus	Recording	B-P Amp (µV)		LatNPk (ms)		Dist (mm)		Norm B-P Amp	Norm LatNPk	Temp (°C)	
			L	R	L	R	L	R			L	R
Sural	Lower Leg	Lat. Malleolus	**Absent**	5.00	**Absent**	3.60	140	140	>3 µV	<4.6 ms	33.0	30.6
Superficial peroneal (fibular)	Lower leg	Ankle	**Absent**	3.90	**Absent**	3.40	100	100	>3 µV	<4.6 ms	33.1	30.1

Motor nerve conduction

Nerve	Recording	Stimulus	B-P Amp (mV)		LatOn (ms)		CV (m/s)		Dist (mm)		Norm B-P Amp	Norm LatOn	Norm CV	Temp (°C)	
			L	R	L	R	L	R	L	R				L	R
Peroneal (fibular)	Extensor digitorum brevis	Ankle	**Absent**	5.80	**Absent**	4.00	n/a	n/a			>2.5 mV	<6 ms	>40 m/s	33.2	30.7
		Pop. foss—knee	**Absent**	4.70	**Absent**	13.00	n/a	47.5		430				33.1	30.7
Tibial	Abductor hallucis	Ankle	**Absent**	7.60	**Absent**	4.30	n/a	n/a			>4 mV	<6 ms	>40 m/s	33.3	30.5
		Pop. fossa-knee	**Absent**	4.50	**Absent**	13.30	n/a	44.4		400				33.3	30.5
Peroneal (fibular)	Tibialis anterior	Below fibular head	**Absent**	5.10	**Absent**	2.70	n/a	n/a			>3 mV	<4.5 ms	>40 m/s	33.3	30.5
Femoral	Rectus femoris	Inguinal Lig	5.50	6.20	4.90	5.30	n/a	n/a			>3 mV	<6.5 ms		33.2	30.1

H-reflex summary table

Nerve	Stimulus	Recording	Side	M-Wave		H-Wave	
				Lat (ms)	Amp (mV)	Lat (ms)	Amp (mV)
Tibial	Popliteal Fossa	Soleus	L	**Absent**		**Absent**	
Tibial	Popliteal Fossa	Soleus	R	5.7 ms	8.4 mV	32.1 ms	1.3 mV

Needle EMG summary

Side	Muscle	Ins Act.	Fib	PW	Fasc	Other	Number	Recruit	Dur	Dur	Amp	Amp	Poly	Poly	Descript
L	Abductor Hallucis	Norm	1+	1+	0			None							NC
	Extn.Digitorum Brevis	Norm	1+	3+	0			None							NC
	Tibialis Posterior	Norm	0	2+	0			None							NC
	Gluteus Medius	Norm	0	0	0		Norm	Full		Norm		Norm		Norm	NC
	Tibialis Anterior	Norm	1+	2+	0		SMU	Mod	All	2+		Norm	All	2+	NC
	Gastrocnemius, medial head	Norm	0	2+	0	CRD	3–	Mod	Most	1+		Norm		Norm	NC
	Rectus Femoris	Norm	0	0	0		Norm	Full		Norm		Norm		Norm	NC
	Biceps Femoris, short head	Norm	0	1+	0		2–	Mod-R	Many	1+	Few	1+		Norm	NC
	Semitendinosus	Norm	0	0	0		2–	Mod-R	Some	1+	Some	1+		Norm	NC
	Lumbar paraspinals (Low)	Norm	0	0	0		1–	Mod		Norm		Norm		Norm	NC

CRD complex repetitive discharges

On exam there was moderate weakness of right ankle dorsiflexion and right foot eversion. There was reduced sensation to light touch and pinprick in the dorsum of the right foot, including the first web space. The remainder of the neurological exam was normal, specifically: intact power with ankle inversion, knee and hip flexion and extension. The deep tendon reflexes were normal.

Electrodiagnostic studies (see Table 5.8) were done to work-up the differential diagnoses including a right peroneal (fibular) mononeuropathy, a right sciatic mononeuropathy or a right lumbar (particularly L5) radiculopathy.

Motor nerve conduction studies of the right peroneal (fibular) nerve demonstrated normal CMAP amplitude when recording both the extensor digitorum brevis (EDB) and the tibialis anterior (TA) muscles, stimulating at the ankle (for the EDB) and below fibular head sites (for both EDB and TA). For the EDB and TA, the CMAP amplitude was markedly reduced (drop >50%, implicating conduction block) when stimulating above the fibular head/at the popliteal fossa. The right superficial peroneal (fibular) sensory response was absent. The right tibial motor responses showed normal amplitude, distal latency and conduction velocity. The right sural response was also normal.

Needle EMG demonstrated abundant fibrillation (and often positive sharp wave) potentials in the right TA, EDB and peroneous longus muscles with decreased recruitment of motor unit potentials (which were normal in size and configuration), firing at a moderately fast to rapid rate. Findings were normal in the right tibial-innervated muscles including the medial gastrocnemius, tibialis posterior and abductor hallucis, as well as sciatic-innervated (peroneal/fibular divison) muscles like the short head of the biceps femoris. More proximal right L5/S1-innervated muscles, such as the semitendinosus and gluteus medius displayed normal findings.

In this case, *the electrodiagnostic findings are consistent with a subacute right common peroneal (fibular) mononeuropathy, localizable at the fibular head, axon loss in character but also with prominent focal demyelination manifested by complete conduction block (and segmental conduction velocity slowing) at the fibular head recording both EDB and TA, severe in degree electrically. These findings are further supported by absence of the right superficial peroneal (fibular) sensory response, in the context of normal sural (sensory) and tibial motor responses. In addition, supportive needle EMG findings include active/ongoing denervation changes in peroneal (fibular)-innervated muscles supplied by both deep and superficial branches, with sparing of the tibial-innervated, and more proximal non-peroneal (non-fibular)-innervated L5/S1-innervated muscles. It is too soon in the timeline to be considered a chronic lesion since the MUAPs are still normal in size and configuration (not yet remodeled and larger) despite the reduced recruitment pattern seen.*

Tibial Neuropathy (at the Tarsal Tunnel)

A 30 year old dancer presented with 3 months of progressive pain and burning paresthesia on the sole of her left foot, noticing the onset of these at the end of a very busy performance season. She does not recall any definite antecedent accident or injury to the left foot, and there is no visible swelling or skin color changes in the affected area. The symptoms appear to be aggravated with prolonged time spent on her feet, especially when dancing. Although when pain becomes severe it may make her walk "funny", she denies any significant limb weakness.

Examination findings are most notable for numbness intermixed with hyperalgesic/dysesthetic distortion of pinprick perception throughout the plantar aspect of her left foot. Pain symptoms of similar quality and distribution appear to be triggered with lightly tapping over an area slightly posterior and inferior to the right medial malleolus. She also demonstrates some weakness with abduction of toes of the left foot. Deep tendon reflexes, including the left ankle jerk are all intact. Gait is notable for slight antalgic features on the left.

Electrodiagnostic studies (see Table 5.9) were done to workup the differential diagnoses which included a left tibial mononeuropathy at the tarsal tunnel (i.e. tarsal tunnel syndrome), versus a

Table 5.8 Case electrodiagnostic data

Sensory nerve conduction

Nerve	Stimulus	Recording	B-P Amp (μV)		LatNPk (ms)		CV (m/s)		Dist (mm)		Norm B-P Amp	Norm LatNPk	Norm CV	Temp (°C)	
			L	R	L	R	L	R	L	R				L	R
Sural	Lower Leg	Lat. Malleolus		13.52		4.04		n/a		140	>4 μV	<4.6 ms	>40 m/s		32.1
Superficial peroneal (fibular)	Lower Leg	Ankle	5.60	**Absent**	3.30	**Absent**	n/a	n/a	100	100	>4 μV	<4.6 ms		31.7	31.5

Motor nerve conduction

Nerve	Recording	Stimulus	B-P Amp (mV)		LatOn (ms)		CV (m/s)		Dist (mm)		Norm B-P Amp	Norm LatOn	Norm CV	Temp (°C)	
			L	R	L	R	L	R	L	R				L	R
Peroneal (fibular)	Extensor digitorum brevis	Ankle	3.91	3.41	4.65	5.75	n/a	n/a			>2.5 mV	<6 ms	>40 m/s	32.7	31.1
		Pop Foss—Knee	3.38	**0.39**	14.00	17.45	46.0	**37.6**	430	440				32.8	31.0
		Below Fibular Head		2.97		13.90		45.4		370					31.0
Tibial	Abductor hallucis	Ankle		5.38		3.95		n/a			>4 mV	<6 ms	>40 m/s		30.4
		Pop Fossa—Knee		4.10		12.55		51.2		440					30.6
Peroneal (fibular)	Tibialis anterior	Below Fib Head	3.87	3.10	2.30	2.25	n/a	n/a			>3 mV	<4.5 ms	>40 m/s	32.3	30.8
		Pop Fossa—Knee	3.65	**0.80**	4.40	5.05	47.6	**35.7**	100	100				32.0	30.9

F-wave side-to-side comparison table

Nerve	Stimulus	Recording	F-Waves	
			Lat (ms)	
			L	R
Tibial	Ankle	Abductor hallucis		44.20

H-reflex summary table

Nerve	Stimulus	Recording	Side	M-Wave		H-Wave	
				Lat (ms)	Amp (mV)	Lat (ms)	Amp (mV)
Tibial	Popliteal Fossa	Soleus	Right	4.0 ms	10.6 mV	30.3 ms	2.7 mV

Needle EMG summary

Side	Muscle	Ins Act.	Fib	PW	Fasc	Other	Number	Recruit	Dur	Dur	Amp	Amp	Poly	Poly.	Descript
R	Abductor Hallucis	Norm	0	0	0		1–	Mod-V		Norm		Norm		Norm	NC
	Extensor Digitorum Brevis	1+	2+	0	0		3–	Mod-R		Norm		Norm		Norm	NC
	Tibialis Posterior	Norm	0	0	0		Norm	Full		Norm		Norm		Norm	NC
	Tibialis Anterior	1+	2+	1+	0		3–	Mod-R		Norm		Norm		Norm	NC
	Peroneus Longus	1+	1+	1+	0		3–	Mod-R		Norm		Norm		Norm	NC
	Gastrocnemius, medial head	Norm	0	0	0		Norm	Full		Norm		Norm		Norm	NC
	Rectus Femoris	Norm	0	0	0		Norm	Full		Norm		Norm		Norm	NC
	Biceps Femoris, short head	Norm	0	0	0		Norm	Full		Norm		Norm		Norm	NC
	Semitendinosus	Norm	0	0	0		Norm	Full		Norm		Norm		Norm	NC
	Gluteus Medius	Norm	0	0	0		Norm	Full		Norm		Norm		Norm	NC

Table 5.9 Case electrodiagnostic data

Sensory nerve conduction

Nerve	Stimulus	Recording	B-P Amp (μV)		LatNPk (ms)		CV (m/s)		Dist (mm)		Norm B-P Amp	Norm LatNPk	Norm CV	Temp (°C)	
			L	R	L	R	L	R	L	R				L	R
Sural	Lower Leg	Lat. Malleolus	15.98		3.94		n/a		140		>6 μV	<4.4 ms	>41 m/s	31.8	
Superficial peroneal (fibular)	Lower Leg	Ankle	16.36		3.42		n/a		100		>6 μV	<4.4 ms		31.1	
Med. Plantar	Med. Sole	Ankle	11.20	24.02	**7.0**	3.08	n/a	n/a	110	110	>5.3	<6.8		31.5	30.3

Motor nerve conduction

Nerve	Recording	Stimulus	B-P Amp (mV)		LatOn (ms)		CV (m/s)		Dist (mm)		Norm B-P Amp	Norm LatOn	Norm CV	Temp (°C)	
			L	R	L	R	L	R	L	R				L	R
Peroneal (fibular)	EDB	Ankle	5.90		3.90		n/a				>3 mV	<5.5 ms	>41 m/s	31.0	
		Pop Foss—Knee	5.59		11.45		50.3		380					30.9	
Tibial	AH	Ankle	**7.50**		**7.70**		n/a				>8 mV	<5.8 ms	>41 m/s	30.8	
		Pop Fossa—Knee	**7.25**		15.70		48.1		385					30.6	
Tibial	ADQP	Ankle	6.50	13.45	**7.80**	3.15	n/a	n/a			>4 mV	<6 ms	>41 m/s	30.1	30.5

F-wave side-to-side comparison table

Nerve	Stimulus	Recording	F-waves	
			Lat (ms)	
			L	R
Tibial	Ankle	AH	56.10	

H-reflex summary table

Nerve	Stimulus	Recording	Side	M-Wave		H-Wave	
				Lat (ms)	Amp (mV)	Lat (ms)	Amp (mV)
Tibial	Pop Fossa	Soleus	Left	3.9 ms	15.4 mV	27.5 ms	4.7 mV

Needle EMG summary

Side	Muscle	Ins Act.	Fib	PW	Fasc	Other	Number	Recruit	Dur	Dur	Amp	Amp	Poly	Poly.	Descript
L	Abductor Hallucis	1+	1+	0	0		2–	Rapid	Many	1+	Some	1+	Few	1+	NC
	Extensor digitorum brevis	Norm	0	0	0		Norm	Full		Norm		Norm		Norm	NC
	Abductor Digiti Quinti Pedis	1+	1+	0	0		2–	Rapid	Some	1+	Some	1+		Norm	NC
	Flex. Digitrum Longus	Norm	0	0	0		Norm	Full		Norm		Norm		Norm	NC
	Tibialis Anterior	Norm	0	0	0		Norm	Full		Norm		Norm		Norm	NC
	Gastrocnemius, medial head	Norm	0	0	0		Norm	Full		Norm		Norm		Norm	NC
	Rectus Femoris	Norm	0	0	0		Norm	Full		Norm		Norm		Norm	NC
	Gluteus Medius	Norm	0	0	0		Norm	Full		Norm		Norm		Norm	NC

EDB extensor digitorum brevis, *AH* abductor hallucis, *ADQP* Abductor digiti quinti pedis left tibial mononeuropathy at another level/site, a left lumbosacral (particularly S1) radiculopathy, or early manifestation of a generalized large fiber peripheral polyneuropathy.

Nerve conduction studies disclosed significant prolongation of the peak/distal latency of the left medial plantar mixed nerve response, as well as distal latency of the left tibial motor responses recording the abductor hallucis (AH) and the abductor digiti quinti pedis (ADQP) muscles. Other sensory and motor nerve conduction responses (including the left tibial H-reflex response, and contralateral tibial/plantar responses) were within normal limits. Needle EMG of left lower limb disclosed mild-to-moderate chronic motor axon loss changes in the AH and ADQP muscles, with normal findings in other muscles (including extensor digitorum brevis). Both AH and ADQP also demonstrated some fibrillation potentials.

In this case, *the electrodiagnostic findings are consistent with a left tibial mononeuropathy at or distal to the tarsal tunnel, compatible with a clinical diagnosis of left tarsal tunnel syndrome. This lesion would be considered at least moderate in degree electrically, especially considering the degree of distal/peak latency prolongation of the medial plantar mixed nerve response and the distal latency prolongation of the tibial motor responses recording the AH (medial plantar nerve supplied) and ADQP (lateral plantar nerve supplied), plus the denervation changes exclusively appreciated in these two muscles.*

Femoral Neuropathy

History of Presentation and Exam Findings

A 50-year-old woman complained of persistent right leg weakness and difficulty walking 3 months after a total hip replacement surgery via an anterior approach. Immediately following surgery, the patient noticed weakness on right knee extension with the inability to lock the knee when standing to prevent buckling of the leg. Despite physical therapy, the weakness did not improve over time, now accompanied by numbness and "pins and needles" paresthesia in the anterior thigh and medial leg on the right.

Examination revealed mildly reduced muscle bulk in the right quadriceps, with strength reduced particularly with right knee extension (MRC grade 2/5), noting normal strength in all other muscle groups, but reduced sensation to light touch, temperature and pinprick in the right anterior thigh, medial knee and medial calf area. There was an absent right knee jerk, but all other deep tendon reflexes were normal.

Electrodiagnostic studies (see Table 5.10) were done to work up the differential diagnoses which included a right femoral neuropathy, and less likely a lumbar plexopathy or lumbar radiculopathy (especially L2–L4 nerve root lesions).

Nerve conduction studies demonstrated an absent right femoral motor response recording rectus femoris, and an absent right saphenous sensory response. Additional routine nerve conduction studies of the lower extremity including peroneal (fibular) motor, tibial motor, as well as sural and superficial peroneal (fibular) sensory responses were normal.

The needle EMG showed abundant fibrillation and positive sharp wave potentials in the right quadriceps (rectus femoris and vastus lateralis muscles), with only a few to some rapidly-firing large and polyphasic MUAPs in each of these two muscles. The iliacus, adductor longus, lumbar paraspinal muscles, as well as the muscles below the knee were all normal on needle EMG.

In this case, *the electrodiagnostic findings are consistent with a subacute on early chronic right femoral mononeuropathy, predominantly axon loss in character and severe in degree electrically, localizable at or distal to the inguinal ligament (i.e. distal to the branch supplying the*

Table 5.10 Case electrodiagnostic data

Sensory nerve conduction studies

Nerve	Stimulus	Recording	B-P Amp (μV)		LatNPk (ms)		CV (m/s)		Dist (mm)		Norm B-P Amp (μV)	Norm LatNPk (ms)	Norm CV (m/s)	Temp (°C)	
			L	R	L	R	L	R	L	R				L	R
Sural	Lower leg	Lateral malleolus		14		3.6		48		140	>6	<4.4	>41		30.8
Superficial peroneal (fibular)	Lower leg	Dorsolateral ankle		9.4		2.5		46		100	>6	<4.4	>41		31.0
Saphenous	Medial calf	Medial/anterior ankle	10.3	**Absent**	2.6	**Absent**	42	**Absent**		140	>4	<4.6	>41		31.1

Motor nerve conduction studies

Nerve	Recording	Stimulus	B-P Amp (mV)		LatOn (ms)		CV (m/s)		Dist (mm)		Norm B-P Amp (mV)	Norm LatOn (ms)	Norm CV (m/s)	Temp (°C)	
			L	R	L	R	L	R	L	R				L	R
Tibial	AH	Ankle		6.7		2.9					>4	<6	>40		31.8
		Pop Foss-knee		6.4		12.3		40.8		385					
Peroneal (fibular)	EDB	Ankle		3.0		4.0					>2.5	<6	>40		31.8
		Popliteal fossa		2.8		11.6		50.0		380					
Femoral	Rectus femoris	Middle of inguinal area	3.5	**Absent**	4.3	**Absent**		**Absent**			>3	<6.5	>40		30.2

F-wave studies

Nerve	Stimulus	Recording	F-waves Lat(ms)	
			L	R
Tibial	Ankle	AH		49.7

Needle EMG summary

Side	Muscle	Ins Act	Fib	PW	Fasc	Other	Number	Recruit	Dur	Dur	Amp	Amp	Poly	Poly	Descript
R	Iliacus	0	0	0	0			Norm		Norm		Norm		Norm	NC
	Vastus lateralis	1+	2+	2+	0		3–	Rapid	Few	1+	Few	1+	Few	1+	NC
	Rectus femoris	1+	3+	2+	0		3–	Rapid	Some	1+	Few	1+	Some	1+	NC
	Gastrocnemius, medial head	0	0	0	0			Norm		Norm		Norm		Norm	NC
	Tibialis anterior	0	0	0	0			Norm		Norm		Norm		Norm	NC
	Extensor digitorum brevis	0	0	0	0			Norm		Norm		Norm		Norm	NC
	Adductor longus	0	0	0	0			Norm		Norm		Norm		Norm	NC
	Lumbar paraspinals (Mid)	0	0	0	0			Norm		Norm		Norm		Norm	NC

EDB extensor digitorum brevis, *AH* abductor hallucis

iliacus muscle). This is supported by the findings of an absent right femoral motor response (recording rectus femoris) and an absent right saphenous response, and evidence of marked active/ongoing denervation with early chronic motor axon loss changes in the rectus femoris and vastus lateralis muscles only.

References

1. Sternbach G. The carpal tunnel syndrome. J Emerg Med. 1999;17(3):519–23.
2. Chen P-C. A Bayesian network meta-analysis: comparing the clinical effectiveness of local corticosteroid injections using different treatment strategies for carpal tunnel syndrome. BMC Musculoskel Disord. 2015;16:363. https://doi.org/10.1186/s12891-015-0815-8.
3. Newington L. Carpal tunnel syndrome and work. Best Pract Res Clin Rheumatol. 2015;29:440e453.
4. Vasiliadis HS. Treatment of carpal tunnel syndrome. A systematic review and meta-analysis. PLoS One. 10(12):e0143683. https://doi.org/10.1371/journal.pone.0143683.
5. Ellis R. Is there a relationship between impaired median nerve excursion and carpal tunnel syndrome? A systematic review. J Hand Ther. 2017;30:3e12.
6. Yi-Ming Ren MD. Efficacy, safety, and cost of surgical versus nonsurgical treatment for carpal tunnel syndrome. Medicine. 2016;95:40.
7. Yunoki M. Importance of recognizing carpal tunnel syndrome for neurosurgeons: a review. Neurol Med Chir (Tokyo). 2017;57:172–83.
8. Lim YH. Median nerve mobilization techniques in the treatment of carpal tunnel syndrome: a systematic review. J Hand Ther. 2017;30:397e406.
9. Bekhet AH. Efficacy of low-level laser therapy in carpal tunnel syndrome management: a systematic review and meta-analysis. Lasers Med Sci. 2017;32:1439–48.
10. Hermiz SJ. Evidence-based medicine: current evidence in the diagnosis and management of carpal tunnel syndrome. Plast Reconstr Surg. 2017;140:1
11. Ballestero-Pérez R. Effectiveness of nerve gliding exercises on carpal tunnel syndrome: a systematic review. J Manipulative Physiol Therap. 2017;40(1).
12. Mediouni Z. Is carpal tunnel syndrome related to computer exposure at work?. JOEM. 2014;56(2).
13. Smeraglia F. Endoscopic cubital tunnel release: a systematic review. Br Med Bull. 2015;116:155–63. https://doi.org/10.1093/bmb/ldv049.
14. Jonathan Robert Staples MD. Cubital tunnel syndrome: current concepts. J Am Acad Orthop Surg. 2017;25:e215–24.
15. Ren Y-M. Open versus endoscopic in situ decompression in cubital tunnel syndrome: a systematic review and meta-analysis. Int J Surg. 2016;35:104e110.
16. Anderson JC. Common fibular nerve compression anatomy, symptoms, clinical evaluation, and surgical decompression. Clin Podiatr Med Surg. 2016;33:283–91.
17. Bregman PJ. Current diagnosis and treatment of superficial fibular nerve injuries and entrapment. Clin Podiatr Med Surg. 2016;33:243–54.
18. Doneddu PE. Tarsal tunnel syndrome: still more opinions than evidence. Status of the art. Neurol Sci. 2017;38:1735–9. https://doi.org/10.1007/s10072-017-3039-x.
19. Tladi MJ. Schwannoma and neurofibroma of the posterior tibial nerve presenting as tarsal tunnel syndrome: review of the literature with two case reports. Foot. 2017;32:22–6.
20. Casazza GC. Systematic review of facial nerve outcomes after middle fossa decompression and transmastoid decompression for bells's palsy with complete facial paralysis. Otol Neurol. 2018;39:1311–8.
21. Nicholas S. Andresen. Facial nerve decompression. Curr Opin Otolaryngol Head Neck Surg. 2018;26:280–5.

Polyneuropathies

6

Megha Chetan Dhamne and John A. Morren

Introduction

Polyneuropathy (often also referred to as peripheral neuropathy) is a broad term that encompasses conditions characterized by a generalized disorder of peripheral nerves. By fairly conservative estimates, it affects 1–3% of the population, with incidence increasing with age to 3–5% above the age of 50 years [1]. Most commonly, patients present with sensory symptoms such as numbness or paresthesia starting in the toes/feet (i.e. following a length-dependent pattern). Common causes of polyneuropathy include diabetes mellitus, chronic alcoholism, nutritional deficiencies such as vitamin B12 and immune-mediated conditions. Leprosy or Hansen's disease is still considered among the leading causes of polyneuropathy worldwide, albeit rare in most developed countries. Each of these have distinct clinical and electrophysiological features. Hence a systematic and practical approach is needed for cost-effective diagnosis and early recognition of treatable forms of polyneuropathy.

M. C. Dhamne
Department of Neurology, Dr. L H Hiranandani Hospital, Mumbai, Maharashtra, India
e-mail: megha.dhamne@hiranandanihospital.org

J. A. Morren
Neuromuscular Center, Neurological Institute, Cleveland Clinic, and Cleveland Clinic Lerner College of Medicine of Case Western Reserve University, Cleveland, OH, USA
e-mail: morrenj@ccf.org

Classification of Polyneuropathy

Polyneuropathies may be classified based on:

1. Pathogenesis
2. Temporal evolution
3. Type of nerve fibers involved/modalities affected
4. Pattern of neuropathy

Pathogenesis

Based on the pathogenesis, polyneuropathies can be divided into:

1. Axon loss polyneuropathies
2. Demyelinating polyneuropathies
3. Nodopathies/Paranodopathies

Polyneuropathies are traditionally classified into axon loss (axonal) or demyelinating according to whether the pathologic process primarily affects the axon itself or the Schwann cell myelin sheath. Electrophysiological studies are helpful in determining whether the neuropathy is axonal or demyelinating. Peripheral nerves are surrounded by an incomplete blood-nerve barrier. Additionally, the length of the nerve is an important factor in the vulnerability of axons to injury. Microtubules are used as molecular tracks to guide delivery of cargoes (such as

N. Galvez-Jimenez et al. (eds.), *Electrodiagnostic Medicine*,
https://doi.org/10.1007/978-3-030-74997-2_6

newly synthesized proteins, lipids, RNA, and organelles) to different parts of the axon. Axonal transport is bidirectional and is essential for the nutrition of axons. An intact microtubule network is required for the clearance of damaged organelles by cellular degradation. Disturbance in the axonal transport or alterations in the cytoskeleton by various insults such as toxins, metabolic alterations, vitamin deficiencies, and inflammation causes peripheral axonal neuropathies. Improving these mechanisms may facilitate regeneration of axons and are explored as potential therapeutic targets in axonal neuropathies. Inherited axonal neuropathies include those that are a result of defective genes that influence axonal transport (example: MFN2, DYNC1H1, HSPB1) [2].

Integrity of the myelin sheath is essential for effective nerve function. Disorders of the Schwann cells/myelin sheath cause demyelinating neuropathies which may be either hereditary or acquired. The pathologic hallmark of acquired inflammatory demyelinating polyradiculoneuropathies is segmental demyelination that may begin at the nodes of Ranvier, usually extending to the internodal area and accompanied by lymphocytic infiltration [3]. Acute inflammatory demyelinating polyradiculoneuropathy (AIDP) and chronic inflammatory demyelinating polyradiculoneuropathy (CIDP) are the commonest acquired inflammatory demyelinating polyradiculoneuropathies. Determining whether the underlying polyneuropathy is demyelinating is crucial as this is a potentially treatable neuropathy. Autoantibodies have been implicated in the pathogenesis of acquired demyelinating neuropathy such as anti-GQ1B antibodies in Miller Fisher syndrome. Defective genes encoding for structural myelin proteins are implicated in the pathogenesis of inherited demyelinating neuropathies [e.g. PMP22 deletion causing Hereditary Neuropathy with liability to Pressure Palsies (HNPP)].

Nodopathies are disorders of the nodal/paranodal region including channelopathies affecting those sites. Some toxic, hereditary and immune mediated conditions cause a physiological conduction failure at the nodes of Ranvier resulting in a transient slowing or conduction block. Patients often show a quick clinical recovery. A notable example of this is a recently described entity, early reversible conduction failure (ERCF) in "axonal" Guillain–Barré syndrome (GBS) [4].

Temporal Evolution

Peripheral neuropathies may be classified depending on their time course as acute (days ~4 weeks), sub-acute (~4–8 weeks) and chronic (> ~8 weeks) (see Table 6.1). Acute polyneuropathies include GBS and its variants [for e.g. Acute Inflammatory Demyelinating Polyradiculoneuropathy (AIDP), Acute Motor Axonal Neuropathy (AMAN), Acute Motor and Sensory Axonal Neuropathy (AMSAN), Miller Fisher syndrome (MFS)], as well as less common enti-

Table 6.1 Classification of polyneuropathies by temporal course

Acute	Subacute	Chronic
GBS and variants (AMAN, AMSAN, MFS, PCB, AMAN/AMSAN with reversible conduction failure, AIDP)	Subacute GBS	Chronic axon loss polyneuropathy
Acute porphyria	Mononeuritis multiplex (MNM)	CIDP and variants
Acute thallium toxicity		Paraproteinemic neuropathy
Acute diphtheria		Hereditary neuropathies (CMT, HNPP)

Abbreviations: *GBS* Guillain–Barré syndrome, *AMAN* acute motor axonal neuropathy, *AMSAN* acute motor and sensory axonal neuropathy, *MFS* Miller Fisher syndrome, *PCB* pharyngeal-cervical-brachial variant, *AIDP* acute inflammatory demyelinating polyradiculoneuropathy, *CIDP* chronic inflammatory demyelinating polyradiculoneuropathy, *CMT* Charcot-Marie Tooth disease, *HNPP* hereditary neuropathy liable to pressure palsies ties like acute porphyria. Subacute neuropathies include subacute GBS, and mononeuritis multiplex due to vasculitis. Chronic neuropathies are either due to axon loss or demyelination. Chronic Inflammatory Demyelinating Polyradiculoneuropathy (CIDP) and porphyria are among those which may have a relapsing and remitting course [5].

Type of Modality Affected/Type of Nerve Fiber Affected

1. Modalities affected—motor/sensory/autonomic
2. Type of nerve fiber affected—large fiber/small fiber

Polyneuropathy is clinically suspected based on the characteristic pattern of sensory and/or motor involvement. Most polyneuropathies involve both sensory and motor fibers. Initially a patient may have only sensory symptoms. Sensory symptoms may be classified as positive (increased or hyperfunction of the sensory pathways) or negative (due to decreased or lack of function of sensory pathways) [6]. Positive sensory symptoms include tingling or prickling sensation. Patients often describe it as a sensation of "pins and needles", "ants crawling sensation", "bunched up socks under the toes" or an "electric shock-like" sensation. Negative sensory symptoms include numbness or loss of sensation to touch or temperature. Sensory loss in the feet may go unrecognized in very slowly progressive neuropathies such as hereditary neuropathy, diabetic polyneuropathy or in the elderly. Loss of proprioception may cause gait imbalance leading to increased falls, especially at night or in dim light.

Pain when present, may be extremely severe and the most disabling symptom. Pain may be the heralding symptom in ischemic and some inflammatory neuropathies or small fiber neuropathy. Dysesthesias, hyperalgesia, and allodynia are terms used to describe abnormal sensations. *Dysesthesia* is an unpleasant abnormal sensation, whether spontaneous or evoked. *Hyperalgesia* (increased perception of painful sensation) is an increased sensitivity to a stimulus that is normally painful. *Allodynia* is an increased painful response to a normally innocuous stimulus.

Common autonomic symptoms are orthostatic light-headedness, heat or cold intolerance, bloating, constipation, diarrhea, urinary retention, or change in the frequency of urination and sexual dysfunction. Diabetic neuropathy, acute porphyric neuropathy, GBS, amyloid neuropathy and other small fiber neuropathies may have autonomic involvement.

Nerve fibers are generally categorized by fiber size into large-diameter, myelinated fibers and small-diameter unmyelinated fibers. Motor fibers are large-diameter myelinated fibers while autonomic fibers are small, unmyelinated *c*-fibers. Sensory fibers are either large diameter fibers that carry sensation of vibration and joint position (proprioception) or small thinly myelinated A-delta fibers that carry sensation of somatic pain and temperature. It is important to recognize clinically and electrophysiologically the type of nerve fiber involved as the causes of each are varied. A large fiber neuropathy may cause muscle weakness, tingling or numbness, with sensory ataxia due to loss of proprioception. Small fiber neuropathy causes loss of pain and temperature sensation, and/or autonomic dysfunction. It manifests as a "painful" neuropathy. Patients complain of "burning pain", *dysesthesia, hyperalgesia* and *allodyni*a.

Small fiber neuropathy most commonly presents as a length dependent neuropathy, with a loss of pain and temperature sensation in a glove-stocking distribution. Sometimes patients may present with focal, asymmetric symptoms as mononeuritis multiplex or with a proximal sensory impairment as in sensory ganglionopathy. Causes of small fiber neuropathy include diabetes mellitus/prediabetes ± metabolic syndrome, hypothyroidism, vitamin B12 deficiency, vitamin B6 excess, excessive alcohol, celiac disease, collagen vascular diseases, HIV, sarcoidosis, chemotherapy, amyloidosis and hereditary causes. Despite extensive work up, 30–50% patients with small fiber neuropathy are labelled as "idiopathic". Diagnosis of small fiber neuropathy requires a detailed history, physical examination, a skin biopsy to evaluate for the intraepidermal nerve fiber density and/or Quantitative Sudomotor

Axon Reflex Test (QSART). Small fiber neuropathy is not detected on EMG. EMG in this setting is usually done to look for or rule out a large fiber neuropathy, that may be coexisting, based on clinical features [7].

Typically, a large fiber neuropathy is a mixed sensorimotor neuropathy. Some large fiber neuropathies may present as predominantly motor or pure motor neuropathies. Patient presents with pure weakness, and no or minimal sensory symptoms. Upper motor neuron (UMN) type weakness suggests disease of the spinal cord, brainstem or higher in the corticospinal tract or motor cortex. Lower motor neuron (LMN) weakness localizes the lesion to anterior horn cell (AHC) (e.g. spinomuscular atrophy, progressive muscular atrophy), nerve roots, plexus, peripheral nerves, or neuromuscular junction. A thorough clinical evaluation and EMG is crucial for the localization of the cause of muscle weakness along the neuroaxis.

Pattern of Polyneuropathy

The pattern of neuropathy is determined based on the distribution of motor and sensory involvement. The most commonly encountered neuropathy is distal, symmetric axonal sensory/sensorimotor neuropathy. However, it is important to recognize atypical patterns such as non-length dependence, asymmetry, upper limb predominance, predominantly motor neuropathy as these may be potentially treatable neuropathies.

The pattern of neuropathy is assessed as:

1. **Length dependent/Non-length dependent**
2. **Symmetric/Asymmetric**

It is useful to identify the pattern of polyneuropathy first as length dependent or non-length dependent. The next step is to assess if the weakness and/or the sensory deficits are symmetrical or asymmetrical in distribution.

Length Dependent Polyneuropathy

Axon loss polyneuropathies are often length dependent. This is because the distal-most nerve fibers which are generally thinner are most vulnerable to the underlying insult. Some acquired demyelinating neuropathies are classically distal, (e.g. distal acquired demyelinating neuropathy), as are many hereditary polyneuropathies.

Distal Symmetric Polyneuropathy

Distal symmetric polyneuropathy (DSP) is one of the commonest basis of referral for electrodiagnostic testing. DSP may be a large fiber and/or a small fiber neuropathy. Diabetes mellitus and/or impaired glucose tolerance accounts for 32–53% of cases. Other causes of DSP include hereditary, metabolic, nutritional (e.g. B12 deficiency), alcohol/toxic/drug-related, infectious (HIV, leprosy), inflammatory, autoimmune, paraproteinemia-related and paraneoplastic. Despite a thorough evaluation, the cause may remain idiopathic in approximately 30% of cases.

Diabetes mellitus is the commonest cause of chronic axon loss length dependent sensorimotor polyneuropathy in the United States, affecting up to 50% patients with type 1 and type 2 diabetes mellitus. However, only 10–15% of patients with neuropathy due to diabetes mellitus may be symptomatic. The occurrence of neuropathy in diabetes mellitus correlates with the duration of diabetes, glycemic control, and presence of microvascular ischemia with nephropathy and retinopathy [8]. Electrophysiologic studies commonly show features of axonal degeneration and at least subtle segmental demyelination. The reason for slow conduction velocity was believed to be due to loss of fast-conducting large fibers or an alteration at the nodes of Ranvier. Conduction block or temporal dispersion are not found, however the degree of slowing or increase in distal latency may almost reach demyelinating criteria. These findings have to be interpreted with caution, as it needs to be differentiated from chronic inflammatory demyelinating neuropathy (CIDP) to avoid unnecessary immune therapy [9].

Inherited (Hereditary) Polyneuropathies

Inherited polyneuropathies are diverse group of disorders, both clinically and genetically and may present with systemic features or central nervous system involvement. They are often overlooked as the cause of chronic length dependent, motor predominant or sensorimotor polyneuropathy. A positive family history is useful but may be difficult to obtain as patients may have a normal lifespan with or without minimal disability. Some hereditary polyneuropathies may have an acute/subacute onset. They may have fairly specific characteristics, for e.g.: (1) myelin protein zero (MPZ) mutation phenotype, is sometimes accompanied by an Adie pupil or bulbar involvement; (2) PMP22 deletion, leading to hereditary neuropathy with liability to pressure palsies (HNPP); (3) septin 9 (SEPT9) mutation, presenting with attacks of brachial plexopathy; (4) androgen receptor (AR) mutation, causing spinal bulbar muscular atrophy (Kennedy's disease) and (5) mitofusin 2 (MFN2) mutation, presenting with sudden-onset optic neuropathy [10].

Inherited polyneuropathies may be classified broadly to include:

1. Hereditary motor sensory neuropathy (HMSN), or Charcot-Marie-Tooth disease
2. Hereditary sensory autonomic neuropathy (HSAN) or hereditary sensory neuropathy (HSN)
3. Distal hereditary motor neuronopathy (dHMN), affecting the lower motor neurons. It overlaps phenotypically and genetically with HMSN
4. Hereditary brachial plexus neuropathy (HBPN),
5. Hereditary neuropathy with liability to pressure palsies (HNPP), presenting as recurrent mononeuropathies, often at compressible sites

Distal Acquired Demyelinating Symmetric (DADS) Neuropathy

Distal acquired demyelinating symmetric (DADS) neuropathy is another rare distal symmetric demyelinating neuropathy that should be differentiated from the axonal neuropathy and hereditary neuropathy. Katz et al., 2000 [11] described patients with DADS neuropathy presenting with chronic length-dependent, distal symmetric sensory symptoms with sensory ataxia due to loss of proprioception and vibration. Muscle weakness when present, is confined to the distal muscles (toes, ankles, fingers and wrists), thus differentiating it from the more common clinical presentation of proximal and distal weakness in chronic inflammatory demyelinating neuropathy (CIDP). Two-thirds of patients with DADS neuropathy harbour a monoclonal gammopathy, which is almost exclusively IgM monoclonal protein (called DADS-M). More than 90% are men with onset in the sixth decade or later. In most series, one half to two-thirds patients with DADS-M neuropathy patients may express anti-myelin associated glycoprotein antibodies (anti-MAG antibodies). MAG is a glycoprotein localized to the periaxonal membranes of myelin forming Schwann cells. Patients with DADS-M neuropathy with anti-MAG antibodies either do not respond or respond poorly to immunomodulating therapies [12].

Non-length Dependent Polyneuropathies

After determining that the pattern of polyneuropathy is non-length dependent, it may be further classified as symmetric vs asymmetric based on the distribution of weakness and/or sensory findings (see Table 6.2).

Neuropathies with Symmetric, Predominantly Proximal Weakness

The importance of identifying predominantly proximal, symmetric weakness cannot be overemphasized as this identifies an important subset of patients with potentially treatable acquired demyelinating neuropathies. This clinical pattern is the hallmark of acute and chronic acquired inflammatory demyelinating polyradiculoneuropathies (AIDP and CIDP), and their variants. GBS is the acute acquired polyradiculoneuropathy which incorporates demyelinating (AIDP) and axonal (AMAN and AMSAN) variants. Clinically, patients present with ascending paralysis with areflexia and minimal sensory involvement (except for AMSAN). Acute porphyric neuropathy mimics GBS. However, it occurs during porphyric attacks and usually after exposure of provocating factors, commonly medications (e.g. dapsone, isoniazid, metronidazole, tricyclic antidepressants, anti-epleptics).

Table 6.2 Non-length dependent polyneuropathies

Proximal symmetric weakness	Predominant upper extremity weakness	Asymmetric weakness
• Acute: • GBS and variants • Acute Porphyric Neuropathy# • Toxic neuropathy • Tick paralysis • Chronic: • CIDP and variants • Paraproteinemic neuropathy	• Acute porphyric neuropathy • Lead intoxication neuropathy • CIDP variants: • MMN with CB • MADSAM	• Proximal asymmetric weakness: • Polyradiculoplexopathy: • DLSRPN • Infectious (TB, HIV, Lyme) • Malignant infiltration • Familial brachial plexopathy • Distal asymmetric weakness: • Motor neuropathy • Multiple mononeuropathies: • Entrapment • Inherited (HNPP) • MNM: Infectious (leprosy, HIV) • Vasculitis • Paraneoplastic • CIDP variants: • MADSAM, • MMN with CB

Abbreviations: *GBS* Guillain Barré syndrome, *CIDP* chronic inflammatory demyelinating polyradiculoneuropathy, *MMN with CB* multifocal motor neuropathy with conduction block, *MADSAM* multifocal acquired demyelinating sensory and motor neuropathy, *HNPP* hereditary neuropathy with liability to pressure palsies, *DLSRPN* diabetic lumbosacral radiculoplexus neuropathy, *MNM* mononeuritis multiplex

#Acute porphyric neuropathy may be asymmetric but classically resembles GBS

Guillain–Barré syndrome (GBS)

GBS is the most common and the most severe acute paralytic polyneuropathy, with about 100,000 people worldwide developing the disorder every year. The incidence increases with age and is slightly more frequent in males than females. Approximately 70% patients have a history of upper respiratory or gastrointestinal infection, trauma, surgery, or vaccination within 4 weeks prior to the onset of weakness. Under the umbrella term of GBS are several recognisable variants with distinct clinical and pathological features (Table 6.3). Patients present with ascending paralysis, symmetric weakness and areflexia. Cranial nerve involvement, autonomic dysfunction and/or respiratory failure may occur. Cerebrospinal fluid (CSF) examination typically shows albuminocytological dissociation. Weakness is monophasic and deficits rapidly progress to reach a nadir usually by 2 weeks with no progression beyond 4 weeks. The severe form of GBS with respiratory failure is seen in 20–30% [13]. Recovery may take months to years.

Table 6.3 Clinical and electrophysiological variants of Guillain–Barré syndrome (GBS)

1. Acute inflammatory demyelinating polyradiculoneuropathy (AIDP)
2. Acute motor axonal neuropathy (AMAN)
3. Acute motor sensory axonal neuropathy (AMSAN)
4. Miller Fisher syndrome (MFS)
5. Bickerstaff brainstem encephalitis (BBE)
6. Pharyngo-cervico-brachial variant (PCB)
7. Paraparetic variant
8. Facial diplegia variant
9. Pure sensory GBS
10. Pure autonomic failure variant
11. Reversible conduction failure (nodopathy) (RCF)

Chronic inflammatory demyelinating polyradiculoneuropathy (CIDP)

CIDP is the commonest chronic immune-mediated polyradiculoneuropathy. The pathologic features of CIDP described by Dyck were "onion bulb" formation, perivascular inflammatory infiltrates and segmental demyelination in teased fibers [14]. Apart from the temporal course (>8 weeks), CIDP differs from GBS in the following ways: (1) GBS is a monophasic illness while CIDP is relapsing-remitting or slowly progressive; (2) patients may or may not have a prior history of infection or a trigger; (3) Cranial nerve palsies, autonomic dysfunction or respiratory failure rarely occurs in CIDP; (4) CIDP is steroid responsive. Sometimes it may present acutely like GBS. CSF in CIDP shows albuminocytological dissociation, with cell count <10/mm^3. CSF pleocytosis suggests a co-infection such as HIV. Most patients with CIDP respond to immunomodulatory therapy. CIDP variants are outlined in Table 6.4.

Although very rare, CIDP has been shown to be associated with several malignancies: lung (typically small cell carcinoma), ovary, and uterus, colon, pancreas, and Hodgkin's lymphoma.

Paraproteinemic polyneuropathy

Paraproteinemic polyneuropathies are a heterogenous group of polyneuropathies associated with an abnormally elevated monoclonal (M) protein (see Table 6.5). Typically, the neuropathy associated is a length dependent axon loss sensory/sensorimotor polyneuropathy. However, demyelinating polyneuropathy can also occur. Distal acquired demyelinating sensory (DADS) neuropathy is seen with IgM monoclonal gammopathy of undetermined significance (MGUS), while a CIDP-like presentation is seen in patients with IgA/IgG MGUS, or plasma cell dyscrasias including osteosclerotic myeloma and POEMS (Polyneuropathy, Organomegaly, Endocrinopathy, Monoclonal protein, Skin changes) syndrome- the associated M protein is typically IgG or IgA, but the light chain type is almost always lambda. Other plasma cell dyscrasias; namely, multiple myeloma, Waldenstrom's macroglobulinemia, POEMS, primary amyloidosis are commonly associated with an axon loss distal symmetric sensorimotor polyneuropathy (see Table 6.6). The underlying plasma cell dyscrasia is treated with chemotherapy and/or radiation therapy (surgical resection may be done for solitary plasmacytomas). Resistant cases are treated with autologous stem cell transplantation [15].

Table 6.4 Chronic inflammatory demyelinating polyradiculoneuropathy (CIDP) variants

1. Multifocal acquired demyelinating sensory and motor neuropathy (MADSAM) or Lewis-Sumner syndrome
2. Multifocal motor neuropathy with conduction block (MMN with CB or MMNCB)
3. Distal acquired demyelinating symmetric neuropathy (DADS)
4. Chronic immune sensory polyradiculopathy (CISP)
5. Chronic ataxic neuropathy with ophthalmoparesis, M protein, cold agglutinins and disialosyl ganglioside antibodies (CANOMAD)

Table 6.5 Polyneuropathy associated with MGUS

Type of neuropathy	Monoclonal protein
Distal acquired demyelinating symmetric neuropathy (DADS neuropathy), Rarely asymmetric neuropathy	IgM, ~50% have anti-MAG antibody, ~15% have anti-GD1b and GQ1b antibodies
Distal symmetric sensorimotor axonal neuropathy	IgG or IgA
CIDP—MGUS	IgG or IgA

Table 6.6 Plasma cell dyscrasias and polyneuropathy

Type of neuropathy	Plasma cell dyscrasia	Monoclonal protein
Distal symmetric sensory > motor neuropathy	Waldenstrom's macroglobulinemia	Monoclonal spike >3 g/dl IgM Anti-MAG +
Distal sensory > motor neuropathy	Multiple myeloma	Kappa light chains
Demyelinating, motor predominant neuropathy, CIDP-like	Osteosclerotic myeloma	Often IgG or IgA, or elevated lambda light chains
Demyelinating sensorimotor neuropathy, CIDP-like	POEMS	Often IgG or IgA, or elevated lambda light chains (often elevated VEGF levels also)
Distal symmetric sensorimotor neuropathy	Primary light chain amyloidosis	Lambda light chains predominate

CIDP Chronic inflammatory demyelinating polyradiculoneuropathy; *POEMS* Polyneuropathy, Organomegaly, Endocrinopathy, Monoclonal protein, Skin changes; *MAG* myelin-associated glycoprotein; *VEGF* Vascular endothelial growth factor

Upper Limb Predominant Weakness

When a patient presents with acute/subacute upper limb predominant weakness, distally with a wrist drop, lead neuropathy should be suspected. A more slowly progressive course with asymmetric hand/arm weakness with sensory symptoms suggests a MADSAM neuropathy, while pure motor weakness without sensory features point towards MMN with CB. These are rare variants of CIDP that typically respond well to immune therapy. MMN with CB needs to be differentiated from motor neuron disease. Asymmetric weakness in the hands is also seen in myopathies like inclusion body myositis (IBM) and anoctamin 5 myopathy. Rarely, neuromuscular junction transmission disorders like myasthenia gravis may present with hand weakness.

Asymmetric Weakness

Distal asymmetric weakness should alert the neurologist to consider radiculopathies (particularly affecting C8-T1 or L5-S1 roots), multiple mononeuropathies (including lead toxicity-related radial neuropathy that may present with wrist drop), or rarely motor neuron disease, or acute porphyric neuropathy. Mononeuropathies may be demyelinating as in MMN with CB, compressive or entrapment neuropathies, and hereditary as in HNPP, or axonal as in infectious, infiltrative, or mononeuritis multiplex (often vasculitic). Patients with HNPP may or may not have a family history. These patients typically present with multiple entrapment neuropathies, including those of ulnar, median and common peroneal (fibular) nerves.

An asymmetric weakness with axon loss characteristics on electrodiagnostic studies is seen in mononeuritis multiplex. This is a potentially treatable condition and hence should not be missed. Causes are summarized in Table 6.7.

The clinical presentation of mononeuritis multiplex is distinctive. It typically presents as a painful subacute, stepwise, asymmetric, large fiber sensorimotor polyneuropathy. Weakness and sensory loss is in the distribution of multiple peripheral nerves of the lower and upper extremity but when advanced it may be less focal and more symmetrical/confluent. It may then be difficult to differentiate it from the common distal sensorimotor neuropathy. A comprehensive array of tests should be done to investigate for the causes of mononeuritis multiplex. If identified early and the underlying disease is treated appropriately then full recovery is possible, although it may take months to years.

Table 6.7 Etiology of mononeuritis multiplex

• Vasculitis—primary, secondary
• Infections—HIV, hepatitis B and C, leprosy, Lyme disease
• Diabetes mellitus
• Cancer associated conditions—Paraneoplastic, direct tumor invasion with intraneural spread (lymphoma, B cell leukemia, carcinoid tumor), chronic graft vs host disease (GVHD)
• Infiltrative—neurosarcoidosis, amyloidosis
• Cryoglobulinemia

Radiculopathies are an important differential that is commonly encountered in routine electrodiagnostic studies. Polyradiculoplexopathies such as diabetic lumbosacral or cervical plexopathy present with proximal lower or upper extremity asymmetric weakness respectively. An important differential is familial brachial plexopathy (hereditary neuralgic amyotrophy, as seen with mutations in the SEPT9 gene) that may present with unilateral or bilateral upper limb weakness.

Determining the Underlying Etiology: Asking the Right Questions Related to the Past Medical/Surgical, Medication, Family and Social History

Past medical history of diabetes mellitus, or metabolic syndrome are risk factors for distal symmetric axonal polyneuropathy. Cancer may be associated with polyneuropathy due to the chemotherapeutic medications, direct invasion into the nerves or plexus, late effects of radiation, or as a paraneoplastic syndrome. A positive family history suggests a possible inherited cause for the chronic slowly progressive polyneuropathy, especially if the patient has foot deformities like hammer toes and high arches. Screening the other family members with EDX, and/or genetic testing is sometimes carried out for establishing the inheritance pattern and counselling the patient and his/her family. Alcohol is another common cause of distal symmetric neuropathy and a history of the duration, and amount of alcohol intake needs to be specifically obtained. Exposure to toxins (accidental, or occupational exposure) and medications (e.g. chemotherapy, antibiotics like isoniazid and metronidazole) needs to be looked into thoroughly. Vitamin B12 deficiency is a common cause of distal symmetric axonal neuropathy in patients who are vegetarians or vegans, and those after bariatric surgery.

Electrodiagnostic Studies in Polyneuropathy

Nerve conduction studies (NCS) and needle electromyographic studies (EMG) aid in the classification and differentiation of peripheral neuropathies. The distinction between axon loss and demyelinating neuropathies has diagnostic and prognostic implications. The routine electrodiagnostic evaluation of patients with suspected polyneuropathy includes sensory NCS, motor NCS, F-wave studies, H-wave studies and needle electrode examination (NEE). A wide variability exists amongst neurophysiologists regarding the use of electrodiagnostic examination techniques, reference values, interpretation of individual tests, and criteria for diagnosis and classification of peripheral neuropathy. However, the basic approaches are similar in most laboratories.

Electrodiagnosis of Axonal Polyneuropathies

Axonal or "axon loss" polyneuropathy is the commonest type of polyneuropathy encountered in clinical practice and in the electrodiagnostic lab. These are primarily associated with Wallerian or axonal degeneration, sometimes referred to as "dying back" neuropathy. When studied electrophysiologically, this is reflected as reduced motor and sensory amplitude and area. A reduced compound muscle action potential (CMAP) amplitude is seen in an axon loss polyneuropathy and it correlates closely with muscle weakness. CMAP amplitude or area may also be reduced from a conduction block in acquired demyelinating neuropathies due to segmental demyelination located between the site of stimulation and the recorded muscle (failure of the impulse to travel across the point of conduction block), a presynaptic neuromuscular junction disorder such as Lambert Eaton myasthenia gravis (LEMS) and myopathies. Weakness in demyelinating neuropathies is due to interruption or block of conduction along the motor nerves, which is reflected as slowed conduction or conduction block along the nerves. While all fibers contribute to the CMAP amplitude and area, only the fastest conducting fibers contribute to the conduction velocity and the latency measured by routine NCS. Hence mild slowing of conduction velocity (CV) and distal latency occur with loss of the largest or the fastest conducting axons in an axon loss polyneuropathy. However, marked slowing will not occur because even the slowest nerve fibers conduct at ~35 m/s. With a random drop out of fibers in axon loss polyneuropathies there is: (1) reduced CMAP and sensory nerve action potential (SNAP) amplitude (and area), (2) mild slowing of conduction velocity; and (3) mild prolongation of distal latency. In severe axon loss neuropathy with preservation of few fastest fibers, CMAP amplitude decreases markedly with preservation of conduction velocity and distal latency. With loss of almost all axons including the fastest fibers, the conduction velocity may drop down to as low as ~35 m/s with reduced CMAPs. However, reduction in the CV or prolongation of distal latency will not be in the demyelinating range [CV <70% lower limit of normal (LLN) and distal latency >130% upper limit of normal (ULN)].

Different patterns on NCS and EMG are seen in axonal polyneuropathy, depending on (1) Whether axon loss is acute/subacute or chronic; (2) Whether it involves motor and/or sensory fibers and (3) Distribution of polyneuropathy: length dependent or non-length dependent and symmetric or asymmetric. Acute axonal polyneuropathies include inflammatory neuropathies (rare variants of GBS—AMAN: acute motor axonal motor neuropathy, AMSAN: acute motor sensory axonal neuropathy) and metabolic neuropathies: acute porphyria and critical illness neuropathy. Electrodiagnosis of acute axonal inflammatory neuropathies (AMAN and AMSAN) will be discussed under electrodiagnosis GBS and its variants. Subacute axonal neuropathies include the asymmetric mononeuritis multiplex, seen for example in vasculitides. Therefore, asymmetry on electrodiagnostic studies should alert the electromyographer to consider vasculitic neuropathy as this is potentially treatable. The other differential for an asymmetric pattern in an axon loss neuropathy is an underlying or a superimposed radiculopathy. In a review of patients referred for EDX testing at an academic neurology department, NCS/EMG resulted in alternative diagnoses in 43% of suspected cases, most often lumbar radiculopathy (18%) [16].

We will discuss here the electrodiagnosis of more commonly encountered chronic axonal length dependent distal symmetric polyneuropathy (DSP). In DSP, greater clinical and electrophysiological changes are seen distally in the nerves of the lower extremity before they affect the upper extremity nerves. Since the neuropathy is chronic, enough time has passed for Wallerian degeneration to occur. Hence, both SNAP and CMAP amplitudes are reduced. Sensory axons are generally involved earlier and more severely affected than motor axons.

Sensory NCS, particularly in the lower extremity are more sensitive than motor NCS in the detection of peripheral neuropathy [17]. Patients may have minimal or no sensory symptoms but have decreased sensory responses or absent SNAPs. The earliest sign of an axon loss polyneuropathy is absent or decreased sensory nerve action potential (SNAP) amplitude of distal nerves in the lower extremity. The commonly studied sensory responses in the lower extremity are those of the sural and superficial peroneal (fibular) sensory nerves. The demonstration of low amplitude or absent sural SNAPs and normal radial SNAP improves the diagnostic accuracy of axonal polyneuropathy, although recent evidence supports the use of sural SNAP amplitude alone [18, 19]. The sensory nerves that are routinely examined (e.g. sural and superficial peroneal (fibular) sensory nerves) are proximal to the sites affected very early in distal polyneuropathy. The utility of more distal sensory nerves; plantar sensory/mixed and dorsal sural nerves have been studied in improving the diagnostic yield of early or subclinical polyneuropathy. However, their routine use in DSP is limited due to the absence of plantar nerve responses in healthy individuals over the age of 40–50 years, technical difficulties in the recording, and damage in entrapment neuropathies of the foot, particularly tarsal tunnel syndrome [20]. Dorsal sural nerve, the distal continuation of the sural nerve in the foot that supplies the lateral border of the foot, is easily accessible to nerve conduction techniques because of its superficial location and is less prone to damage by local trauma or entrapment compared to the medial plantar and interdigital nerves. However, it may be absent in healthy individuals, have a lower SNAP amplitude (dorsal sural nerve SNAP amplitude was found to be 50–73% lower than that of the sural nerve, using antidromic recording) and has anatomic variability of its branches, limiting its use in routine evaluation of distal symmetric polyneuropathies [21, 22]. Sural SNAPs may be absent with increasing age in up to 24% of healthy individuals >70 years of age, and 40% in >80 years age. More recent studies showed that sural SNAPs can be obtained, albeit with reduced amplitude in 98–100% of healthy elderly individuals. Tavee et al. showed that absence of sural SNAP response before the age of 75 years of age should be regarded as abnormal. She proposed the lower limit of normal (LLN) for sural amplitudes as 3 μV for individuals aged 60–69 years and 1 μV for those aged 70–74 years [23]. Lo et al. showed that even though superficial peroneal (fibular) nerve is at equal distance to the sural nerve, it is more involved in peripheral neuropathy (88.5% abnormalities for superficial peroneal (fibular) nerve, compared to 75% for sural nerve in patients with peripheral neuropathy) [24].

The only abnormality on NCS in early or mild polyneuropathy may be reduced or absent sensory responses in the lower extremity. Motor NCS may be completely normal. NEE may show evidence of active/ongoing denervation (abnormal spontaneous activity—fibrillation, positive sharp wave potentials) and decreased recruitment limited to the intrinsic foot muscles only.

As the polyneuropathy progresses further, axon loss involves the motor nerve fibers with reduction in the CMAP amplitude seen on NCS along with a reduced/absent SNAP response of sensory nerves of the lower extremity, including sural and superficial peroneal (fibular) nerves. SNAPs and CMAPs of lower extremity nerves are affected while those in the upper extremity are normal or less affected.

In a severe axon loss neuropathy, sensory responses are absent in the lower extremity, motor responses are reduced to absent and there is now involvement of distal nerves in the upper extremity with reduced to absent sensory and motor responses in the median and ulnar nerves before it affects the radial nerves. As discussed earlier, with moderate to severe axon loss neuropathy, there may be secondary demyelination-type changes, including mild slowing of conduction velocity and prolongation of distal latency due to loss of large diameter, fastest-conducting nerve fibers.

Active/ongoing motor axon loss changes occur generally after ~3 weeks of axonal injury or insult and reinnervation takes months. Hence the changes seen in NCS and EMG may guide us to understand the chronicity of the underlying polyneuropathy. EMG in acute—subacute polyneuropathy may show only denervation potentials (positive sharp waves and fibrillations), while more long-standing neuropathies will show changes of reinnervation/motor unit remodelling. Often, with routine EMG studies, we observe a combination of denervation–reinnervation changes which suggests that the neuropathy is subacute on chronic. In very slowly progressive long-standing neuropathies, reinnervation occurs in pace with denervation. EMG may show reinnervation, with little or no active/ongoing denervation. Decreased recruitment may be the only finding in very acute neuropathies even before any changes are seen on NCS. Reinnervation occurs when there is primary regrowth of the axons or collateral sprouting. This is a very slow process and takes months to years. When reinnervation occurs (within months after axon loss), the motor unit action potentials (MUAPs) become longer in duration, higher in amplitude and show polyphasia. Long duration, high amplitude polyphasic MUAPs are not seen in acute neuropathies. When present, they always imply a chronic neuropathy that has been present for at least a few weeks to months or longer. EMG follows a similar pattern of length dependent changes as seen on NCS, with muscles of the foot (intrinsic foot muscles) and distal leg (for e.g. tibialis anterior, tibialis posterior and gastrocnemius muscles) being involved earlier in a length dependent axonal polyneuropathy. Only when the polyneuropathy is relatively severe, the muscles above the knee (quadriceps, and hamstrings) are affected and the small muscles of the hand will also show evidence of denervation–reinnervation. Any asymmetric findings should alert the neurologist to search for a superimposed radiculopathy/plexopathy or mononeuritis multiplex in the appropriate clinical setting. In the lower extremity, L5 and S1 radiculopathies are the commonest radiculopathies encountered. These should be taken into consideration while evaluating for polyneuropathy. Thus, a proximal L5-innervated muscle (e.g. gluteus medius) and a proximal S1-innervated muscle (e.g. short head of biceps femoris) is routinely sampled while performing EMG for polyneuropathy. Denervation–reinnervation changes in these proximal muscles with relatively unaffected/less affected nearby muscles (e.g. the quadriceps) outside those L5-S1 myotomes would suggest an underlying chronic L5 and/or S1 radiculopathy.

Role of Electrodiagnostic Studies in Diabetes Mellitus

Diabetes (including prediabetes) is the commonest cause of chronic distal symmetric sensory or sensorimotor polyneuropathy (DSP). Electrodiagnostic studies may not be required for evaluation of every distal symmetric polyneuropathy. Review of family history and screening tests for diabetes, vitamin B12 deficiency and monoclonal gammopathy should be assessed in almost every case of polyneuropathy. According to the latest AANEM policy statement [25], EDX testing in a patient with diabetic polyneuropathy is likely to be of low yield when:

1. Symptoms and physical findings are mild
2. Clinically, distal symmetric sensory/sensorimotor polyneuropathy is evident
3. There is a known cause (e.g. diabetes mellitus)
4. There is little suspicion of a coexisting etiology for neuropathy

The potential goals of pursuing electrodiagnosis in diabetes mellitus is to define the extent, severity and prognosis of the neuropathy and identify changes that would define an alternate/additional diagnosis. Diabetes affects both large and small nerve fibers. As discussed earlier, the first abnormalities in NCS in DSP are seen in the distal sensory nerves with absent or reduced plantar (mixed nerve), sural and/or superficial sensory SNAP amplitudes. As larger nerve fibers are lost, conduction velocity decreases and distal latency, as well as F-wave latency increases (in the axon loss range). As the disease progresses, motor nerves are affected similarly. EMG shows denervation in distal muscles of the foot and leg. Polyneuropathy remains in the mild stage in most cases. However, it may progress to involve more proximal muscles in a glove-stocking pattern. In addition to abnormal electrodiagnostic studies in the lower extremities, upper extremity nerves commonly show abnormalities such as entrapment neuropathies: carpal tunnel syndrome and ulnar neuropathy in particular. NCS correlate with the clinical severity of the disease. The challenge in the electrodiagnosis of diabetic neuropathy is when there are atypical presentations or there is a clinical suspicion of CIDP in a patient with severe diabetic polyneuropathy. NCS may show absent distal sensory and motor responses in the lower and upper extremity or severe slowing or even conduction block which may raise the possibility of a superimposed primary demyelinating disorder. In diabetes mellitus, NCS change slowly over years, so a more rapid decline should raise concerns about the adequacy of glycemic control, or another superimposed neuropathy, especially CIDP [26]. The electrophysiological features that favor CIDP over DM are:

1. Features of substantial demyelination (partial or complete motor conduction block, or abnormal temporal dispersion) in at least two nerves.
2. Distal CMAP duration prolongation in at least one nerve and at least one other demyelinating parameter in ≥ 1 nerve.

Another classic form of diabetic neuropathy is diabetic lumbosacral radiculoplexoneuropathy (DLRPN) or diabetic amyotrophy. This is an asymmetric neurogenic process and it associated with pain and weight loss. Femoral motor and sensory nerve responses are absent or reduced in amplitude. Femoral sensory i.e. saphenous nerve study is technically difficult, especially in obese individuals. However, when absent unilaterally, it may suggest a lumbar plexopathy or femoral neuropathy rather than an L2-L4 radiculopathy. EMG shows denervation–reinnervation changes in the muscles innervated by the femoral nerve (quadriceps, iliopsoas) and obturator nerve (adductor longus).

Nutritional Deficiency and Polyneuropathy

Polyneuropathy is seen in 25% patients with vitamin B12 deficiency. Electrodiagnostic studies have shown various subtypes based on NCS: 76% axon loss peripheral neuropathy, while 24% with demyelinating features. Rare cases of demyelinating neuropathy with conduction block and also an acute sensorimotor axon loss polyneuropathy have been reported. Vitamin B12 levels may be normal [27]. Hence the need to test for the metabolites, methylmalonic acid (MMA) ± homocysteine in patients with borderline levels of B12, to confirm the diagnosis of B12 deficiency.

B6 (pyridoxine) deficiency causes distal symmetric axon loss polyneuropathy. On the other hand, B6 toxicity affects the dorsal root ganglion (sensory neuronopathy) leading to sensory ataxic polyneuropathy. Nerve conduction studies show widespread absent sensory responses with preserved or mildly affected motor responses.

Toxic Polyneuropathies

Electrophysiologic studies in polyneuropathies due to neurotoxic exposure are rather non-specific. Very few may have characteristic electrophysiologic features. However, it is important to recognize these as improvement may be seen once the exposure to a particular toxin is reduced or eliminated. The most common pattern of toxic neuropathy seen on NCS is distal symmetric sensory/sensorimotor neuropathy, as seen with exposure to vincristine, chronic arsenic poisoning and ethyl alcohol. Sensory predominant distal polyneuropathy or a sensory neuronopathy is classically seen in patients with thallium toxicity, or with drugs/agents such as pyridoxine, platinum-based chemotherapy, styrene or thalidomide. Lead toxicity, dapsone and L-tryptophan may cause mononeuritis multiplex. Lead toxicity may present with an isolated wrist drop or a finger drop. Exposure to dapsone may resemble mononeuritis multiplex, however this is a motor predominant polyneuropathy. Organophosphorus poisoning may have two different neuropathic manifestations: rapidly progressive early distal motor axonal polyneuropathy (within 2–3 weeks) or a delayed distal sensorimotor axonal polyneuropathy. Nitrofurantoin polyneuropathy may present with rapid onset respiratory failure with painful paresthesias and progressive limb weakness mimicking GBS with an acute motor/sensorimotor axonal polyneuropathy (AMAN or AMSAN). Predominantly motor neuropathies with conduction slowing may be seen with amiodarone, disulfiram, acute arsenic exposure and n-Hexane exposure. The acute presentation of these polyneuropathies may resemble GBS and hence a careful history of exposure to various toxins and medications will guide the treating neurologist make appropriate treatment decisions in patients not responding to plasmapheresis or intravenous immunoglobulin for suspected GBS.

Differential Diagnosis of Distal Symmetric Polyneuropathy

Many inherited polyneuropathies and DADs neuropathy also present with distal symmetric neuropathic features. Axonal inherited polyneuropathy may be difficult to distinguish from a severe distal symmetric polyneuropathy due to metabolic or toxic insult. Clinical features (e.g. high plantar arches, hammer toes, childhood onset) with a motor predominant distal polyneuropathy and family history if present, may be clues to an inherited polyneuropathy. DADs is a distal demyelinating polyneuropathy which will be discussed in the section on electrodiagnosis of demyelinating neuropathies. An important consideration while performing electrodiagnostic studies of polyneuropathy is motor neuron disease and radiculopathies, particularly when there is any asymmetry found on clinical or electrodiagnostic tesing. Abnormal sensory studies rule out or lowers the possibility of amyotrophic lateral scleroris (ALS). In the absence of sensory abnormalities, it is difficult to distinguish a pure motor axonal polyneuropathy (albeit a rare condition) from an anterior horn cell disease or a polyradiculopathy. Topographical distribution of changes seen in NEE provide some clues: active/ongoing and chronic denervation changes in distal muscles symmetrically would suggest an axonal polyneuropathy while in ALS, these changes are seen asymmetrically in both proximal and distal muscles, often accompanied by fasciculation potentials and motor unit instability features. Denervation–reinnervation changes due to radiculopathy are restricted to the muscles innervated by the affected nerve root (supplied by different peripheral nerves).

Electrodiagnosis of Demyelinating Polyneuropathies

It is very important to recognize features of demyelination during electrophysiological studies as demyelinating polyneuropathies are potentially treatable polyneuropathies. Mononeuropathies, such as entrapment mononeuropathies often show features of focal demyelination (at site of entrapment) on NCS. When a patient has evidence of primary demyelination on NCS, the differential diagnosis is narrowed as shown in Table 6.8. CIDP is the most common chronic demyelinating neuropathy. Inherited demyelinating polyneuropathies are rare, typically have onset in childhood and may have central nervous system involvement.

Table 6.8 Demyelinating polyneuropathies

Symmetric
Hereditary
• Hereditary sensorimotor neuropathy type I (Charcot–Marie-Tooth 1)
• Hereditary sensorimotor neuropathy type III (Dejerine-Sottas)
• Hereditary sensorimotor neuropathy type IV (Refsum disease)
• Krabbe disease
• Metachromatic leukodystrophy
• Adrenoleukodystrophy
• Cockayne syndrome
• Niemann-Pick disease
• Cerebrotendinous xanthomatosus
Acquired
• Acute inflammatory demyelinating polyradiculoneuropathy (AIDP)
• Chronic inflammatory demyelinating polyradiculoneuropathy (CIDP)
• CIDP associated with paraproteinemia (e.g.- IGA/IgG MGUS, Osteosclerotic myeloma, POEMS), malignancy (lymphoma)
• CIDP variants: particularly distal acquired demyelinating symmetric neuropathy (DADS)
Asymmetric
Mononeuropathies
• Entrapment or compression neuropathy
• Hereditary neuropathy with liabilty to pressure palsies (HNPP)
CIDP variants
• Multifocal motor neuropathy with conduction block (MMN with CB)
• Multifocal acquired demyelinating sensory and motor neuropathy (MADSAM)

Myelin is essential for saltatory conduction along the nerves. Loss of myelin results in slowing of conduction. Electrophysiologically, demyelination is determined by the following:

- Slowing of conduction (prolongation of peak/distal latencies, slowing of nerve conduction velocity, prolongation/absence of F-wave latency)
- Conduction block
- Temporal dispersion of Compound Muscle Action Potential (CMAP) configuration

The electrodiagnostic hallmark of acquired demyelination is conduction block and temporal dispersion of M-wave/CMAP configurations. Secondary axon loss may be seen in severe demyelinating polyneuropathy with reduction in CMAP amplitudes.

Electrodiagnosis of Acute Inflammatory Demyelinating Polyradiculoneuropathy (AIDP)

Electrophysiologic studies play an important role in the diagnosis of GBS, classification of the subtypes and in establishing prognosis. Albuminocytological dissociation in cerebrospinal studies or abnormal NCS may not be demonstrable in the first few days of the illness as demyelination is segmental or patchy. This makes the diagnosis challenging. Early diagnosis is important, however, because early treatment has been shown to improve outcomes.

In the first few days, nerve conduction studies are normal despite clinical weakness. Prolonged or absent late responses: particularly, F-wave latency and tibial H-reflex are the earliest findings on nerve conduction studies. Wilbourn et al. studied the electrodiagnostic findings in the first week of illness in GBS. He reported an absent tibial H-reflex in 97% of patients with early GBS. Other abnormal early electrodiagnostic findings were: abnormal F-wave (84%), combination of abnormal sensory responses in the upper extremity with a normal sural response (67%) and evidence of demyelination (slow conduction velocity, prolonged distal latency, conduction block and temporal dispersion). Although very sensitive, an absent tibial H-reflex, by itself is non-specific. However, along with an abnormal F-wave, abnormal upper extremity SNAP and normal sural SNAP, these findings are characteristic of early demyelinating GBS or AIDP. Hence, Wilbourn suggested that the tibial H-reflex is the most sensitive test for early GBS and should be a part of the standard NCS protocol for GBS. If multiple nerves are tested, a definitive diagnosis of AIDP is possible in half of the patients but not until the fifth day after the onset of symptoms [28].

Normal peripheral nerve conduction study with an abnormal F-wave (absent or slow) as an isolated finding was seen in 10–30% of patients in early GBS [29]. Absent or reduced F-waves with preserved distal CMAPs is used to assess demyelination in the proximal segments. At least four mechanisms account for the selectively abnormal F-wave in early GBS: (1) demyelinating conduction block in the proximal segment (if normal distal CMAPs), (2) proximal axonal degeneration (3) physiological conduction failure causing a proximal conduction block (4) impaired excitability of the motor neuron.

A-wave (axon reflex) is seen in demyelinating polyneuropathies, often in the first several days of illness in GBS. Hence, A-waves may also be utilized as a marker of early demyelination.

"Sural sparing" pattern in GBS

"Sural sparing" pattern is described in acute and chronic demyelinating neuropathies. Definition of "abnormal sural pattern" is variable and different patterns have been studied in GBS. It was first described by Bromberg and Albers in 1993 as "abnormal median normal sural" and shown to be 100% specific for AIDP and CIDP versus motor neuron disease and diabetes mellitus polyneuropathy [30]. Al-Shekhlee et al., in their 2005 paper described it as "normal or relatively preserved sural sensory nerve action potential (SNAP) compared with at least two abnormal SNAPs in the upper limb" [31]. Sural sparing (abnormal ulnar/normal sural response) has been found to be most specific in distinguishing GBS from its mimics in a multicenter study [32]. Sural sparing was seen in both demyelinating and axonal forms of GBS [33]. Rajabally et al., in 2016 reconfirmed the usefulness of "absent median present sural" and "absent median normal sural" patterns with sensitivities of 27.8% and 19.4% respectively, with specificity of 100% for AIDP vs axonal GBS, regardless of the criteria used to define GBS. Ulnar and radial patterns were not helpful [34].

When distal NCS are normal in a patient with suspected GBS, electrophysiological studies at the Erb's point (site at the brachial plexus, located 2–3 cm above the clavicle) have been shown to be very helpful in the diagnosis of early GBS, as it reflects the condition of proximal nerves. The NCS at Erb's point may show prolonged latency, low motor amplitude or conduction block (>50% amplitude drop). This may be the only abnormal parameter in early GBS and is relatively easy to study [35]. Technical difficulties are encountered in achieving a supramaximal stimulus due to the deeper location of the brachial plexus and patient's body habitus, including effects of obesity or large neck girth.

Acute inflammatory demyelinating polyradiculoneuropathy (AIDP) is electrophysiologically characterized by conduction slowing, conduction block and temporal dispersion. Due to loss of myelin, nerve conduction velocity is either markedly slow or blocked. Slowing of nerve conduction is associated with marked slowing of conduction velocity (<70% LLN) and/or prolongation of distal motor latency (>130% ULN) and prolongation of late responses—F-wave latency (>130% ULN). SNAPs are often low or absent (outside of sural sparing). CMAPs are reduced in amplitude depending on the site of demyelination that produces a conduction block and/or temporal dispersion. Conduction block is defined as obtaining a response at a proximal site of stimulation with a drop in CMAP amplitude or area >50% when CMAP duration increase is <30%. Temporal dispersion is defined as >30% increased duration of proximal CMAP compared to the distal CMAP.

80% of patients with AIDP have evidence of nerve conduction slowing or conduction block at some point of their illness although up to 20% will have normal conduction studies. The sites of demyelinating conduction slowing, and block are patchy or segmental, the most affected regions are: terminal segment distal to the wrist, common sites of entrapment neuropathy and proximal nerve segments including spinal roots. The relative deficiency of the blood-nerve barrier at the proximal nerve roots may make these more vulnerable for the immune attack in GBS. Distal demyelination affects both sensory and motor nerves, with absent sensory responses and evidence of reduced CMAP amplitude at distal and proximal stimulation sites. This may mimic acute motor/+ sensory axonal neuropathy (AMAN/AMSAN). Proximal demyelination at nerve roots is reflected as normal distal sensory and motor responses with abnormal F-wave studies. Erb's point or axillary stimulation is helpful in these cases to look for evidence of additional demyelination at proximal sites. Electrodiagnostic studies involving proximal extremity nerves, facial nerve studies and blink responses provide additional evidence of demyelination. These studies may be particularly useful in the first 2 weeks of the illness when the nerve conduction study of the distal nerves may fail to demonstrate demyelination.

Sequential electrodiagnostic abnormalities in patients with AIDP were described by Albers et al., in 1985. Abnormal median sensory response with relative sparing of sural response ("sural sparing") was the earliest finding observed during the first 2 weeks. The earliest abnormality seen on needle EMG was decreased recruitment of motor unit action potentials (MUAPs), with no change in configuration or evidence of abnormal spontaneous activity. Early presence of relatively large amplitude MUAPs may be seen due to selective loss of small MUAPs. However, this should not be considered as evidence of chronicity. Abnormal spontaneous activity occurs between the second and the fourth week of illness, in both proximal and distal muscles. Myokymic discharges can be seen transiently during the first 3 weeks but not subsequently in most cases. Among early abnormalities seen otherwise is increased percentage of polyphasic MUAPs at about the fourth week in both proximal and distal muscles [36]. Prominent fibrillation potentials in the paraspinal muscles in the first 2–3 weeks should raise the possibility of acute porphyric polyneuropathy that often mimics AMAN/AMSAN.

Clinical recovery in GBS precedes that of NCS abnormalities. Restoration of demyelinating conduction block begins with remyelination resulting in temporal dispersion.

Electrodiagnosis of AMAN/AMSAN

Three patterns of nerve conduction abnormalities are described in axonal GBS [37]:

1. Simple axonal degeneration (at least ~50%)
2. Transient conduction block/slowing in the motor nerve terminals (early reversible conduction failure) (~20%)
3. Absent F-waves as an isolated conduction abnormality (~12%)

Acute motor axonal neuropathy (AMAN) occurs due to axonal degeneration and the electrophysiological correlate is limited to widespread severely reduced CMAP amplitudes. When sensory responses are also affected, it is defined as acute motor and sensory axonal neuropathy (AMSAN). More recently, some patients with AMAN and AMSAN have been shown to demonstrate a transient conduction block/slowing due to nodal dysfunction mimicking demyelination. Recovery is quick and without evidence of remyelination (abnormal temporal dispersion). This has been referred to as reversible conduction failure (RCF) [38]. It is thought to be due to antiganglioside antibodies attacking the nodes of Ranvier by a complement mediated immune attack. This causes a transient dysfunction of the Na+/K+ channels at the nodes and may not progress to axonal degeneration. The conduction failure improves quickly within a few weeks without the otherwise typical evidence of remyelination, so that there is no temporal dispersion demonstrated. RCF can be recognized only by serial nerve conduction studies. It is not included in the current electrodiagnostic criteria of GBS. A new criterion for GBS has been proposed by Rajabally et al. 2015 to incorporate reversible conduction failure by a single NCS study [39].

Electrodiagnostic Findings in Other Variants of GBS

Pharyngeal–cervical-brachial variant of GBS is a subtype of axonal GBS. Miller Fisher syndrome shows axonal neuropathy with decreased CMAPs and SNAPs. Demyelinating forms are less reported. RCF has been reported in patients with MFS and MFS/GBS overlap syndrome [40]. Facial motor and blink responses may be abnormal. Loss of the H-reflex may be the earliest finding due to involvement of Ia afferent fibers. EMG may show fibrillation potentials in the facial muscles in addition to the limb muscles.

Pure sensory GBS shows abnormal SNAPs with absent or reduced amplitude and normal or slightly slow sensory conduction velocity. Motor conduction studies are normal. Low SNAPs are generally found to be reversible.

Electrodiagnostic Studies in Chronic Inflammatory Demyelinating Polyradiculoneuropathy (CIDP)

As we discussed earlier, demyelinating polyneuropathy is diagnosed by evidence of conduction slowing, and in the case of acquired etiologies: conduction block with or without temporal dispersion. It is important to determine whether chronic (>8 weeks) polyneuropathy has features consistent with chronic inflammatory demyelinating polyradiculoneuropathy (CIDP) as this is a potentially treatable polyneuropathy. The diagnosis can be very challenging in a patient with underlying long-standing severe axonal diabetic polyneuropathy with markedly reduced/absent lower extremity sensory and motor responses.

CMAP amplitude in primary demyelinating polyneuropathy

CMAP amplitudes are typically normal or slightly reduced in primary demyelinating polyneuropathies. However, if markedly reduced, it is difficult to determine whether this is due to axon loss or demyelination. Decrease in CMAP amplitude is due to either (1) axon loss (2) conduction block (3) abnormal temporal dispersion. A linear correlation was found between the decrease in amplitude and slowing of conduction in the majority of motor as well as sensory nerves, which was steeper in the axonal than in demyelinating polyneuropathies [41, 42]. However, a more frequent and a larger decrease in mean amplitude was found in sensory and motor nerves in demyelinating neuropathies, contrary to the belief that axon loss results in greater decrease in CMAP and SNAP amplitudes. Thus, a pathophysiological basis of electrodiagnosis may be missed by just looking at the CMAP and SNAP amplitudes. Tankisi et al., in 2007 demonstrated that a more pronounced decrease in SNAP or CMAP amplitude in demyelinating neuropathies was due to abnormal temporal dispersion or distal conduction block. Part of the explanation for more pronounced decrease in CMAPs in demyelinating neuropathies is also because motor fibers are generally more affected in demyelinating neuropathies while sensory fibers are generally more affected in axonal neuropathies [42].

Conduction slowing is suggestive of demyelinating polyneuropathy

A nerve is composed of slow and fast conducting fibers. Distal latency and conduction velocity are essentially the same measurement, they differ only by a multiplication factor (i.e. distance) and represent the conduction of the fastest conducting fibers in a nerve. Demyelination affecting these fastest conducting fibers results in slowing of conduction. Slowing of conduction velocity may also be evident in patients with axonal polyneuropathy if the fastest conducting fibers are affected. However, the conduction velocity in such situations typically does not fall into the demyelinating range (70% of lower limit of normal). This is because normal myelinated fibers do not conduct slower than this. Hence greater slowing of conduction on NCS suggests a primary demyelinating process. Only in extremely rare cases of regenerating nerve fibers, after a complete axonal injury (e.g. nerve transection) can conduction velocities be reduced in the demyelinating range. When conduction velocity is reduced, other features of NCS are taken into consideration, such as CMAP amplitude, conduction block, and temporal dispersion to help the electromyographer determine with certainty whether the underlying process is primary demyelinating or axonal.

An absence or prolongation of mean latency of the F-wave is among the most common features in acute and chronic demyelinating neuropathies. It reflects conduction slowing due to demyelination of the proximal nerve segment.

Temporal dispersion

Temporal dispersion (Fig. 6.1) results from an abnormally increased range of conduction velocities amongst individual nerve fibers, leading to decreased amplitude with increased duration of CMAP or SNAP, especially with longer recording distances [43]. Caliandro et al., in 2007 found that CMAP amplitude and temporal dispersion are more sensitive electrophysiologic parameters than conduction velocity to determine moderate demyelination. Conduction velocity is reduced only when myelin damage is severe as it decreases when both large and small axons are affected [44].

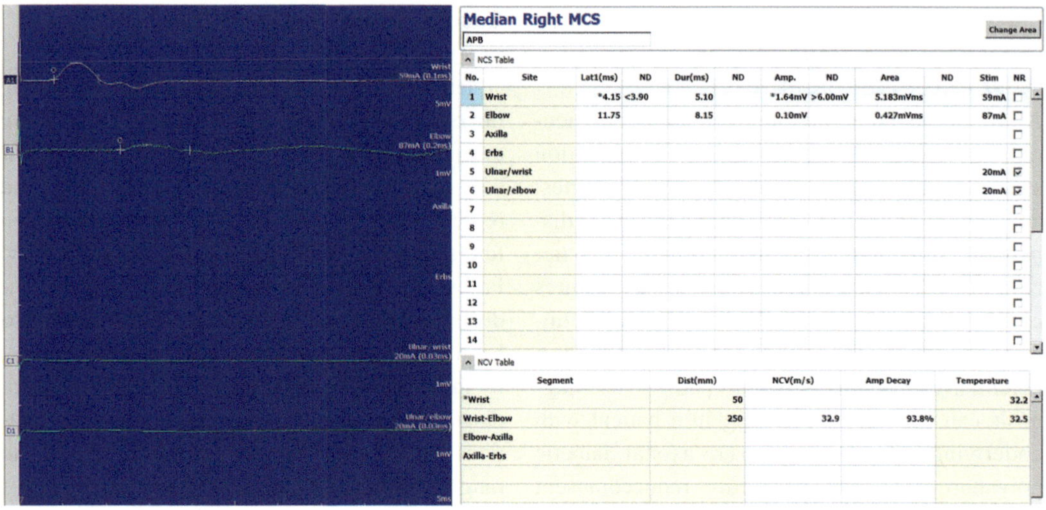

Fig. 6.1 Temporal dispersion in the right median motor nerve conduction study in a patient with CIDP. It is more pronounced at the proximal recording site (elbow), compared to the distal site at the wrist

Conduction block

Conduction block (see Fig. 6.2) and temporal dispersion are electrophysiologic hallmarks of acquired demyelination. A sufficient number of motor axons have to be blocked to result in a CMAP drop which can be caused by either conduction block or abnormal temporal dispersion. Conduction block along the motor or sensory nerve results in interruption of transmission of impulse across the nerve, resulting in a reduced CMAP/SNAP amplitude and area. Verifying that a drop in CMAP amplitude/area between the distal and proximal stimulation site is due to a true conduction block can be very challenging. The CMAP is the summation of nearly synchronous muscle fiber action potentials recorded from a muscle. Demyelination amplifies the effect of normal phase cancellation causing a further drop in amplitude/area of the proximal CMAP. Therefore, diagnostic criteria are necessary to distinguish between reduction in CMAP amplitude due to conduction block versus abnormal temporal dispersion.

From studies in normal subjects, CMAP amplitude and area normally does not decrease by more than 20% and CMAP duration increase by more than 15%, when recorded from the typical distal and proximal stimulation sites (e.g. wrist to elbow, ankle to knee). These studies imply that a drop of >20% in proximal CMAP area/amplitude defines conduction block and increase in CMAP duration >15% signifies abnormal temporal dispersion. The effects of temporal dispersion are increased for more proximal stimulation sites such as Erb's point or axilla. Hence, the cut off values for motor conduction block are doubled to >40% drop in proximal CMAP area or amplitude in the absence of temporal dispersion (<30% increase in CMAP duration). However, a drop in proximal CMAP amplitude/area of <20% over a very short segment should not be disregarded as it may imply an underlying conduction block. Currently the criteria of more than 50% drop in CMAP area or amplitude between proximal and distal stimulation sites best defines conduction block, regardless of the amount of temporal dispersion [45]. CMAP area rather than CMAP amplitude is the preferred measure for evaluating conduction block.

Errors in recording a conduction block may be due to the following physiological or technical factors:

1. Temperature
2. Stimulus site
3. Supramaximal stimulus
4. Movement of stimulating electrode
5. Martin–Gruber anastomosis

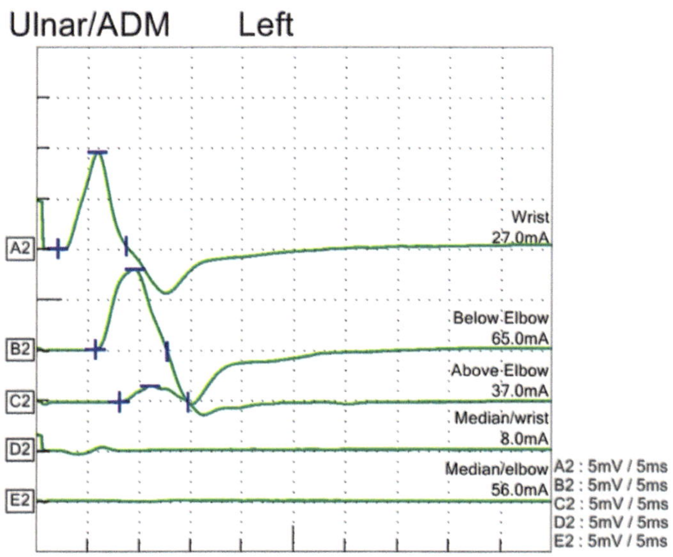

Motor Nerve Conduction

Nerve	Recording	Stimulus	B-P Amp (mV)		LatOn (ms)		CV (m/s)		Dist (mm)		Norm B-P Amp	Norm LatOn	Norm CV	Temp (C)	
			L	R	L	R	L	R	L	R				L	R
Ulnar/ADM	ADM	Wrist	9.80		2.20		n/a		50		> 7 mV	< 3.1 ms	> 50 m/s	32.7	
		Below Elbow	8.10		5.90		56.8		210					32.8	
		Above Elbow	**1.70**		8.20		51.7		310					32.7	
		Median/wrist	NR		NR		n/a							32.7	
		Median/elbow	NR		NR		n/a							32.7	

Fig. 6.2 Left ulnar motor study shows a decrease in the CMAP amplitude >50% at the proximal recording site at above elbow, compared to the distal recording site at below elbow. There is no temporal dispersion, hence this drop in CMAP amplitude is due to a true conduction block across the elbow

The limb that is being studied for NCS should be appropriately warmed if necessary, to achieve a limb temperature ideally >37 °C (hands should be >33 °C and feet >30 °C as per European Federation of Neurological Societies/Peripheral Nerve Society (EFNS/PNS) Joint Task Force, 2010 [46]. Conduction block may be missed in cold temperatures. Lower stimulus intensity at deeper sites such as Erb's point, and popliteal fossa may erroneously result in reduced CMAPs. If supramaximal stimulus is not applied to obtain a maximum CMAP response by increasing the stimulus intensity by further 20% after a maximum CMAP response is obtained, then a reduced CMAP response may be seen. This may be spuriously interpreted as a true conduction block. Care must be taken to avoid recording a volume conducted CMAP from the neighbouring motor nerves. This is important while recording the median nerve at the wrist and at proximal stimulation sites where multiple nerves are in the vicinity of each other. A Martin–Gruber anastomosis between the proximal median or anterior interroseous nerve and ulnar nerve may occasionally produce a "pseudo" conduction block between the proximal and distal ulnar stimulating sites. This has to be differentiated from a true conduction block by appropriate "crossover" studies.

Sensory studies

Sensory nerve action potentials (SNAPs) have low amplitude and short duration. Hence, the effect of normal temporal dispersion is amplified in sensory nerves. Demyelination causes further increase in temporal dispersion and conduction slowing/block. This makes the use of sensory NCS less reliable in assessing demyelination in peripheral neuropathies. However, significant slowing on sensory NCS is suggestive of demyelination. Absence of responses in the commonly studied distal sensory nerves in both lower and upper extremities is seen in severe axonal as well as demyelinating neuropathy and makes the distinction between them unreliable based only on sensory studies. The Ad Hoc Subcommittee of the American Academy of Neurology AIDS Task Force (1991) Criteria recognized sensory nerve conduction velocity <80% LLN as being supportive of CIDP [47]. Acute and chronic acquired inflammatory demyelinating neuropathies have segmental demyelination with "sural sparing" that is classically described in demyelinating polyneuropathies. Thus, the sensory nerve conduction studies play an important role in combination with motor nerve conduction studies in the diagnosis of CIDP (Table 6.9).

Supportive criteria

(A) Elevated CSF protein with cell counts <10/mm^3
(B) Magnetic resonance imaging showing gadolinium enhancement and/or hypertrophy of the cauda equina, lumbosacral or cervical nerve roots, or the brachial or lumbosacral plexuses
(C) Nerve biopsy showing unequivocal evidence of demyelination and/or remyelination in >5 fibers by electron microscopy or in >6 of 50 teased fibers
(D) Clinical improvement following immunomodulatory treatment

Diagnostic categories

- **Definite CIDP**: Clinical criteria 1 A or B and 2 and EDX criteria 1; or Probable (electrophysiology) CIDP + at least 1 Supportive criterion or Possible (electrophysiology) CIDP + at least 2 Supportive criteria
- **Probable CIDP:** Clinical criteria 1 A or B and 2 with EDX criteria 2; or Possible (electrophysiology) CIDP + at least 1 Supportive criterion
- **Possible CIDP:** Clinical criteria 1 A or B and 2 with EDX criteria 3

Distal demyelination

CMAP duration is defined as the distance from the onset of the first negative deflection to return to baseline of the last negative deflection. The terminal positive deflection is not included [49]. Methods that do not include the later negative components of the CMAP may fail to accurately measure the duration of the desynchronised CMAP. Prolongation of distal CMAP duration or dispersion of distal CMAP duration was proposed as a new electrodiagnostic criteria for diagnosis of CIDP by the EFNS/PNS task force in 2010 to recognize distal demyelination. A cutoff value of 9 ms duration of distal CMAP duration was proposed in the earlier criteria and later the limits were specified for different nerves as: median ≥6.6 ms, ulnar ≥6.7 ms, peroneal (fibular) ≥7.6 ms, and tibial ≥8.8 ms [48]. While distal motor latency reflects conduction along the fastest conducting motor fibers, distal CMAP duration depends on the temporal dispersion between the slow and fast motor fibers distally within the nerve. It is a useful marker of distal demyelination.

Needle EMG in CIDP shows changes of secondary axonal degeneration in the proximal and distal muscles of the upper and lower extremity. Evidence of chronic motor axon loss is seen in these muscles in the form of long duration, large amplitude, polyphasic motor unit action potentials (MUAPs), often with active/ongoing denervation features comprising fibrillation and/or positive sharp wave potentials.

CIDP Variants

Multifocal motor neuropathy with conduction block (MMNCB or MMN)

Conduction block at non-entrapment sites along the motor nerve is the electrophysiological hallmark of MMN. Sensory nerves are typically not affected. Motor conduction block is not specific for MMN. It may be seen in other acquired demyelinating and entrapment neuropathies. Other features of acquired demyelination such as temporal dispersion with prolongation of distal latency, slowing of conduction velocity and prolongation of F-wave latency may be present. CMAP area/amplitude drop (between proximal and distal stimulation sites) of >50% defines

Table 6.9 Clinical and electrodiagnostic criteria for CIDP [48]

Clinical
1. Inclusion criteria
(a) Typical CIDP
Chronically progressive, stepwise, or recurrent symmetric proximal and distal weakness and sensory dysfunction of all extremities, developing over at least 2 months; cranial nerves may be affected; and
Absent or reduced tendon reflexes in all extremities
(b) Atypical CIDP (still considered CIDP but with different features)
One of the following, but otherwise as in (a) (tendon reflexes may be normal in unaffected limbs):
Predominantly distal (distal acquired demyelinating symmetric, DADS) or
Asymmetric [multifocal acquired demyelinating sensory and motor neuropathy (MADSAM), Lewis–Sumner syndrome] or
Focal (e.g., involvement of the brachial or lumbosacral plexus or of one or more peripheral nerves in one upper or lower limb)
Pure motor or
Pure sensory (including chronic immune sensory polyradiculopathy affecting the central process of the primary sensory neuron)
(2) Exclusion criteria
Borrelia burgdorferi infection (Lyme disease), diphtheria, drug or toxin exposure probably to have caused the neuropathy
Hereditary demyelinating neuropathy
Prominent sphincter disturbance
Diagnosis of multifocal motor neuropathy
IgM monoclonal gammopathy with high titre antibodies to myelin-associated glycoprotein
Other causes for a demyelinating neuropathy including POEMS syndrome, osteosclerotic myeloma, diabetic and non-diabetic lumbosacral radiculoplexus neuropathy. PNS lymphoma and amyloidosis may occasionally have demyelinating features
Electrodiagnostic
1. Definite
At least one of the following:
(a) Motor distal latency prolongation ≥50% above ULN in two nerves (excluding median neuropathy at the wrist from carpal tunnel syndrome), or
(b) Reduction of motor conduction velocity ≥30% below LLN in two nerves, or
(c) Prolongation of F-wave latency ≥30% above ULN in two nerves (≥50% if amplitude of distal negative peak CMAP <80% of LLN values), or
(d) Absence of F-waves in two nerves if these nerves have distal negative peak CMAP amplitudes ≥20% of LLN + ≥1 other demyelinating parameter in ≥1 other nerve, or
(e) Partial motor conduction block: ≥50% amplitude reduction of the proximal negative peak CMAP relative to distal, if distal negative peak CMAP ≥ 20% of LLN, in two nerves, or in one nerve + ≥1 other demyelinating parameter in ≥1 other nerve, or
(f) Abnormal temporal dispersion (>30% duration increase between the proximal and distal negative peak CMAP) in ≥2 nerves, or
(g) Distal CMAP duration (interval between onset of the first negative peak and return to baseline of the last negative peak) increase in ≥1 nerve (median ≥6.6 ms, ulnar ≥6.7 ms, peroneal (fibular) ≥7.6 ms, tibial ≥8.8 ms) + ≥1 other demyelinating parameter in ≥1 other nerve.
2. Probable
• ≥30% amplitude reduction of the proximal negative peak CMAP relative to distal, excluding the posterior tibial nerve, if distal negative peak CMAP ≥20% of LLN, in two nerves, or in one nerve + ≥1 other demyelinating parameter in ≥1 other nerve.
3. Possible
• As in "definite" but in only one nerve.

Motor conduction block is not considered in the ulnar nerve across the elbow and at least 50% amplitude reduction between Erb's point and the wrist is required for probable conduction block. Temperatures should be maintained to at least 33°C at the palm and 30°C at the external malleolus

CMAP compound muscle action potential, *ULN* upper limit of normal values, *LLN* lower limit of normal values conduction block, regardless of the presence of temporal dispersion. CMAP area is the preferred measure for evaluating conduction block than CMAP amplitude. An abrupt drop in CMAP over a short segment also signifies a conduction block. When the distal CMAP amplitude is <1 mV, it is not useful to define the presence of focal conduction block in MMN. There are two reasons for this—

1. The effects of normal temporal dispersion are magnified with very few fibres, giving a false positive proximal CMAP drop, thus erroneously giving the impression of a conduction block.
2. IVIG has not been shown to be useful in nerves with distal CMAP <1 mV, probably because such low CMAPs represent marked secondary axon loss (late stage of MMN) [45].

Conduction block is most frequently present in the upper extremity nerves at non-entrapment sites. It may be missed on routine NCS if present in proximal nerve segments (plexus, or root) or when associated with significant secondary axonal loss. When conduction block is more proximal, both the routine proximal and distal CMAP will be normal. When a conduction block is distal to the distal stimulation site along the motor nerve, both the proximal and distal CMAPs are reduced in amplitude and this mimics an axon loss motor neuropathy or motor neuron disease. Identification of conduction block along very proximal or distal segments can be challenging for the electromyographer. Prolongation of F-wave latency favors demyelination in the absence of an easily identifiable conduction block or other indicators of demyelination. In exceptional cases, only proximal conduction block may be present, hence more proximal segments of motor nerve should be studied (e.g. stimulating axilla, Erb's point or cervical root). Needle electrode examination shows abnormal spontaneous activity with presence of fibrillation potentials ± fasciculation potentials, in addition to decreased motor unit recruitment manifested by large motor unit potentials.

Technical difficulties may arise due to inability to use a supramaximal stimulus at the Erb's point due to the large amount of subcutaneous tissue. In the lower extremity, caution is warranted with stimulation of the tibial nerve at the popliteal fossa as the stimulus may not be supramaximal to the deeper location of the nerve at this site, erroneously resulting in a reduction in CMAP amplitude. It is emphasized that the electromyographer should thoroughly search for the presence of a motor conduction block as MMN is a potentially treatable neuropathy that mimics Amyotrophic Lateral Sclerosis (ALS). Conduction block is not an absolute requirement for diagnosis if other features of demyelination are present. In a series of MMN patients, only 31% had conduction block; 44% had temporal dispersion, and 94% had other electrodiagnostic features of demyelination with superimposed axonal degeneration [50]. Response to treatment with IV immunoglobulin was no different with/without the conduction block. Presence of anti-ganglioside antibodies in high titers is rather specific for MMN but not an absolute requirement for diagnosis of MMN (anti-GM1 antibodies are absent in approximately 50% of MMN patients).

By definition, MMN affects more than one motor nerve, clinically and electrophysiologically. However rarely conduction block may be seen in only one motor nerve, with a very good response to immunotherapy. An axonal phenotype of MMN, multifocal axonal motor neuropathy (MAMN) has been described in a small series of patients, lacking overt conduction block, ± elevated titers of anti-GM1 antibodies, but responded very well to IV immunoglobulin therapy just like MMN [51]. MMN should be differentiated from other asymmetric neuropathies: e.g. mononeuritis multiplex and MADSAM.

Multifocal acquired demyelinating sensory and motor neuropathy (MADSAM)

NCS show features consistent with acquired demyelination as in CIDP. However motor and sensory nerves are affected in an asymmetric manner. These include prolongation of F-wave latency (>130% ULN), distal latency (>150% ULN), slowing of nerve conduction velocity (<70% LLN), conduction block, temporal dispersion and increase in distal CMAP duration. Mononeuritis multiplex and MMN remain important differentials. Mononeuritis multiplex is an axon loss polyneuropathy affecting multiple nerves in an asymmetric fashion. These features also overlap with HNPP which should be considered especially in patients who are young, have a history of recurrent multifocal entrapment neuropathies and a positive family history.

Distal acquired demyelinating symmetric neuropathy (DADS)

NCS shows widespread slowing in distal sensory and motor nerves of the lower extremity. Distal latencies are markedly prolonged, resulting in short terminal latency index (TLI) which is the electrodiagnostic hallmark of DADs neuropathy. Short TLI can reliably distinguish DADs with anti MAG antibodies (anti-MAG neuropathy) from CIDP and other chronic demyelinating neuropathies [52]. Conduction block is uncommon.

Other Demyelinating Polyneuropathies

Monoclonal gammopathy with undetermined significance (MGUS)

If a patient with CIDP-like pattern on EDX does not respond to standard line of care, the treating provider should reconsider the diagnosis, work up for an alternative cause such as paraproteinemic neuropathy. Two patterns of demyelinating neuropathies are seen in patients with MGUS. DADs neuropathy is an IgM MGUS associated neuropathy with (or without) anti-MAG antibodies with distal weakness, prominent hand tremor and predominant distal demyelination manifested by prolonged distal latencies. CIDP-MGUS (non-IgM) essentially has the same clinical and electrophysiological characteristics as CIDP, with patients typically having an IgA or IgG M protein. Patients with MGUS have a risk of lymphoproliferative malignancies and hence should be followed up regularly. Neuropathy associated with lymphoma and osteosclerotic myeloma, as opposed to multiple myeloma may also present like CIDP. It responds to treatment of the underlying malignancy.

Inherited Polyneuropathies

Neurophysiologic studies are very helpful in distinguishing inherited from acquired demyelinating neuropathies. Lack of temporal dispersion and conduction block with very slow (and uniform) conduction velocities in the range of 20–30 m/s on motor NCS is suggestive of an inherited demyelinating neuropathy.

CMT-IA (caused by PMP22 duplication) is characterized by widespread, uniform conduction slowing, which remains stable over decades; conduction block is unusual, and when found, probably reflects superimposed nerve entrapment. A lack of profound conduction slowing does not exclude a diagnosis of CMT-IA. Neurologic disability correlates more closely with reduced motor amplitudes (a marker of axonal loss) than with slowed conduction velocities. Substantial phenotypic and electrophysiologic variability can occur within families. There is marked slowing of conduction velocity, usually below 75% of the lower limit of normal. Since slowing is uniform in all nerves, conduction block or temporal dispersion is not seen. Slowing can also be demonstrated in the upper extremities, which may or may not be weak clinically. Velocities as low as 20–25 m/s are seen in patients with CMT1A. CMT-1B may have even slower velocities, 15 m/s or less [10].

CMT-X, an X-linked neuropathy is caused by a mutation of the gene for connexin 32 protein and is characterized by nonuniform conduction slowing. In CMT-X, conduction slowing may be "intermediate" between CMT-1 and CMT-2 (axonal form) with velocities of 30–40 ms. Furthermore, in CMT-X there can be multifocal, segmental demyelination with temporal dispersion and conduction block that simulates CIDP [10]. Females with the mutation may have modest conduction slowing, and many such patients have been misclassified as having CMT-2. CMT-X always should be considered in any inherited neuropathy without male-to-male transmission.

Conduction velocity parameters in the forearm have been used to classify inherited neuropathies to help select the genetic test for inherited neuropathies. Sensory studies are typically abnormal with low or absent amplitudes. Some secondary axonal loss is expected causing reduction in the CMAPs and concurrent disability.

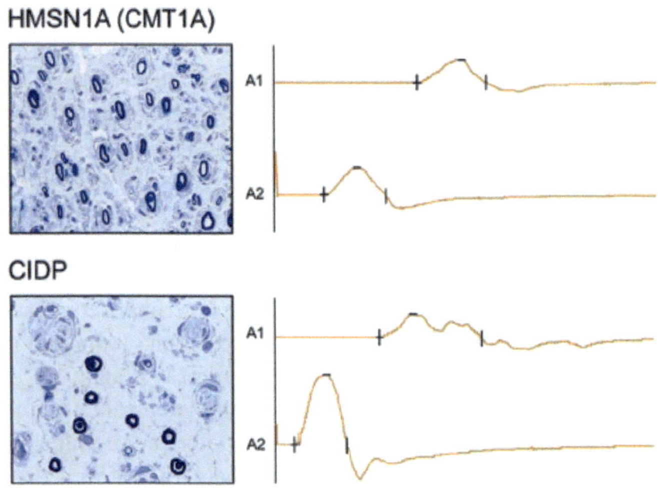

HMSN1A (CMT1A) — Left Ulnar; Recording site: Abductor digiti minimi

Stimulus site	Lat1 ms	Dur ms	Amp mV	Area mVms	Temp °C
A1: Elbow	18.7	8.9	5.2	57.4	35.0
A2: Wrist	6.3	8.2	6.3	28.2	35.0

Segment	Dist mm	Diff ms	CV m/s
Elbow-Wrist	294	12.4	24
Wrist-Abductor digiti minimi	66	6.3	---

CIDP — Left Ulnar; Recording site: Abductor digiti minimi

Stimulus site	Lat1 ms	Dur ms	Amp mV	Area mVms	Temp °C
A1: Elbow	13.9	13.5	1.975	13.56	34.5
A2: Wrist	2.6	6.8	5.626	24.10	34.3

Segment	Dist mm	Diff ms	CV m/s
Elbow-Wrist	362	11.3	32
Wrist-Abductor digiti minimi	65	2.6	---

Fig. 6.3 Inherited neuropathy vs CIDP ([10]—*used with permission*). Nerve conduction study in inherited neuropathy (hereditary motor and sensory neuropathy-HMSN1A) shows uniform demyelinating slowing, without conduction block or temporal dispersion as seen below in chronic acquired demyelinating polyradiculoneuropathy (CIDP). These electrophysiological differences can be explained by the different pathological findings in the two. Nerve biopsy in HMSN1A reveals uniform myelin lamella collagen thickening (onion bulbs) with PMP22 duplications; while in CIDP there are onion bulbs seen; the latter produces variable conduction velocities between fibers with observed dispersion and potential conduction blocks

Nerve conduction studies are helpful in early diagnosis and prognostication in patients with CMT.

Demyelinating neuropathy in the absence of dispersion and conduction block favors an inherited etiology (particularly CMT-1) over acquired etiology (e.g. CIDP), as illustrated in Fig. 6.3.

Unlike CIDP, DADS neuropathy associated with IgM MGUS is difficult to differentiate from inherited neuropathy due to their common clinical features, prominent distal weakness, and NCS showing uniform slowing with absence of temporal dispersion and conduction block. Also, the prevalence of IgM monoclonal protein in the general population increases with age >50 years and anti-MAG antibody, hence, it may be difficult to determine if an abnormal M protein is the cause of the neuropathy. NCS may allow this distinction as DADS neuropathy shows preferential distal slowing in conduction velocities, while conduction velocities are equally slow proximally and distally in inherited neuropathies. Specifically, the TLI = (1/distal motor latency [milliseconds] × (distal conduction distance [millimeters]/distal motor conduction velocity [meters/second]) less than 0.26 is seen in IgM MAG-associated DADS neuropathy whereas hereditary demyelinating neuropathies generally have a TLI >0.26.

Small fiber and autonomic testing is helpful in patients with suspected hereditary sensory and autonomic neuropathies.

Hereditary neuropathy with liability to pressure palsies (HNPP) is characterized by segmental slowing at common points of compression and by prolonged distal motor latencies. However, conduction block is found only in a minority of patients.

Electrodiagnostic Examination Techniques and Protocol for Evaluation of Polyneuropathy

The goal of electrodiagnostic studies is to confirm the presence of a polyneuropathy, assess the type of nerve fibers involved (sensory and/or motor), pattern, chronicity (and possibly tempo), pathophysiology (primarily axonal vs demyelinating) and its severity.

Sensory NCS

Antidromic versus orthodromic stimulation may be employed when performing sensory NCS. Antidromic stimulation (stimulating proximally, recording distally) generally produces a higher SNAP amplitude (due to the proximity to the recording electrodes), and tends to be less painful. However, orthodromic stimulation (stimulating distally, recording proximally) generally produces a lower SNAP amplitude, and tends to be more painful.

H-reflex response is obtained when a low submaximal stimulus of long duration is applied to a motor nerve. This selectively activates the Ia fibers. The tibial H-reflex response is an electrical correlate of the S1-mediated deep tendon reflex (ankle jerk).

Motor NCS

Motor NCS are critical in the assessment of polyneuropathy. Similar to the sensory NCS, the differences in the techniques of motor NCS are due to the use of surface vs needle stimulation electrodes and use of different recording electrodes. The different recording electrodes affect the compound muscle action potential (CMAP) amplitude. Surface recording using the "belly-tendon" method is preferred, where the active electrode is over the muscle belly and the reference electrode is over the tendon insertion point.

F-wave response, a late motor response that is recorded after a CMAP with supramaximal stimulus to a motor nerve assesses the proximal nerve segments. It travels through the entire length of the nerve including the distal segment.

Axon (A) reflex is an intermediate or late response seen during routine F-wave recording. This is a small motor response identical in latency and configuration that occurs between the M- and the F-responses. It occurs from ephaptic spread from one nerve fiber to another and proximal re-excitation at a point of inflammation and demyelination. Axon reflexes are typically seen in reinnervated nerves, especially when a submaximal stimulus is given.

Needle electrode examination (NEE) or electromyography (EMG)

NEE/EMG evaluates the extent of denervation and reinnervation in the muscles due to primary or secondary axon loss. This may be done by semi-quantitative (qualitative) or quantitative methods. Semi-quantitative technique includes assessment of insertional activity, spontaneous activity and recruitment pattern of motor units, while quantitative techniques use motor unit potential analysis, including turn–amplitude analysis.

Factors influencing NCS in the electrophysiology lab need to be considered prior to assessing the results of the NCS. These are:

1. Age:
   Sensory nerve conduction velocities (NCVs) are slower at birth and reach adult values by age 5 years. This is explained by incomplete myelination of sensory nerves that is completed by 5 years of age. Sensory NCVs start declining at the age of 20 years, by 1 m/s until 55 years. Thereafter the decline occurs by 3 m/s per decade.
2. Height:
   Increased height is associated with lower SNAP amplitudes, prolonged distal latency and slower conduction velocity. This is partly attributed to cooler distal limb temperatures and smaller axonal diameter of distal nerves in taller individuals.
3. Temperature:
   Cooler temperatures slow down nerve conduction and prolong the distal latencies, while increasing the sensory and motor amplitudes. This is due to longer duration of opening of sodium channels. To reduce the confounding effect of temperature, the limb should be appropriately warmed (hands should be at least >32 °C and feet >30 °C), if necessary.

Nerve Conduction Study

Before starting nerve conduction study, the limb to be tested is appropriately warmed to ensure the desired limb temperature as aforementioned. Sensory NCS, motor NCS, F-wave response and H-reflex responses are typically performed on one side in the lower and upper extremity. This is followed by needle electrode examination. Most commonly, surface electrodes are used to record the sensory and motor nerve action potentials.

Nerve conduction studies are generally performed on the most symptomatic extremity. Sensory nerve conduction studies in the lower extremity: sural and superficial sensory nerve studies are usually performed first. Then peroneal (fibular) motor response is recorded at the extensor digitorum brevis muscle (EDB). If reduced, then proximal studies are recorded at the tibialis anterior muscle. The tibial motor response is recorded distally at the abductor hallucis brevis (AH) muscle along with the F-wave response. In most polyneuropathies and radiculopathies (C8-T1 in the upper limb, and L5-S1 in the lower limb), F-responses are prolonged or even absent. F-response prolongation or absence may be the earliest and the only finding in GBS, as demyelination occurs at the nerve roots. Finally, the tibial/soleus H-reflex is performed. Prolonged H-reflex latency is seen in S1 radiculopathy, lumbosacral plexopathy, sciatic or tibial neuropathy or axonal polyneuropathy. It is useful in the assessment of very early polyneuropathy.

For any abnormal nerve conductions, an identical study is performed on the opposite side. Thereafter, routine distal motor and sensory studies are performed in the upper extremity. In a clinically suspected length dependent axonal polyneuropathy (pain or tingling or weakness in bilateral toes or feet or gait abnormality), upper extremity nerve conduction studies may not necessarily be performed if all the lower extremity nerve conduction studies are normal (absent sural sensory nerve action potential above the age of 75 years or absent H-reflex above 60 years is considered normal for age), and demyelinating or a pure sensory neuropathy or sensory ganglionopathy is not suspected. The routine nerve conduction studies performed in the upper extremity for clinically suspected distal symmetric length dependent axonal polyneuropathy are median motor nerve conduction study recorded at the abductor pollicis brevis muscle and ulnar motor nerve conduction study recorded at the abductor digiti minimi muscle, along with the ulnar motor F-wave response. Sensory nerves studied are median sensory at digit II, ulnar sensory at digit V and superficial radial sensory nerve at the snuff box. Radial sensory response is spared in local entrapment neuropathies such as median neuropathy at the wrist (carpal tunnel syndrome) or ulnar neuropathy at the elbow. Hence a reduced radial sensory response, with a reduced median and ulnar sensory response is likely due to an underlying axonal polyneuropathy, with reduced or absent sural and superficial peroneal (fibular) sensory responses. Reduced sensory responses in the upper extremity with an intact sural sensory response in the lower extremity suggests a demyelinating polyneuropathy. Further studies are then directed to find more evidence of a demyelinating polyneuropathy. If motor amplitudes are low, test for Lambert Eaton myasthenic syndrome by exercising muscles for 10 s, followed by a single stimulation post exercise.

If a demyelinating neuropathy (GBS, CIDP) is suspected, additional studies are performed involving the motor nerves of the upper extremity in addition to the routine motor and sensory nerves in the lower and upper extremity, along with the F-wave response and H-reflex response as discussed above. The ulnar motor nerve is stimulated at five points instead of routine three-point stimulation; namely at wrist, below elbow, above elbow, axilla and Erb's point. A more extensive search is carried out to find evidence of demyelinating neuropathy, especially so in cases where all routine distal sensory and motor responses in the lower and upper extremity are absent. In such cases it may be worthwhile to study additional proximal nerves of the upper extremity (musculocutaneous, axillary nerves) or facial motor nerves and blink responses.

Electromyography

The EMG approach is similar to the NCS approach in the assessment of axonal polyneuropathy. Needle EMG is performed first in the muscles of the lower extremity. Muscles on the contralateral side are sampled to check for symmetry or confirming a focal abnormality on the tested side. An axonal polyneuropathy is typically length-dependent and symmetric. So, the most distal muscles, extensor digitorum brevis (EDB), abductor hallucis (AH) and abductor digiti quinti pedis (ADQP) muscles will be affected early. Needling these muscles is often very painful and abnormalities seen in EMG in these intrinsic foot muscles may be otherwise seen in normal subjects as well even without an underlying polyneuropathy due to repetitive trauma from walking or running and use of foot wear. Hence if intrinsic foot muscles are needled in the evaluation of polyneuropathy, the chronic motor axon loss changes seen should be interpreted with caution. Muscles routinely studied are tibialis anterior, tibialis posterior, medial gastrocnemius, vastus lateralis, and gluteus medius. If any abnormality is seen in one muscle, a root search is also performed by sampling more proximal muscles as these will not be affected in a typical length-dependent, axonal polyneuropathy unless the polyneuropathy is severe. Hence, a proximal L5 muscle, e.g. gluteus medius and a proximal S1 muscle, e.g. biceps femoris short head or gluteus maximus may be studied routinely if tibialis anterior (distal L5 muscle) and medial gastrocnemius muscle (distal S1 muscle) shows evidence of active/ongoing or chronic motor axon loss. Check for symmetry by sampling corresponding muscles on the contralateral side.

After sampling the lower extremity, if abnormalities are found in the proximal muscles of the thigh (vastus lateralis, semitendinosus), distal muscles of the upper extremity (first dorsal interroseous, abductor digiti minimi, abductor pollicis brevis, extensor indicis proprius and flexor pollicis longus) are sampled to look for evidence of active or chronic motor axon loss. If a demyelinating polyneuropathy is the question, then proximal muscles in the upper extremity (e.g. deltoid, biceps, triceps) and proximal muscles in the lower extremity (e.g. gluteus medius and maximus) are sampled including the cervical and lumbosacral paraspinal muscles. A major role of needle EMG in a demyelinating neuropathy is to assess the amount of secondary axon loss and the severity of the axon loss. If proximal muscles are predominantly involved along with the distal muscles, this supports a non-length dependent pattern of neuropathy. As discussed earlier, proximal predominance is seen in demyelinating neuropathies (AIDP, CIDP) and porphyria (particularly with involvement of paraspinal muscles). Contralateral muscles in each limb is compared to assess for symmetry.

In mild polyneuropathies, or early polyneuropathies with normal NCS, the only abnormalities may be found in the intrinsic foot muscles. Loss of only a few axons may result in fibrillation potentials that are easily seen in EMG, but this may cause little or no appreciable change on routine distal motor and sensory nerve conduction studies. Hence in the evaluation of polyneuropathy, needle EMG is very sensitive in identifying early changes.

EMG also helps in identifying other possible differentials, superimposed radiculopathy, anterior horn cell disease or a myopathy.

Recommended Nerve Conduction Study Protocol for Polyneuropathy

Routine sensory studies

1. Sural, recording at the ankle
2. Superficial peroneal (fibular), recording at the ankle
3. Median sensory, recording at digit II
4. Ulnar sensory, recording at digit V
5. Radial sensory, recording at the snuff box

Routine motor studies

1. Peroneal (fibular), recording extensor digitorum brevis and stimulating at the ankle, below fibular neck, and lateral popliteal fossa. If low or absent responses, peroneal (fibular) motor study is performed recording the tibialis anterior and stimulating at below fibular head and lateral popliteal fossa
2. Tibial, recording abductor hallucis brevis and stimulating ankle and popliteal fossa
3. Median, recording abductor pollicis brevis and stimulating wrist and antecubital fossa
4. Ulnar, recording abductor digiti minimi and stimulating wrist, below elbow and above elbow

Late responses

1. F-wave responses: tibial and ulnar
2. Tibial/Soleus H-reflexes

Additional studies:

If clinical suspicion of asymmetry (e.g. mononeuritis multiplex), then the contralateral side is also studied.

If a demyelinating polyneuropathy is suspected, then the ulnar nerve is stimulated at five points: wrist, below and above elbow, axilla and Erb's point. Additional proximal motor or facial motor nerve with blink responses may be studied for more evidence of demyelination.

Case 1

A 58-year-old Caucasian female was seen in the neuromuscular clinic for numbness in her hands and feet that started 5 years ago. She first noticed tingling in the tips of toes and fingers on either side. After a year, she had tingling and numbness "everywhere", including her head, face, trunk, arms and legs. Such symptoms have been pretty constant over the past 4 years or so. She endorses generalized fatigue, and gait difficulty with some tendency to fall over the past 1.5 years (mostly has near-falls), no gait assistive device use reported. She is equivocal about the presence of significant muscle atrophy, but suspects some in the shin area, and possibly the forearms bilaterally. She has a past medical history of gastroesophageal reflux disease, irritable bowel disease, depression with anxiety, and hypothyroidism. Neurological examination was remarkable for focal atrophy in the intrinsic foot muscles and distal leg muscles. Strength was reduced moderately in the intrinsic muscles of hand and toe dorsiflexors and plantar flexors, however, in all other muscle groups it was intact. Deep tendon reflexes were reduced to absent throughout. Pinprick sensation was decreased around the ankles bilaterally, while other modalities of sensations were intact.

SUMMARY:

The patient's clinical history is consistent with a polyneuropathy that started 5 years ago, which is now stable. She has sensory symptoms which started distally in the fingers and toes at around the same time. This suggests that we are dealing with a some what non-length dependent polyneuropathy. A chronic non-length dependent polyneuropathy, with reduced or absent deep tendon reflexes should make one think of chronic inflammatory demyelinating polyradiculoneuropathy (CIDP). There is evidence of some motor involvement, limited to the distal muscles as well in both the upper and lower extremities. Typically, in CIDP, proximal muscles are weak too. Based on the history and physical examination, this is a chronic non-length dependent sensorimotor polyneuropathy, predominantly affecting the distal limbs. This may be a distal variant of CIDP.

Nerve conduction studies are performed on the left upper and lower extremities (see Table 6.10). The sural sensory nerve amplitude is normal while that of the median and ulnar sensory nerve is reduced. The radial sensory amplitude is also mildly reduced. This pattern is that of a reduced median and ulnar sensory amplitude with an intact sural sensory response (sural sparing). Motor studies in the lower extremity reveal >50% drop in proximal compared to distal CMAP in the peroneal (fibular) nerve recorded at the extensor digitorum brevis, and the tibial nerve recorded at the abductor hallucis muscle, consistent with a conduction block along the nerves. There is slowing of peroneal (fibular) motor conduction velocity (<70% of LLN). Tibial F-wave latency is marginally delayed (20% above ULN), with absence of the tibial H-reflex response. Looking at the upper extremity motor studies, we find a conduction block (>50% proximal/distal CMAP drop) along the left median nerve, with mild prolongation of its distal latency, and concomitant slowing of motor conduction velocity. Median F-wave latency is prolonged in the demyelinating range (>30% above ULN). The mildly increased median distal motor latency is potentially attributable to carpal tunnel syndrome. The reduction in ulnar CMAP seen with Erb's point stimulation compared to that at the axilla may suggest a true conduction block along the left ulnar motor nerve, with conduction slowing also manifested by a prolonged ulnar F-wave latency (>30% above ULN). Hence, the NCS findings are consistent with a diagnosis of CIDP with features of demyelination in at least $\geq$2 motor nerves as discussed above. The sural sparing pattern is also consistent with CIDP.

The EMG (see Table 6.10) shows at least some chronic motor axon loss changes with large amplitude, long duration, polyphasic MUAPs in

Table 6.10 Case electrodiagnostic data

Nerve conduction studies

Sensory nerve conduction

Nerve	Stimulus	Recording	B-P Amp (μV)		LatNPk (ms)		CV (m/s)		Dist (mm)		Norm B-P Amp	Norm LatNPk	Norm CV	Temp (°C)	
			L	R	L	R	L	R	L	R				L	R
Sural	Lower Leg	Lat. Malleolus	11.72		3.88		n/a		140		>4 μV	<4.6 ms	>40 m/s	30.1	
Median	Wrist	Index	**9.56**		**3.88**		n/a		130		>15 μV	<3.6 ms	>50 m/s	32.7	
Ulnar	Wrist	5th Dig	**4.80**		3.02		n/a		110		>10 μV	<3.1 ms	>50 m/s	33.5	
Radial	Thumb	Forearm	**13.46**		2.00		n/a		100		>14 μV	<2.7 ms	>50 m/s	33.8	

Motor nerve conduction

Nerve	Recording	Stimulus	B-P Amp (mV)		LatOn (ms)		CV (m/s)		Dist (mm)		Norm B-P Amp	Norm LatOn	Norm CV	Temp (°C)	
			L	R	L	R	L	R	L	R				L	R
Peroneal (fibular)	Extensor digitorum brevis (EDB)	Ankle	3.21		3.95		n/a				>2.5 mV	<6 ms	>40 m/s	30.7	
		Pop Fossa–Knee	**0.63**		18.40		**28.4**		410					30.5	
		Below Fibular Head	**0.60**		15.15		**29.5**		330					30.1	
Tibial	Abductor hallucis (AH)	Ankle	12.96		3.30		n/a				>4 mV	<6 ms	>40 m/s	30.5	
		Pop Fossa–Knee	**5.87**		15.65		**34.8**		430					30.4	
Peroneal (fibular)	Tibialis anterior (TA)	Below Fib Head	4.85		1.95		n/a				>3 mV	<4.5 ms	>40 m/s	31.2	
		Pop Fossa–Knee	3.76		6.05		**24.4**		100					31.0	
Median	Abductor pollicis brevis (APB)	Wrist	8.25		**4.10**		n/a		50		>6 mV	<4 ms	>50 m/s	33.9	
		Elbow	**3.54**		9.95		**44.4**		260					33.8	
		Ulnar/wrist	NR		NR		n/a							33.6	
		Ulnar/elbow	NR		NR		n/a							33.6	
Ulnar	Abductor digiti minimi (ADM)	Wrist	**6.59**		2.65		n/a		50		>7 mV	<3.1 ms	>50 m/s	33.9	
		Below elbow	**4.03**		7.30		**49.5**		230					33.9	
		Above elbow	**2.89**		9.50		**48.2**		330					33.9	
		Axilla	**2.21**		13.55		**48.6**		530					33.9	
		Erb's	**0.30**		17.50		**49.2**		730					33.6	
		Post exercise	**6.73**		2.55		n/a							33.8	

(continued)

Table 6.10 (continued)

F-wave side-to-side comparison table

Nerve	Stimulus	Recording	F-Waves Lat (ms) L	F-Waves Lat (ms) R
Tibial/AH	Ankle	AH	**68.50**	
Median/APB	Wrist	APB	**49.30**	
Ulnar/ADM	Wrist	ADM	**42.00**	

H-Reflex summary table

Nerve	Stimulus	Recording	Side	M-Wave Lat (ms)	M-Wave Amp (mV)	H-Wave Lat (ms)	H-Wave Amp (mV)
Tibial	Pop Fossa	Soleus	Left	5.9 ms	8.5 mV	**NR**	

Electromyography

Needle EMG summary

Side	Muscle	IInsertional Activity	Fibrillation Potentials	Positive Sharp Wave Potentials	Fasciculation Potentials	Other	Number	Recruitment	Duration	Duration	Amplitude	Amplitude	Polyphasia	Polyphasia	Description
L	1st Dorsal Interosseous	Norm	0	0	0		Norm	Full		Norm		Norm		Norm	NC
	APB	Norm	0	0	0		1–	Mod-V		Norm		Norm		Norm	NC
	Flex.Pollicis Longus	Norm	0	0	0		1–	Mod		Norm		Norm	Few	1+	NC
	Extensor Indicis	Norm	0	0	0		Norm	Full		Norm		Norm		Norm	NC
	Pronator Teres	Norm	0	0	0		1–	Mod		Norm		Norm		Norm	NC
	Biceps Brachii	Norm	0	0	0		2–	Mod		Norm		Norm		Norm	NC
	Triceps-Lateral Head	Norm	0	0	0		1–	Mod		Norm		Norm		Norm	NC
	Deltoid, Middle Head	Norm	0	0	0		1–	Mod		Norm		Norm		Norm	NC
	Cervical paraspinal (Low)	Norm	0	0	0		2–	Mod		Norm		Norm		Norm	NC

	Abductor Hallucis	Norm	0	0	0		3–	Mod-V	Many	1+	Some	1+		Norm	NC
	EDB	Norm	1+	0	0		SMU	Rapid	All	1+	All	1+	All	1+	NC
	Flexor Digitorum Longus	Norm	0	0	0		2–	Mod-V	Some	1+	Some	1+	Some	1+	NC
	Tibialis Anterior	Norm	0	0	0		2–	Mod-V	Some	1+	Some	1+	Some	1+	NC
	Gastrocnemius, Medial Head	1+	0	0	0		2–	Mod	Some	1+	Few	1+	Few	1+	NC
	Rectus Femoris	Norm	0	0	0		1–	Mod	Few	1+		Norm	Few	1+	NC
	Tensor Fascia Lata	Norm	0	0	0		1–	Mod	Few	1+	Few	1+		Norm	NC
	Lumbar paraspinal (Low)	Norm	0	0	0		2–	Mod		Norm		Norm		Norm	NC

the lower extremity muscles. There are almost no active/ongoing motor axon loss changes seen in the form of fibrillation or positive sharp wave potentials. Accordingly, the secondary axon loss is relatively mild and this is a predominantly demyelinating polyneuropathy.

IMPRESSION:

There is electrodiagnostic evidence of an acquired, chronic, non-length dependent sensorimotor predominantly demyelinating polyneuropathy, compatible with a diagnosis of chronic inflammatory demyelinating polyneuropathy (CIDP).

Case 2

A 50-year-old left-handed Caucasian female with a history of scoliosis (s/p corrective surgery at childhood), presented to the neuromuscular clinic for evaluation of progressive generalized weakness. She reported having numbness and tingling in her feet over the past ~3 years with imbalance and a couple of falls in the past year. She also noted muscle twitching in her arms at night and cramps in her hands and feet. Her mother had similar symptoms with weakness in the legs, and she died at the age of 76 years. No other family member had similar problems.

Examination was notable for thinning of distal legs and ankles and high arched feet on both sides. She was also noted to have bilateral foot drop which she recollected as being there since her childhood, requiring bracing. Muscle strength was moderately reduced proximally in the upper and lower extremity. Distally, her finger abductors and ankle dorsiflexors were much weaker. Her ankle reflex was absent, knee jerks were trace and the deep tendon reflexes in the upper extremity were very reduced. Sensations were markedly reduced to all modalities in a glove-stocking pattern. No palpable nerves were appreciated.

SUMMARY:

This is a 50-year-old lady with chronic/longstanding foot drop and at least moderate generalized weakness with sensory involvement and reduced to absent deep tendon reflexes. Clinically, this suggests a polyneuropathy with both motor and sensory involvement, predominating distally, causing bilateral foot drop and hand weakness. The pattern of sensory involvement is also distal/length-dependent. Some clinical features such as atrophy of the distal leg muscles, high arched feet and scoliosis with onset likely in the childhood and a positive family history suggest an underlying hereditary polyneuropathy. The mother being affected points towards a possible autosomal dominant inherited polyneuropathy. It is not uncommon in longstanding inherited polyneuropathy for patients to present late at this age (in 40s–50s) with worsening of their symptoms. Clinically distal areflexia/reduced reflexes globally also suggest an underlying demyelinating polyneuropathy.

Looking at the nerve conduction studies (see Table 6.11), the sensory responses are all absent in the lower and the upper extremities. This strongly supports a diagnosis of polyneuropathy. Motor nerve conduction studies reveal an absent peroneal (fibular) motor response recorded at the extensor digitorum brevis muscle and a severely reduced motor amplitude when recorded from the tibialis anterior muscle, together with a markedly reduced motor conduction velocity (15.9 m/s) and prolonged distal latency (7.15 ms) which is in the demyelinating range. The tibial motor response is also absent. In the upper extremity, the median motor response recorded at the abductor pollicis brevis muscle reveals a markedly prolonged distal latency (13.55 ms), and reduced motor conduction velocity (17.1 m/s) with a severely reduced motor amplitude. The ulnar motor response is absent. Such markedly reduced motor conduction velocities and prolonged distal motor latencies, without evidence of acquired demyelination (conduction block and temporal dispersion) are suggestive of an inherited demyelinating polyneuropathy. Needle electrode examination is most notable for widespread marked chronic (without significant active/ongoing) motor axon loss changes in the lower and upper limbs, with features generally conforming to a length-dependent patern as well (see Table 6.11).

IMPRESSION:

There is electrodiagnostic evidence of a chronic, length-dependent, sensorimotor, predominantly demyelinating poly neuropathy, with marked secondary chronic axon loss features. Findings compatible with a hereditary etiology

Table 6.11 Case electrodiagnostic data

Nerve conduction study

Sensory nerve conduction

Nerve	Stimulus	Recording	B-P Amp (μV)		LatNPk (ms)		CV (m/s)		Dist (mm)		Norm B-P Amp	Norm LatNPk	Norm CV	Temp (°C)	
			L	R	L	R	L	R	L	R				L	R
Sural	Lower leg	Lat. Malleolus	**NR**		**NR**		n/a		140		>4 μV	<4.6 ms	>40 m/s	32.1	
Superficial peroneal (fibular)	lower leg	Ankle	**NR**		**NR**		n/a		100		>4 μV	<4.6 ms		32.0	
Median	Wrist	Index	**NR**		**NR**		n/a		130		>15 μV	<3.6 ms	>50 m/s	33.6	
Ulnar	Wrist	5th Dig	**NR**		**NR**		n/a		110		>10 μV	<3.1 ms	>50 m/s	33.7	
Radial	Thumb	Forearm	**NR**		**NR**		n/a		100		>14 μV	<2.7 ms	>50m/s	33.7	

Motor nerve conduction

Nerve	Recording	Stimulus	B-P Amp (mV)		LatOn (ms)		CV (m/s)		Dist (mm)		Norm B-P Amp	Norm LatOn	Norm CV	Temp (°C)	
			L	R	L	R	L	R	L	R				L	R
Peroneal (fibular)	Extensor digitorum brevis (EDB)	Ankle	**NR**		**NR**		n/a				>2.5 mV	<6 ms	>40 m/s	31.7	
		Pop Foss–Knee	**NR**		**NR**		n/a							31.6	
Tibial	Abductor hallucis (AH)	Ankle	**NR**		**NR**		n/a				>4 mV	<6 ms	>40 m/s	31.6	
Peroneal (fibular)	Tibialis anterior (TA)	Below Fib Head	**0.95**		**7.15**		n/a				>3 mV	<4.5 ms	>40 m/s	31.4	
		Pop Fossa–Knee	**0.75**		13.45		**15.9**		100					31.5	
Median	Abductor pollicis brevis (APB)	Wrist	**0.39**		**13.55**		n/a		50		>6 mV	<4 ms	>50 m/s	34.0	
		Elbow	**0.35**		27.60		**17.1**		240					34.0	
		Post exercise	**0.37**		**15.40**		n/a							33.9	
Ulnar	Abductor digiti minimi (ADM)	Wrist	**NR**		**NR**		n/a		50		>7 mV	<3.1 ms	>50 m/s	34.0	

H-Reflex summary table

Nerve	Stimulus	Recording	Side	M-Wave		H-Wave	
				Lat (ms)	Amp (mV)	Lat (ms)	Amp (mV)
	Pop Fossa	Soleus	Left	**NR**		**NR**	

(continued)

Table 6.11 (continued)

Electromyography															
Needle EMG summary															
Side	Muscle	Ins Act.	Fib	PW	Fasc	Other	Number	Recruit	Dur	Dur	Amp	Amp	Poly	Poly.	Descript
L	1st Dorsal Interosseous	Norm	0	1+	0		2–	Mod-R	Many	1+	Many	1+	Some	1+	NC
	APB	Norm	0	0	0		3–	Rapid	Many	1+	Many	1+	Some	2+	NC
	Flexor Pollicis Longus	Norm	0	0	0		3–	Rapid	Many	1+	Many	1+	Some	1+	NC
	Pronator Teres	Norm	0	0	0		2–	Mod-R	Some	1+	Few	1+	Some	1+	NC
	Extensor Digitorum	Norm	0	0	0		2–	Mod-V	Some	1+	Some	1+	Some	1+	NC
	Biceps Brachii	Norm	0	0	0		2–	Rapid	Some	1+	Some	1+		Norm	NC
	Triceps-Lateral Head	Norm	0	0	0		1–	Mod	Few	1+	Few	1+	Some	1+	NC
	Deltoid, Middle Head	Norm	0	0	0		1–	Mod-R	Some	1+	Some	1+		Norm	NC
	Abductor Hallucis	1–	0	0	0			None							Atrophy
	EDB	1–	0	0	0			None							Atrophy
	Flexor Digitorum Longus	1–	0	0	0		SMU	Rapid	All	1+	All	1+		Norm	NC
	Tibialis Anterior	1–	0	0	0		3–	Rapid	Most	2+		1+		Norm	NC
	Gastrocnemius, Medial Head	1–	0	0+	0		SMU	Rapid	All	2+	All	1+		Norm	NC
	Rectus Femoris	1–	0	0	0		3–	Rapid	All	2+	All	1+	Many	2+	NC
	Tensor Fascia Lata	Norm	0	0	0		3–	Rapid	Most	1+	Most	1+		Norm	NC

include uniform conduction velocity slowing, as well as conspicuous absence of conduction blocks and/or temporal dispersion of M-wave configurations.

References

1. Hanewinckel R, Drenthen J, van Oijen M, Hofman A, van Doorn PA, Ikram MA. Prevalence of polyneuropathy in the general middle-aged and elderly population. Neurology. 2016;87(18):1892–8.
2. Prior R, Van Helleputte L, Benoy V, Van Den Bosch L. Defective axonal transport: a common pathological mechanism in inherited and acquired peripheral neuropathies. Neurobiol Dis. 2017;105:300–20.
3. Asbury AK, Arnason BG, Adams RD. The inflammatory lesion in idiopathic polyneuritis. Its role in pathogenesis. Medicine (Baltimore). 1969;48(3):173–215.
4. Uncini A, Kuwabara S. Nodopathies of the peripheral nerve: an emerging concept. J Neurol Neurosurg Psychiatry. 2015;86(11):1186–95.
5. Barohn RJ, Amato AA. Pattern-recognition approach to neuropathy and neuronopathy. Neurol Clin. 2013;31(2):343–61.
6. Apfel SC, Asbury AK, Bril V, Burns TM, Campbell JN, Chalk CH, et al. Positive neuropathic sensory symptoms as endpoints in diabetic neuropathy trials. J Neurol Sci. 2001;189(1–2):3–5.
7. Terkelsen AJ, Karlsson P, Lauria G, Freeman R, Finnerup NB, Jensen TS. The diagnostic challenge of small fibre neuropathy: clinical presentations, evaluations, and causes. Lancet Neurol. 2017;16(11):934–44.
8. Pasnoor M, Dimachkie MM, Kluding P, Barohn RJ. Diabetic neuropathy. Part 1: Overview and symmetric phenotypes. Neurol Clin. 2013;31(2):425–45.
9. Callaghan BC, Cheng HT, Stables CL, Smith AL, Feldman EL. Diabetic neuropathy: clinical manifestations and current treatments. Lancet Neurol. 2012;11(6):521–34.
10. Klein CJ, Duan X, Shy ME. Inherited neuropathies: clinical overview and update. Muscle Nerve. 2013;48(4):604–22.
11. Katz JS, Saperstein DS, Gronseth G, Amato AA, Barohn RJ. Distal acquired demyelinating symmetric neuropathy. Neurology. 2000;54(3):615–20.
12. Kissel JT, Mendell JR. Neuropathies associated with monoclonal gammopathies. Neuromuscul Disord. 1996;6(1):3–18.
13. Willison HJ, Jacobs BC, van Doorn PA. Guillain-Barre syndrome. Lancet. 2016;388(10045):717–27.
14. Peltier AC, Donofrio PD. Chronic inflammatory demyelinating polyradiculoneuropathy: from bench to bedside. Semin Neurol. 2012;32(3):187–95.
15. Rison RA, Beydoun SR. Paraproteinemic neuropathy: a practical review. BMC Neurol. 2016;16:13.
16. Cho SC, Siao-Tick-Chong P, So YT. Clinical utility of electrodiagnostic consultation in suspected polyneuropathy. Muscle Nerve. 2004;30(5):659–62.
17. Gilliatt RW, Sears TA. Sensory nerve action potentials in patients with peripheral nerve lesions. J Neurol Neurosurg Psychiatry. 1958;21(2):109–18.
18. Barnett C, Perkins BA, Ngo M, Todorov S, Leung R, Bril V. Sural-to-radial amplitude ratio in the diagnosis of diabetic sensorimotor polyneuropathy. Muscle Nerve. 2012;45(1):126–7.
19. Rutkove SB, Kothari MJ, Raynor EM, Levy ML, Fadic R, Nardin RA. Sural/radial amplitude ratio in the diagnosis of mild axonal polyneuropathy. Muscle Nerve. 1997;20(10):1236–41.
20. Reeves ML, Seigler DE, Ayyar DR, Skyler JS. Medial plantar sensory response. Sensitive indicator of peripheral nerve dysfunction in patients with diabetes mellitus. Am J Med. 1984;76(5):842–6.
21. Killian JM, Foreman PJ. Clinical utility of dorsal sural nerve conduction studies. Muscle Nerve. 2001;24(6):817–20.
22. Kural MA, Karlsson P, Pugdahl K, Isak B, Fuglsang-Frederiksen A, Tankisi H. Diagnostic utility of distal nerve conduction studies and sural near-nerve needle recording in polyneuropathy. Clin Neurophysiol. 2017;128(9):1590–5.
23. Tavee JO, Polston D, Zhou L, Shields RW, Butler RS, Levin KH. Sural sensory nerve action potential, epidermal nerve fiber density, and quantitative sudomotor axon reflex in the healthy elderly. Muscle Nerve. 2014;49(4):564–9.
24. Lo YL, Xu LQ, Leoh TH, Dan YF, Tan YE, Nurjannah S, et al. Superficial peroneal sensory and sural nerve conduction studies in peripheral neuropathy. J Clin Neurosci. 2006;13(5):547–9.
25. AANEM policy statement on electrodiagnosis for distal symmetric polyneuropathy. Muscle Nerve. 2018;57(2):337–9.
26. Dyck PJ, Albers JW, Andersen H, Arezzo JC, Biessels GJ, Bril V, et al. Diabetic polyneuropathies: update on research definition, diagnostic criteria and estimation of severity. Diabetes Metab Res Rev. 2011;27(7):620–8.
27. Huang CR, Chang WN, Tsai NW, Lu CH. Serial nerve conduction studies in vitamin B12 deficiency-associated polyneuropathy. Neurol Sci. 2011;32(1):183–6.
28. Gordon PH, Wilbourn AJ. Early electrodiagnostic findings in Guillain-Barre syndrome. Arch Neurol. 2001;58(6):913–7.
29. Kuwabara S, Ogawara K, Mizobuchi K, Koga M, Mori M, Hattori T, et al. Isolated absence of F-waves and proximal axonal dysfunction in Guillain-Barre syndrome with antiganglioside antibodies. J Neurol Neurosurg Psychiatry. 2000;68(2):191–5.
30. Bromberg MB, Albers JW. Patterns of sensory nerve conduction abnormalities in demyelinating and axonal peripheral nerve disorders. Muscle Nerve. 1993;16(3):262–6.

31. Al-Shekhlee A, Hachwi RN, Preston DC, Katirji B. New criteria for early electrodiagnosis of acute inflammatory demyelinating polyneuropathy. Muscle Nerve. 2005;32(1):66–72.
32. Derksen A, Ritter C, Athar P, Kieseier BC, Mancias P, Hartung HP, et al. Sural sparing pattern discriminates Guillain-Barre syndrome from its mimics. Muscle Nerve. 2014;50(5):780–4.
33. Umapathi T, Li Z, Verma K, Yuki N. Sural-sparing is seen in axonal as well as demyelinating forms of Guillain-Barre syndrome. Clin Neurophysiol. 2015;126(12):2376–80.
34. Hiew FL, Rajabally YA. Sural sparing in Guillain-Barre syndrome subtypes: a reappraisal with historical and recent definitions. Clin Neurophysiol. 2016;127(2):1683–8.
35. Ye Y, Zhu D, Liu L, Wang K, Huang K, Hou C. Electrophysiological measurement at Erb's point during the early stage of Guillain-Barre syndrome. J Clin Neurosci. 2014;21(5):786–9.
36. Albers JW, Donofrio PD, McGonagle TK. Sequential electrodiagnostic abnormalities in acute inflammatory demyelinating polyradiculoneuropathy. Muscle Nerve. 1985;8(6):528–39.
37. Hiraga A, Kuwabara S, Ogawara K, Misawa S, Kanesaka T, Koga M, et al. Patterns and serial changes in electrodiagnostic abnormalities of axonal Guillain-Barre syndrome. Neurology. 2005;64(5):856–60.
38. Uncini A, Kuwabara S. Electrodiagnostic criteria for Guillain-Barre syndrome: a critical revision and the need for an update. Clin Neurophysiol. 2012;123(8):1487–95.
39. Rajabally YA, Durand MC, Mitchell J, Orlikowski D, Nicolas G. Electrophysiological diagnosis of Guillain-Barre syndrome subtype: could a single study suffice? J Neurol Neurosurg Psychiatry. 2015;86(1):115–9.
40. Umapathi T, Tan EY, Kokubun N, Verma K, Yuki N. Non-demyelinating, reversible conduction failure in Fisher syndrome and related disorders. J Neurol Neurosurg Psychiatry. 2012;83(9):941–8.
41. Caliandro P, Stalberg E, Padua L. In response to "Correlations of nerve conduction measures in axonal and demyelinating polyneuropathies". Clin Neurophysiol. 2008;119(7):1694–5.
42. Tankisi H, Pugdahl K, Johnsen B, Fuglsang-Frederiksen A. Correlations of nerve conduction measures in axonal and demyelinating polyneuropathies. Clin Neurophysiol. 2007;118(11):2383–92.
43. Olney RK, Lewis RA, Putnam TD, Campellone JV Jr. American Association of Electrodiagnostic M. Consensus criteria for the diagnosis of multifocal motor neuropathy. Muscle Nerve. 2003;27(1):117–21.
44. Caliandro P, Stalberg E, La Torre G, Padua L. Sensitivity of conventional motor nerve conduction examination in detecting patchy demyelination: a simulated model. Clin Neurophysiol. 2007;118(7):1577–85.
45. Bromberg MB, Franssen H. Practical rules for electrodiagnosis in suspected multifocal motor neuropathy. J Clin Neuromuscul Dis. 2015;16(3):141–52.
46. Joint Task Force of the E, the PNS. European Federation of Neurological Societies/Peripheral Nerve Society guideline on management of multifocal motor neuropathy. Report of a joint task force of the European Federation of Neurological Societies and the Peripheral Nerve Society – first revision. J Peripher Nerv Syst. 2010;15(4):295–301.
47. Research criteria for diagnosis of chronic inflammatory demyelinating polyneuropathy (CIDP). Report from an Ad Hoc Subcommittee of the American Academy of Neurology AIDS Task Force. Neurology. 1991;41(5):617–618.
48. Van den Bergh PY, Hadden RD, Bouche P, Cornblath DR, Hahn A, Illa I, et al. European Federation of Neurological Societies/Peripheral Nerve Society guideline on management of chronic inflammatory demyelinating polyradiculoneuropathy: report of a joint task force of the European Federation of Neurological Societies and the Peripheral Nerve Society – first revision. Eur J Neurol. 2010;17(3):356–63.
49. Thaisetthawatkul P, Logigian EL, Herrmann DN. Dispersion of the distal compound muscle action potential as a diagnostic criterion for chronic inflammatory demyelinating polyneuropathy. Neurology. 2002;59(10):1526–32.
50. Katz JS, Wolfe GI, Bryan WW, Jackson CE, Amato AA, Barohn RJ. Electrophysiologic findings in multifocal motor neuropathy. Neurology. 1997;48(3):700–7.
51. Katz JS, Barohn RJ, Kojan S, Wolfe GI, Nations SP, Saperstein DS, et al. Axonal multifocal motor neuropathy without conduction block or other features of demyelination. Neurology. 2002;58(4):615–20.
52. Trojaborg W, Hays AP, van den Berg L, Younger DS, Latov N. Motor conduction parameters in neuropathies associated with anti-MAG antibodies and other types of demyelinating and axonal neuropathies. Muscle Nerve. 1995;18(7):730–5.

7 Brachial Plexopathies

Mark A. Ferrante

Introduction

The brachial plexus originates from the spinal cord and advances in an inferolateral direction into the axilla. Its preterminal and terminal nerves supply innervation to the entire upper extremity, as well as to most of the shoulder region. Of the somatic plexuses (cervical, brachial, lumbosacral, coccygeal), brachial plexopathies are most frequent. The incidence of brachial plexopathies exceeds the combined incidences of the others. There are two major reasons for this vulnerability: its greater susceptibility to trauma and its vulnerability to disorders involving adjacent structures (e.g., blood vessels, lymph nodes, and the apex of the lung). Its greater susceptibility to trauma (especially closed traction) reflects its large size, its superficial position, and its location between two highly mobile structures (the neck and arm) (Fig. 7.1) [1–4].

Although the brachial plexus is the largest and most complex structure of the peripheral nervous system (PNS), most brachial plexus disorders are regional [5, 6]. Consequently, regional electrodiagnostic (EDX) assessment is usually sufficient for lesion localization and characterization. Because the sensory axons traversing each brachial plexus region are known [7], the sensory nerve conduction studies (NCS) are particularly important for localizing postganglionic, axon loss lesions. The motor NCS are particularly important for defining lesion severity (and determining the underlying pathology, which is usually axon loss with brachial plexus lesions). The needle EMG study refines the NCS findings, provides temporal information about the lesion (e.g., the rate of progression), defines the degree of reinnervation, and contributes to clinical management and prognosis of the patient. All of these concepts are reviewed in most EDX textbooks [4].

Because the brachial plexus is such a large structure, its complete assessment would be time and cost prohibitive (never mind the unnecessary patient discomfort). Fortunately, most of its disorders involve only a single region of the brachial plexus and, hence, can be easily characterized without a large EDX study [5, 6]. Because most of the disorders affecting the brachial plexus are site specific (Table 7.1), once the lesion has been localized, the differential diagnosis is significantly reduced. In fact, not infrequently, the EDX findings dictate the underlying disorder.

The regional approach used in our EMG laboratories has been previously reviewed [4, 5, 6] and is reviewed again below. This approach requires a thorough understanding of general and regional brachial plexus anatomy. For this reason, this chapter begins with a detailed review of

M. A. Ferrante (✉)
University of Tennessee Health Science Center, Memphis, TN, USA
e-mail: mferrant@uthsc.edu

N. Galvez-Jimenez et al. (eds.), *Electrodiagnostic Medicine*,
https://doi.org/10.1007/978-3-030-74997-2_7

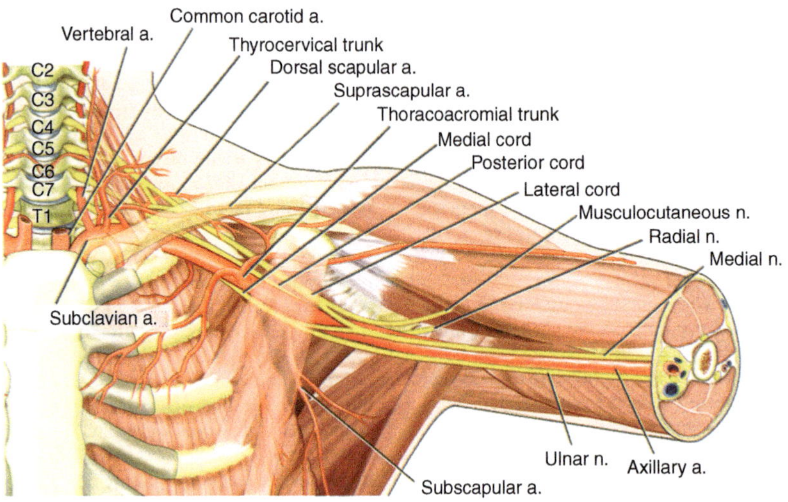

Fig. 7.1 The brachial plexus. The large size, superficial location, and position between the neck and arm contributes to the susceptibility of the brachial plexus to trauma. Diseases of adjacent structures (lung apex, blood vessels, lymph nodes, and clavicle) also render it vulnerable. Reprinted with permission from Ferrante MA. Brachial plexopathies: classification, causes, and consequences. Muscle Nerve 2004;30:547–568

Table 7.1 Site-Specific Brachial Plexus Disorders

Supraclavicular Plexus			
Upper Plexus		**Lower Plexus**	
Classic postoperative paralysis		True neurogenic TOS	
Burner syndrome		Post-median sternotomy brachial plexopathy	
Rucksack paralysis		Pancoast syndrome	
Infraclavicular plexus			
Lateral cord		**Medial cord**	
Axillary lymph node irradiation		Clavicular fractures (midshaft)	
Terminal nerves			
Median terminal nerve	Musculocutaneous terminal nerve	Radial terminal nerve	Axillary terminal nerve
Medial brachial fascial compartment syndrome	Procedures near the coracoid process (iatrogenic)	Crutch palsies	Proximal humeral fractures
			Glenohumeral dislocations

Data compiled from [5, 6]

brachial plexus anatomy, followed by a discussion of the EDX assessment of each of its regions. The chapter concludes with 8 EDX exercises that demonstrate the regional approach outlined in this chapter. We have been using this approach for approximately 25 years and have found it to be quite reliable. Nevertheless, the reader should be aware that there are other, equally effective, approaches.

General Anatomy of the Brachial Plexus

The brachial plexus is composed of connective tissue and neural tissue in an approximate 2 to 1 ratio [8, 9, 10]. The axons composing the brachial plexus—which number in excess of 100,000—represent cytoplasmic extensions from the cell bodies of motor, sensory, and autonomic neurons [11].

The cell bodies of the motor neurons are also referred to as *anterior horn cells* (AHCs) because of their location within the anterior horn of the spinal cord. Each motor neuron gives off a single, peripherally-directed axon. The cell bodies of the sensory neurons are also termed *dorsal root ganglion* (DRG) cells because of their location within DRG. The DRG are located within the intervertebral foramina of the spinal column. Each sensory neuron gives off two axons, one peripherally-directed and one centrally-directed. The centrally-projecting axon is not studied by EDX testing (only the peripherally-directed sensory axon and the DRG cell are assessed by EDX testing). This explains why the sensory responses are spared with radiculopathies (pre-ganglionic lesion).

After the axons exit the spinal column and advance peripherally, they collect into groups called roots. In its traditional formation, the brachial plexus is composed of the C5 through T1 roots. As these collections of axons advance, they repeatedly come together and separate, each time exchanging axons such that each element of the brachial plexus has a unique composition. This intermingling among the various axonal collections produces the brachial plexus elements: 5 roots (C5 through T1), 3 trunks (upper, middle, and lower), 6 divisions (3 anterior and 3 posterior), 3 cords (lateral, posterior, and medial), and 5 terminal nerves (Fig. 7.2). In addition to the 5 terminal nerves, a number of preterminal nerves are given off more proximally. The preterminal and terminal nerves then advance and innervate their end-organs (e.g., muscle fibers and sensory receptors). Because each element is composed of unique sensory and motor axons, disorders affecting individual brachial plexus elements result in localizing clinical features [4].

Distally, once the motor axon enters the muscle that it innervates, it arborizes into a large number of terminal branches, each of which innervates a single muscle fiber via a single neuromuscular junction (NMJ). The number of muscle fibers innervated by a motor axon, termed the *innervation ratio*, is fairly constant for each skeletal muscle. In general, it is inversely proportional to the degree of control required over that muscle. For example, the innervation ratio of the gastrocnemius muscle (an example of a muscle that performs courser movements, such as ankle plantar flexion to peek over a wall) is much greater than that of the first dorsal interosseous muscle (a muscle for which finer control is required, such as during piano playing). Individual sensory axons do not arborize distally; each innervates a single sensory receptor [4].

Elemental Anatomy of the Brachial Plexus

Roots

After the motor and sensory axons exit the spinal cord, they coalesce, forming ventral and dorsal *rootlets*, respectively. The ventral and dorsal rootlets coalesce to form the primary ventral and dorsal roots. The latter traverse the intraspinal canal and enter the intervertebral foramina. Within the intervertebral foramina and just beyond the DRG, the ventral and dorsal roots fuse to form a *mixed spinal nerve*. The adjective, *mixed*, reflects the fact that these elements contain both motor and sensory axons. Just outside the intervertebral foramen, each mixed spinal nerve passes through a gutter located along the superior aspect of the correlating transverse process. Within these gutters, the C5 and C6 mixed spinal nerves are anchored to the transverse process by connective tissue, whereas the C8 and T1 mixed spinal nerves are not. The connective tissue anchoring of the C7 mixed spinal nerve varies. This difference in connective tissue anchoring accounts for the lesion sites occurring with brachial plexus traction injuries. Because traction injuries tend to disrupt axons at their anchorage points, traction involving C5- and C6-derived axons tends to produce ruptures of the C5 and C6 mixed spinal nerves, whereas traction involving the C8- and T1-derived axons tends to produce root avulsion injuries (due to their spinal cord anchorage site). The effect of traction on C7-derived axons depends on their degree of anchorage to the transverse process.

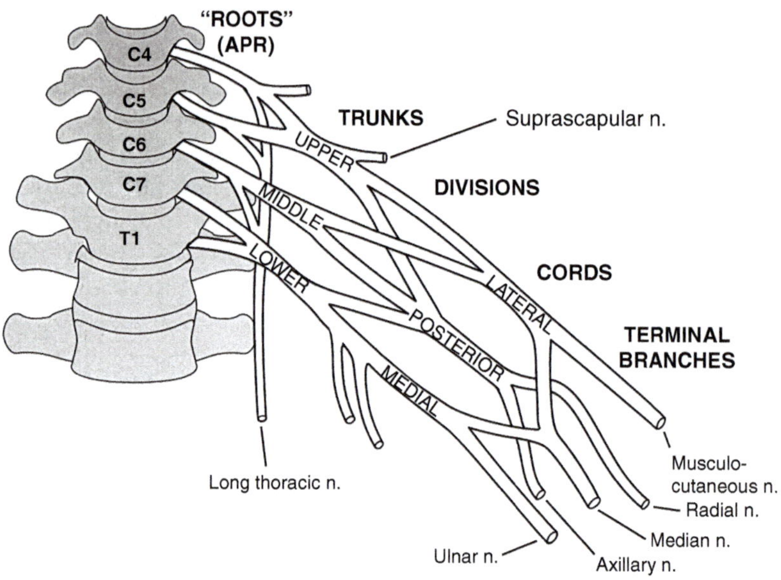

Fig. 7.2 The elements of the brachial plexus. The brachial plexus is composed of 5 roots, 3 trunks, 6 divisions, 3 cords, 5 terminal nerves, and a number of preterminal nerves, two of which are shown in the figure. Reprinted with permission from Ferrante MA, Tsao BE. Brachial plexopathies. In: Katirji B, Kaminski HJ, Ruff RL, editors. Neuromuscular Disorders in Clinical Practice. 2nd ed. New York: Springer;2013:1029–1062).

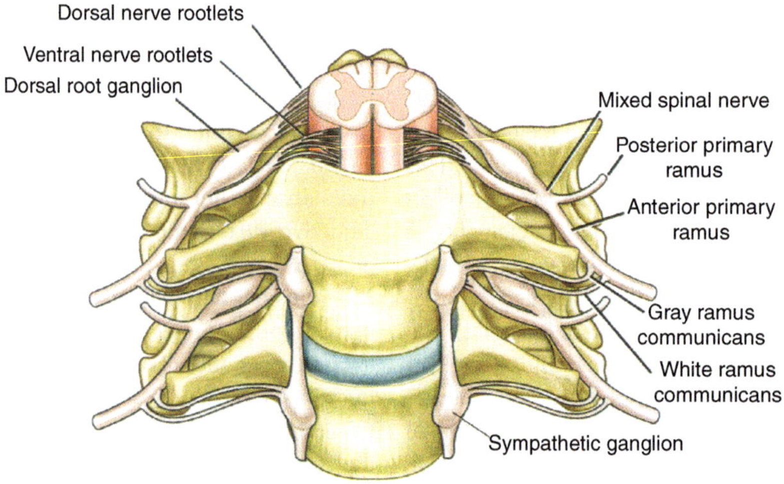

Fig. 7.3 The relationship between the vertebral column and the root elements of the brachial plexus. The dorsal and ventral roots fuse to a mixed spinal nerve, which subsequently divides into a directed branch (the posterior primary ramus) and an anteriorly directed branch (the anterior primary ramus). Reprinted with permission from Ferrante MA. Brachial plexopathies: classification, causes, and consequences. Muscle Nerve 2004;30:547–568

Almost immediately after passing over the transverse process, the mixed spinal nerve divides into a posteriorly directed branch (termed the *posterior primary ramus*) and an anteriorly directed branch (termed the *anterior primary ramus* [APR]) (Fig. 7.3). The C5 through T1 APR exit between the anterior and middle scalene muscles and give off several nerve branches. Some of these APR-derived nerve branches innervate muscles (scalene and longus colli muscles; C5 through C8), whereas others join to form distinct preterminal nerves (the phrenic nerve [C3 through C5 APR], the dorsal scapular nerve [C4 and C5 APR], and the long thoracic nerve [C5 through C7 APR]).

Although most anatomists define the APR elements as the roots of the brachial plexus, most brachial plexologists and other clinicians dealing extensively with brachial plexus disorders consider the roots of the brachial plexus to include all of the structures proximal to the trunk elements. Thus, using this expanded definition, the roots have intraspinal canal, intraforaminal, and extraforaminal segments. Because of the greater clinical utility of the expanded definition, it is used throughout the remainder of this chapter.

Preganglionic sympathetic axons also exit at the level of the APR (from the C5 through T1 APR). These fibers are myelinated and termed *white rami communicantes* (to reflect the whitish hue imparted by the myelination). The preganglionic sympathetic axons enter the nearby sympathetic ganglia. Postganglionic sympathetic axons, which are unmyelinated and, hence, termed *gray rami communicantes*, exit the sympathetic ganglia and enter the C5 through T1 mixed spinal nerves. Because the preganglionic sympathetic fibers supplying the head and neck traverse the C8 and T1 roots on their way to the inferior cervical ganglion, a Horner syndrome may be observed with lesions affecting either of these two roots. Thus, the presence of a Horner syndrome has localizing value.

It is important to realize that there are variations in the root composition of the brachial plexus. As stated above, traditionally, the brachial plexus is composed of axons derived from the C5 through T1 spinal cord segments (i.e., the C5 through T1 roots). Nerve root variations include *expansions* (contributions from C4 or T2) and 1-segment *vertical shifts*. The brachial plexus is termed *prefixed* whenever the C4 contribution is large and the T1 contribution is small, whereas it is termed *postfixed* whenever the C5 contribution is small and the T2 contribution is large [12]. Importantly, because these changes do not affect the internal organization of the brachial plexus, the clinical and EDX features that permit lesion localization are unaffected [7]. In other words, the clinical and EDX features of an upper trunk lesion are identical regardless of whether the upper trunk is composed of C5- and C6-dereived axons (traditional), C4- and C5-derived axons (prefixed), or C6- and C7-derived axons (postfixed).

Trunks

The 3 trunk elements, which are named for their relationship to each other (upper, middle, and lower), are formed from the APR near the lateral borders of the scalene muscles. The C5 and C6 APR join to form the upper trunk, the C7 APR continues as the middle trunk, and the C8 and T1 APR coalesce to form the lower trunk. Due to their superficial course, as they pass through the posterior cervical triangle, these elements are susceptible to trauma. Because the lower trunk lies adjacent to the apex of the lung and also passes next to the subclavian artery, disorders involving either of these two structures may secondarily affect the lower trunk. Trunk anomalies are uncommon. In one report, the middle trunk was of customary formation in 100%, the upper trunk in 90%, and the lower trunk in 95% [13]. The trunk level of the brachial plexus gives off 2 preterminal nerves—the suprascapular nerve (almost immediately upon its formation from the C5 and C6 roots) and the nerve to subclavius. Each trunk terminates by dividing into two divisions, one anterior and one posterior.

Divisions

When the body is oriented in the anatomic position, the division elements lie behind the middle one-third of the clavicle (i.e., they are retroclavicular). The anterior divisions primarily innervate flexors, whereas the posterior divisions primarily innervate extensors. Consequently, the anterior and posterior divisions are not always similar in caliber. The anterior and posterior divisions of the upper trunk are similar in size, the posterior division of the middle trunk is larger (because the C7 root primarily innervates extensor muscles), and the anterior division of the lower trunk is larger (because the C8 and T1 roots primarily innervate flexors) [10]. For this reason, it is at the divisional level of the brachial plexus that the segmental nature of the roots and trunks is lost. In general, there are no preterminal nerves given off at the divisional level.

Cords

The three posterior divisions join to form the posterior cord, the anterior divisions of the upper and middle trunk join to form the lateral cord, and the anterior division of the lower trunk continues as the medial cord. The cords, which are named for their relationship to the axillary artery, are the longest elements of the brachial plexus and are located in the proximal portion of the axilla, near the axillary lymph node chain.

The lateral cord contains C6 and C7 sensory axons and C5 through C7 motor axons. It gives off the lateral pectoral preterminal nerve and the musculocutaneous terminal nerve before terminating as the lateral head of the median nerve. The posterior cord contains C5 through C7 sensory axons and C5 through C8 motor axons. The presence of T1-derived axons occurs less than 5% of the time [9, 14]. The posterior cord gives off the thoracodorsal, the upper subscapular, and the lower subscapular preterminal nerves before terminating as the axillary and radial terminal nerves. The posterior cord provides the sensory axons of the C5 dermatome (via the upper and lower lateral brachial cutaneous nerve branches of the axillary and radial nerves, respectively). The medial cord contains C8 and T1 sensory axons and C8 and T1 motor axons. It gives off the medial pectoral, medial brachial cutaneous, and medial antebrachial cutaneous (MABC) preterminal nerves and the ulnar terminal nerve before terminating as the medial head of the median nerve. The latter joins the lateral head of the median nerve to form the median terminal nerve.

Terminal Nerves

The 5 terminal nerves—musculocutaneous, axillary, median, ulnar, and radial—are located in the distal portion of the axilla. Each originates from a single cord element, except for the median nerve, which originates from two cord elements (medial and lateral cords). Once they exit the axilla, they are no longer considered to be part of the brachial plexus and, at that point, are considered to be upper extremity nerves [5]. Thus, for example, the median nerve axons are termed the terminal median nerve while in the distal axilla and the median nerve after they exit the axilla.

Regional Anatomy of the Brachial Plexus

Because of its large size and the fact that most brachial plexus disorders involve only a portion of the brachial plexus, it is helpful to divide the brachial plexus into smaller regions. These smaller regions of the brachial plexus are also termed plexuses. The initial division is based on the anatomical relationship between the clavicle and the brachial plexus (when the upper extremity is placed in the anatomical position). This relationship allows the brachial plexus to be divided into 3 plexuses: (1) the supraclavicular plexus, which contains the roots and trunks; (2) the retroclavicular plexus, which contains the divisions; and (3) the infraclavicular plexus, which contains the cords and terminal nerves. Not only does this classification have anatomical significance, but it also has clinical significance—supraclavicular plexopathies have a higher incidence and tend to be more severe. Supraclavicular plexopathies tend to be more severe because a greater force is required to produce them and because they are more frequently associated with closed traction injuries [4, 11, 15].

The supraclavicular plexus is further divided into 3 even smaller plexuses. These, like the trunk elements, are named for their relationship to each other: (1) the upper plexus, which consists of the upper trunk and the C5 and C6 roots; (2) the middle plexus, which consists of the middle trunk and the C7 root; and (3) the lower plexus, which consists of the lower trunk and the C8 and T1 roots (Fig. 7.4). This subdivision also has clinical significance—upper plexopathies have the highest incidence, tend to occur in isolation, and most commonly follow trauma (especially closed traction) [7, 16]. For a number of reasons, upper plexopathies tend to be less severe: (1) they are closer to the sensory receptors and muscle fibers that they supply; (2) they are more frequently extraforaminal, which increases the potential for

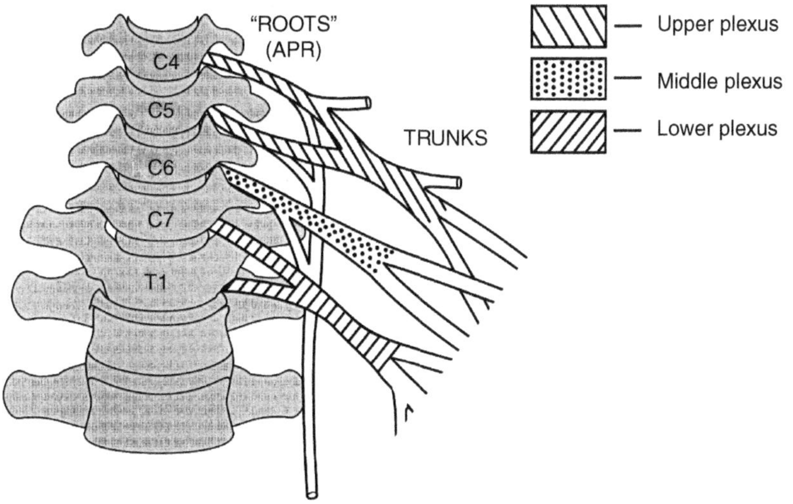

Fig. 7.4 The divisions of the supraclavicular plexus. The supraclavicular plexus is composed of three smaller plexuses, the upper plexus (upper trunk and C5 and C6 roots), the middle plexus (middle trunk and C7 root), and the lower plexus (lower trunk and C8 and T1 roots). Reprinted with permission from Ferrante MA, Tsao BE. Brachial plexopathies. In: Katirji B, Kaminski HJ, Ruff RL, editors. Neuromuscular Disorders in Clinical Practice. 2nd ed. New York: Springer; 2013:1029–1062)

ANTERIOR PRIIMARY RAMI	**C5**	**C6**	**C7**	**C8**	**T1**
Proximal Nerve Innervation					
Rhomboid major/minor (dorsal scapular)					
Supraspinatus (suprascapular)					
Infraspinatus (suprascapular)					
Deltoid (axillary)					
Biceps (musculocutaneous)					
Brachialis (musculocutaneous)					
Radial Nerve Innervation					
Brachioradialis					
Triceps					
Anconeus					
Extensor carpi radialis					
Extensor pollicis brevis					
Extensor indicis					
Median Nerve Innervation					
Pronator teres					
Flexor carpi radialis					
Flexor pollicis longus					
Pronator quadratus					
Abductor pollicis brevis					
Ulnar Nerve					
Flexor carpi ulnaris					
flexor digitorum profundus (D4,D5)					
Abductor digiti minimi					
Adductor polllicis					
First dorsal interosseous					
POSTERIOR PRIMARY RAMI					
Cervical paraspinal muscles					
High thoracic paraspinal muscles					

predominant contribution
sometimes significant contribution
minor contribution

surgical intervention; and (3) the lesions affecting the upper plexus more frequently have a demyelinating component [11]. Middle plexopathies most commonly follow trauma. Lower plexopathies, which have the lowest incidence, also most commonly follow trauma [16]. Due to their location between the upper plexus and the lower plexus, lesions involving the middle plexus rarely occur in isolation. In one large series (n = 417), an isolated middle plexopathy was only observed once [7]. The infraclavicular plexus is not further subdivided. Moreover, infraclavicular plexus lesions do not show significant regional differences in incidence, severity, prognosis, or lesion type [3, 5, 6].

When the brachial plexus is considered regionally (i.e., upper plexus, middle plexus, lower plexus, lateral cord, posterior cord, and medial cord regions), it facilitates communication between physicians, allowing them to regionally localize brachial plexus lesions in the setting of examination limitations (pain; cognitive changes; higher priority injuries), as well as prior to diagnostic testing (e.g., EDX testing).

Brachial Plexus Assessment

Clinical Assessment

Although the focus of this chapter is on the EDX assessment of the brachial plexus, because the EDX examination is an extension of the clinical examination, clinical assessment is briefly discussed. As always, clinical assessment of the brachial plexus begins with a detailed history of the circumstances surrounding the onset of the problem and is followed by a thorough neurological examination. In addition to a detailed assessment of the brachial plexus, the neurological examination must include cervical spinal cord, cervical plexus, spinal accessory nerve, and phrenic nerve assessments. Features of dysautonomia (e.g., sudomotor or vasomotor abnormalities; Horner syndrome) and of proximal brachial plexus involvement (dorsal scapular, phrenic, or long thoracic nerve involvement; Horner syndrome) are sought.

On examination, because most brachial plexopathies involve axon disruption, "negative" deficits, such as weakness and numbness, are expected. Supraclavicular plexopathies produce deficits suggesting involvement of one or more roots, whereas infraclavicular plexopathies produce deficits suggesting involvement of one or more terminal nerves.

With upper plexopathies, the sensory loss involves the C5 and C6 dermatomes, including the lateral aspects of the arm and forearm and the dorsolateral aspect of the hand. The weakness affects the C5 and C6 myotomes, including external humeral rotation, shoulder abduction, forearm flexion and supination, forearm pronation, and forearm extension. Depending on how proximal the lesion is located, weakness involving muscles innervated by the dorsal scapular nerve or the long thoracic nerve may be present. The biceps and brachioradialis muscle stretch reflexes (MSRs) may be hypoactive. With middle plexopathies, the sensory loss and weakness follows a C7 distribution (forearm extension and pronation, radial wrist extension and flexion, and, to a lesser degree, finger extension) and the triceps MSR may be hypoactive. With lower plexopathies, the sensory loss involves the C8 and T1 dermatomes, including the medial aspects of the arm, forearm, and hand; and the weakness involves muscles of the C8 and T1 myotomes. The finger flexor reflex may be affected and, depending on how proximal the lesion lies, a Horner syndrome may be present.

Electrodiagnostic Assessment

Through EDX testing, brachial plexus lesions are localized and characterized. Regarding the latter, their pathophysiology, severity, rate of progression, and degree of reinnervation are defined. These features, in turn, contribute to patient management and treatment, as well as lesion prognostication.

As stated earlier, because most lesions involve only one region of the brachial plexus, a regional approach to lesion localization can be utilized. Because each region of the brachial plexus contains a unique combination of sensory and motor axons, lesions involving a single region of the brachial plexus produce unique clinical and EDX features. The EDX abnormalities reflect the sensory and motor axons traversing each region.

The responses collected during EDX testing represent compound electrical potentials, which are composed of either nerve fiber action potentials or muscle fiber actions potentials. The sensory response represents all of the sensory nerve fiber action potentials elicited by nerve stimulation of the sensory axons. It is also referred to as a compound sensory nerve fiber action potential (SNAP). The motor response represents all of the muscle fiber action potentials elicited by nerve stimulation of the motor axons. It is also referred to as a compound muscle action potential (CMAP). The motor unit action potentials (MUAPs) collected during the needle EMG study represents the muscle fiber action potentials of individual motor units.

The motor axons traversing a specific brachial plexus region determine the CMAP and muscle domains of that region, whereas the sensory axons traversing it dictate its SNAP domain. The unique SNAP, CMAP, and muscle domains of each brachial plexus element are provided (Table 7.2). These domains are easily derived and permit the course of the motor axons through the brachial plexus to be determined.

Table 7.2 The SNAP, CMAP, and Muscle Domains of the Brachial Plexus Regions

	The Upper Plexus	
SNAP Domain^	**CMAP Domain**	**Muscle Domain^^**
LABC (100%)	Musculocutaneous-biceps	Levator scapulae
Median-D1 (100%)	Axillary-deltoid	Rhomboids
S-radial (60%)	Radial-EDC	Serratus anterior
Median-D2 (20%)		Supraspinatus, infraspinatus
Median-D3 (10%)		Biceps, brachialis
		Deltoid, teres minor
		Brachioradialis
		Triceps
		Extensor carpi radialis
		Pronator teres
		Flexor carpi radialis
	The Middle Plexus	
SNAP domain	**CMAP domain**	**Muscle domain**
Median-D2 (80%)		Pronator teres
Median-D3 (70%)		Flexor carpi radialis
S-radial (40%)		Triceps
		Anconeus
		Extensor carpi radialis
		Extensor digitorum communis
		Serratus anterior
	The Lower plexus	
SNAP domain	**CMAP Domain**	**Muscle domain**
Ulnar-D5 (100%)	Ulnar-ADM	Abductor pollicis brevis
MABC (100%)	Ulnar-FDI	Flexor pollicis longus
Median-D3 (20%)	Median-APB	Extensor indicis proprius
	Radial-EI	Extensor pollicis brevis
		Extensor carpi ulnaris
		First dorsal interosseous
		Abductor digiti minimi

(continued)

Table 7.2 (continued)

The Upper Plexus		
SNAP Domain^	**CMAP Domain**	**Muscle Domain^^**
		Adductor pollicis
		Flexor digitorum profundus-4,5
		Flexor carpi ulnaris
	The Lateral Cord	
SNAP domain	**CMAP domain**	**Muscle domain**
LABC (100%)	Musculocutaneous (biceps)	Biceps
Median-D1 (100%)		Brachialis
Median-D2 (100%)		Pronator teres
Median-D3 (80%)		Flexor carpi radialis
	The posterior cord	
SNAP domain	**CMAP domain**	**Muscle domain**
S-radial (100%)	Axillary-deltoid	Latissimus dorsi
	Radial-ED	Deltoid; teres minor
	Radial-EI	Triceps; anconeus
		Brachioradialis
		Extensor carpi radialis
		Extensor digitorum communis
		Extensor pollicis brevis
		Extensor carpi ulnaris
		Extensor indicis proprius
	The Medial Cord	
SNAP Domain	**CMAP Domain**	**Muscle Domain**
Ulnar-D5 (100%)	Ulnar-ADM	Abductor pollicis brevis
MABC (100%)	Ulnar-FDI	Opponens pollicis
Median-D3 (20%)	Median-APB	Flexor pollicis longus
		First dorsal interosseous
		Abductor digiti minimi
		Adductor pollicis
		Flexor digitorum profundus-4,5
		Flexor carpi ulnaris

^ The percentages shown in parentheses represent the frequency with which the sensory responses were abnormal for a specific brachial plexus region. These data imply their dorsal root ganglia (DRG) derivation frequency and permit pathways to be generated.

^^The muscle domains provided are not exhaustive but, rather, reflect those muscles considered most helpful by the author

The Motor Axon Pathways

The motor axons contained within each brachial plexus element can be determined by knowing the root innervation of a muscle. Myotomal charts indicate the root innervations of the muscles and most any anatomy book indicates the specific nerve innervation of the muscles. In this manner, the CMAP and muscle domains for each element are determined. For example, because the deltoid muscle is C5,6-axillary nerve-innervated, the axons innervating the deltoid muscle begin in the C5 and C6 spinal cord segments and end in the axillary nerve. Thus, they must traverse the C5 and C6 roots, the upper plexus, and the posterior cord to reach the axillary nerve. Consequently, the Axillary-Deltoid motor NCS and the needle EMG of the deltoid muscle both assess all of these brachial plexus elements. In summary, the CMAP domain and the muscle domain of a particular brachial plexus region is determined by the motor axons traversing it.

The Sensory Axon Pathways

Similarly, knowledge of the cell bodies of origin of the sensory axons traversing the brachial plexus allows SNAP domains to be determined for each brachial plexus element. In 1995, the DRG of origin for the sensory axons subserving the various upper extremity sensory NCS were reported [7]. This information allowed the SNAP domains for each brachial plexus region, as well as the brachial plexus pathways of the sensory axons subserving each sensory NCS to be determined (Figs. 7.5, 7.6, 7.7, 7.8, 7.9, 7.10, and 7.11). These sensory fiber pathways are discussed here.

The sensory axons composing the lateral antebrachial cutaneous (LABC) nerve emanate from the C6 DRG [7]. Because the LABC nerve is a branch of the musculocutaneous nerve, it can be concluded that the sensory axons must traverse the brachial plexus from the C6 DRG to the musculocutaneous terminal nerve. Consequently, a low amplitude LABC response may be associated with an axon loss lesion involving the C6 DRG, the C6 APR, the upper trunk, the lateral cord, or the musculocutaneous terminal nerve (as well as the musculocutaneous nerve and the LABC nerve).

The median sensory axons innervating the thumb also derive from the C6 DRG [7]. Consequently, a low amplitude median sensory response recording from the thumb (the Median-D1 response) may be observed with an

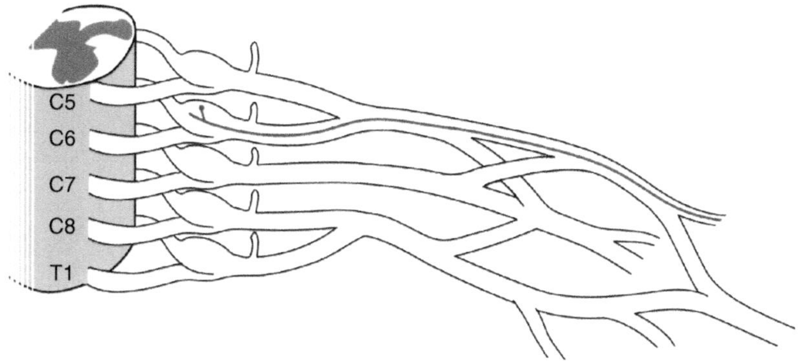

Fig. 7.5 The brachial plexus regions assessed by the lateral antebrachial cutaneous nerve conduction study. Reprinted with permission from Ferrante MA. Comprehensive Electromyography: With Clinical Correlations and Case Studies. New York, Cambridge University Press; 2018

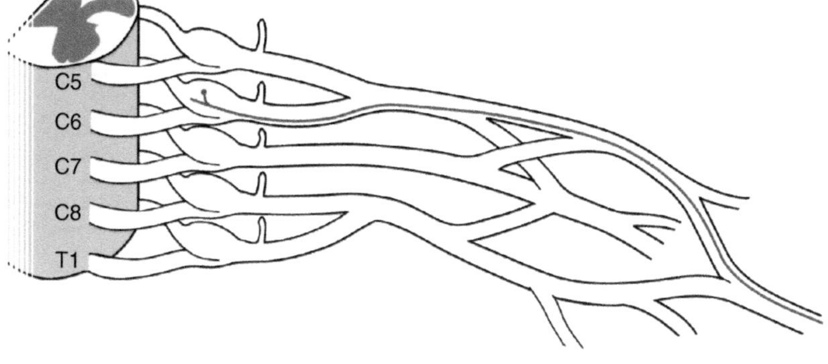

Fig. 7.6 The brachial plexus regions assessed by the median sensory nerve conduction study, recording from the thumb. Reprinted with permission from Ferrante MA. Comprehensive Electromyography: With Clinical Correlations and Case Studies. New York, Cambridge University Press; 2018

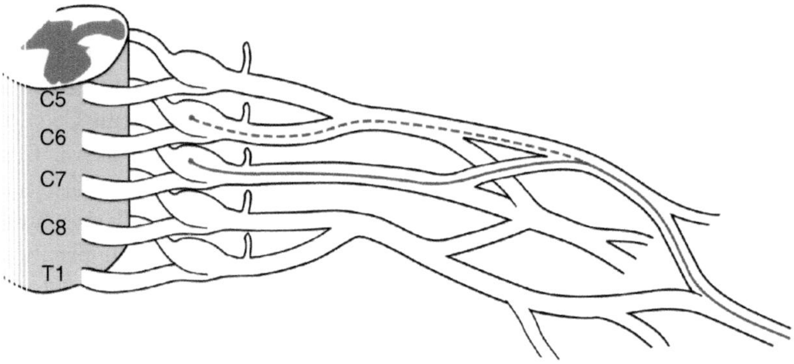

Fig. 7.7 The brachial plexus regions assessed by the median sensory nerve conduction study, recording from the index finger. Reprinted with permission from Ferrante MA. Comprehensive Electromyography: With Clinical Correlations and Case Studies. New York, Cambridge University Press; 2018

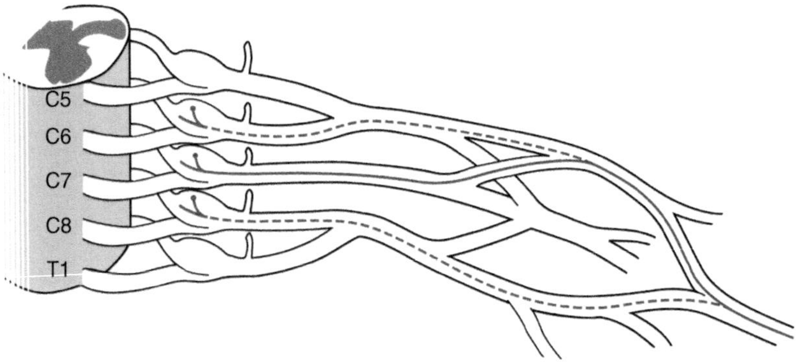

Fig. 7.8 The brachial plexus regions assessed by the median sensory nerve conduction study, recording from the middle finger. Reprinted with permission from Ferrante MA. Comprehensive Electromyography: With Clinical Correlations and Case Studies. New York, Cambridge University Press; 2018

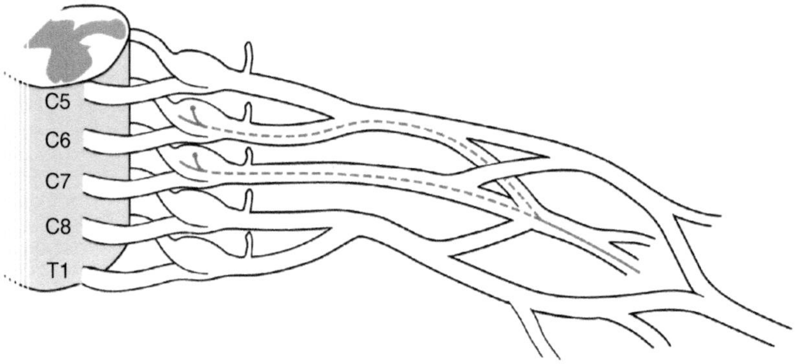

Fig. 7.9 The brachial plexus regions assessed by the superficial radial nerve conduction study. Reprinted with permission from Ferrante MA. Comprehensive Electromyography: With Clinical Correlations and Case Studies. New York, Cambridge University Press; 2018

axon loss lesion involving the C6 DRG, the C6 APR, the upper trunk, the lateral cord, or the median terminal nerve (as well as the median nerve or its sensory branches to the thumb).

The median sensory axons innervating the index finger derive from the C6 DRG and the C7 DRG. In our study, upper plexus lesions affected this response (the Median-D2 response) 20% of the time, mixed upper and middle plexus lesions

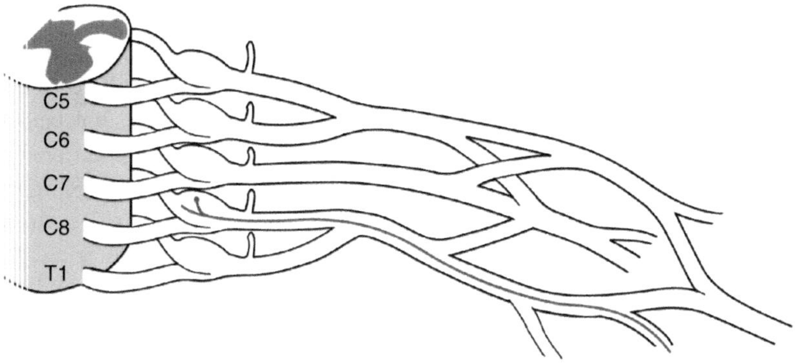

Fig. 7.10 The brachial plexus regions assessed by the ulnar sensory nerve conduction study, recording from the little finger. Reprinted with permission from Ferrante MA. Comprehensive Electromyography: With Clinical Correlations and Case Studies. New York, Cambridge University Press; 2018

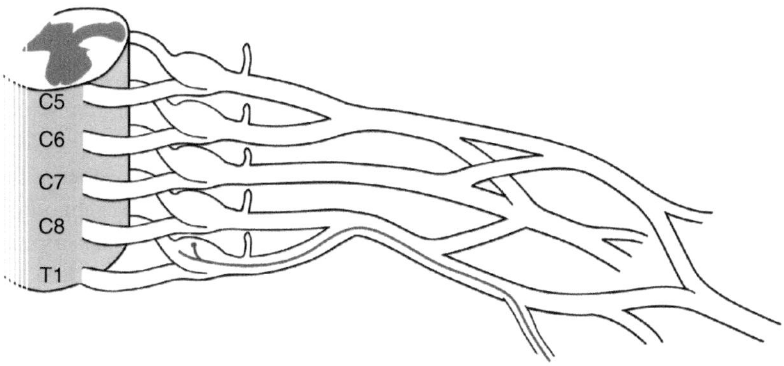

Fig. 7.11 The brachial plexus regions assessed by the medial antebrachial cutaneous nerve conduction study. Reprinted with permission from Ferrante MA. Comprehensive Electromyography: With Clinical Correlations and Case Studies. New York, Cambridge University Press; 2018

affected this response 80% of the time, and lower plexus lesions did not affect it [7]. This indicates that it is not an ideal study to assess the upper plexus, as it is only affected in 20% of cases. Consequently, a low amplitude Median-D2 response may be observed with an axon loss lesion involving the C6 or C7 DRG, the C6 or C7 APR, the upper or middle trunk, the lateral cord, or the median terminal nerve (as well as the median nerve and its sensory branches to the index finger).

The median sensory axons innervating the long finger derive from the C6 DRG, the C7 DRG, and the C8 DRG. In our study, upper plexus lesions affected this response (the Median-D3 response) 10% of the time, mixed upper and middle plexus lesions affected this response 70% of the time, and lower plexus lesions affected it 20% of the time [7]. Consequently, a low amplitude Median-D3 response may be observed with an axon loss lesion involving the C6, C7, or C8 DRG; the C6, C7, or C8 APR; the upper, middle or lower trunk; the lateral or medial cord; or the median terminal nerve (as well as the median nerve and its sensory branches to digit 3). Because of its wide distribution, we infrequently use this sensory NCS.

The sensory axons composing the superficial radial nerve derive from the C6 DRG and the C7 DRG. In our study, upper plexus lesions affected this response (the S-Radial response) 60% of the time, mixed middle and lower plexus lesions affected this response 40% of the time, and lower plexus lesions did not affect it [7]. Consequently, a low amplitude superficial radial response may be observed with an axon loss lesion involving the C6 or C7 DRG, the C6 or C7 APR, the upper or middle trunk, the posterior cord, or the radial terminal nerve (as well as the radial nerve or the superficial radial nerve).

The sensory axons composing the ulnar nerve derive from the C8 DRG [7, 17, 18]. Consequently, a low amplitude ulnar response recording from the fifth digit (the Ulnar-D5 response) may be observed with an axon loss lesion involving the C8 DRG, the C8 APR, the lower trunk, the medial cord, or the ulnar terminal nerve of the brachial plexus (as well as the ulnar nerve or its sensory branches to the fifth digit).

The sensory axons composing the MABC nerve derive from the T1 DRG [7, 9, 17, 18, 19, 20]. Consequently, a low amplitude MABC response may be observed with an axon loss lesion involving the T1 DRG, the T1 APR, the lower trunk, the medial cord, or the MABC preterminal (as well as the MABC nerve more distally).

EDX Assessment of the Brachial Plexus by Region

Introductory Comments

Because of its large size, EDX assessment of the entire brachial plexus is impractical and, fortunately, almost always unnecessary because of the regional involvement of most brachial plexus disorders. Because each part of the EDX examination—sensory NCS, motor NCS, and needle EMG—provides information not provided by the other two parts, each part is mandatory. Although the order of their performance varies among EMG laboratories, we prefer to begin all EDX assessments with the sensory NCS because they are more sensitive to axon loss lesions involving postganglionic PNS structures (i.e., plexus and nerve lesions) than are the motor NCS.

Based on the SNAP domains of the various brachial plexus elements discussed earlier, the pattern of sensory response abnormalities identifies the brachial plexus region involved. In our EMG laboratories, we begin all upper extremity EDX assessments with three screening sensory NCS –Median-D2, S-Radial, and Ulnar-D5. In our EMG laboratories, additional sensory NCS are added to these three screening studies based on the referral diagnosis (i.e., to address those considerations of the referring physician) and based on the clinical features identified prior to the start of the EDX study. From that point forward, the EDX study findings dictate the subsequent studies (i.e., the EDX study is independent).

Localizing Strategies

Sensory NCS

Based on the results of the screening sensory NCS, additional sensory NCS are added. Whenever the amplitude value of the S-Radial or the Median-D2 response is abnormal (both assess C6 or C7 DRG-derived sensory axons), we add the LABC and the Median-D1 NCS because both of these NCS only assess sensory axons derived from the C6 DRG. Thus, their involvement or sparing shortens the list of potential lesion localization sites. For example, whenever the Median-D2 response is reduced in amplitude and either of the other two added sensory NCS is abnormal, the lesion localizes to the lateral cord or upper plexus (i.e., the median nerve and middle plexus sites are excluded). Whenever the S-Radial response is reduced in amplitude and either of the two added sensory NCS is abnormal, the lesion localizes to the upper plexus (the radial nerve and posterior cord localization sites are excluded).

Whenever the amplitude value of the Ulnar-D5 response is abnormal, the MABC NCS is added and, when it is also abnormal, the lesion localizes to the medial cord or lower plexus (i.e., the ulnar nerve localization site is excluded). The amplitudes of the Ulnar-D5 and MABC responses should also be compared to each other. When one of them is affected out of proportion to the other, it may represent a lesion proximal to the lower trunk (e.g., an APR level lesion).

Motor NCS

Following the sensory NCS, the screening motor NCS—Median-APB and Ulnar-ADM—are performed. To these two studies, additional motor NCS are added based on the localizing information derived from the sensory NCS. The motor NCS are important in determining the underlying pathology and, especially, for establishing lesion severity. The severity is determined by comparing the amplitude or negative area under the curve value of the distal response to that of the contralateral, asymptomatic side. The lure to grade lesion severity based on fibrillation potential quantity must be resisted because it is more dependent on the timing of the study than on lesion severity. Following reinnervation via collateral sprouting, the motor responses underestimate lesion severity. To avoid missing significant motor axon loss, the needle EMG study is always performed, even when the motor responses are normal.

The Needle EMG

The needle EMG portion of the EDX study is performed last. Because of the high innervation ratio of most skeletal muscles, the needle EMG can show large numbers of fibrillation potentials when there is no motor NCS evidence (or clinical evidence) of motor axon loss. Thus, it is the most sensitive portion of the EDX examination for identifying motor axon loss. For this same reason, the needle EMG study can demonstrate nerve continuity when there are no perceptible movements clinically.

The needle EMG study not only confirms the impression of the sensory and motor NCS, it further localizes and characterizes the lesion (e.g., its temporal characteristics). It further refines the location of the lesion in those areas of the plexus where distinctions are possible (i.e., where nerve elements join or separate from each other). For example, when the sensory and motor NCS localize the lesion to either the medial cord or the lower plexus, involvement of the extensor indicis muscle on needle EMG eliminates the possibility of a medial cord localization. As another example, the needle EMG study can also differentiate a C6 APR lesion from one involving the upper trunk. The relationship between the acute and chronic changes indicates the rate of progression of the disorder. For example, the presence of large numbers of high amplitude fibrillation potentials indicates a relatively recent process, whereas the presence of long duration MUAPs implies chronicity. Regarding the rate of progression, the presence of large quantities of high amplitude fibrillation potentials (typically with low and medium amplitude fibrillation potentials) and chronic MUAP changes implies that the underlying disorder is rapidly progressive (e.g., amyotrophic lateral sclerosis), whereas the presence of sparse, low amplitude fibrillation potentials and large quantities of long duration, high amplitude MUAPs implies that the underlying disorder is more slowly progressive (e.g., Kennedy disease).

The needle EMG may also disclose focal demyelinating conduction block lesions that are located proximal to the motor NCS performed. For example, whenever the median motor NCS is normal but the needle EMG study of the abductor pollicis brevis muscle shows neurogenic recruitment, a demyelinating conduction block must be present proximal to the elbow stimulation site. This is true because neurogenic recruitment only occurs when APs are unable to traverse the lesion (demyelinating conduction block or axon loss). Because the distal motor response is normal, axon loss is excluded. Thus, the only possibility is demyelinating conduction block. Because the distal motor response is normal, it cannot be distal to the distal stimulation site. Because the distal and proximal motor responses were normal, it cannot be between these two stimulation sites. Consequently, it must be located proximal to the proximal stimulation site.

NCS Assessment of Specific Brachial Plexus Regions

The Upper Plexus

The upper plexus contains motor and sensory axons derived from the C5 and C6 spinal cord segments. The SNAP, CMAP, and muscle domains of the upper plexus are provided (Table 7.2). There are no reliable sensory NCS that assess the C5 sensory fibers of the upper plexus. The LABC and Median-D1 NCS assess its C6 fibers. These two sensory NCS show good correlation with each other and are typically both involved to similar degrees [7]. The S-Radial sensory NCS and the Median-D2 sensory NCS also assess the C6 fibers of the upper plexus, but less frequently (60% and 20%, respectively) [7]. On motor NCS testing, the screening motor NCS are of no value in the EDX assessment of this region. Thus, additional motor NCS must be added whenever an upper plexus lesion is suspected. Both the Musculocutaneous-Biceps NCS and the Axillary-Deltoid NCS assess the upper plexus in its entirety (i.e., the C5 root, the C6 root, and the upper trunk). On needle EMG, additional shoulder girdle and upper extremity muscles are added because the screening muscles do not assess the upper plexus very well.

On sensory NCS, when involved, the S-Radial NCS helps differentiate an upper plexus lesion (involved) from a lateral cord lesion (spared). On motor NCS, the Musculocutaneous-Biceps response may be affected (depending on lesion severity), whereas the Axillary-Deltoid response is spared. When involved, muscles innervated by the dorsal scapular, long thoracic, and suprascapular nerve are helpful in differentiating an APR-level lesion (involved) from an upper trunk lesion (spared). When involved, the C5,6-radial axons are helpful in differentiating upper plexus lesions (involved) from lateral cord lesions (spared).

The Middle Plexus

The middle plexus contains motor and sensory axons derived from the C7 spinal cord segment. The SNAP, CMAP, and muscle domains of the middle plexus are provided (Table 7.2). On sensory NCS testing, the Median-D2, Median-D3, and S-Radial NCS assess its fibers about 80%, 70%, and 40% of the time [7]. There is no motor NCS that solely assesses the middle plexus. We usually perform the Radial-EDC NCS. Because of the overlap between the muscle domains of the upper plexus, the middle plexus, and the lower plexus, a more extensive needle EMG assessment is typically required when localizing lesions to the middle plexus.

On sensory NCS, middle trunk lesions are differentiated from posterior cord lesions by the Median-D2 and the Median-D3 sensory NCS (both are spared with posterior cord lesions). On needle EMG testing, the C6,7-median nerve innervated muscles (e.g., pronator teres; flexor carpi radialis) are helpful to differentiate middle plexus lesions (involved) from posterior cord lesions (spared). The C5,6-radial and the C5,6-axillary nerve-innervated muscles are also helpful in differentiating a middle plexus lesion (spared) from a posterior cord lesion (involved).

The Lower Plexus

The lower plexus contains motor and sensory axons derived from the C8 and T1 spinal cord segments. The SNAP, CMAP, and muscle domains of the lower plexus are provided (Table 7.2). On sensory NCS testing, the Ulnar-D5 and MABC NCS assess its C8 and T1 sensory axons, respectively. With lower trunk involvement, both responses are affected, whereas with C8 APR lesions, the Ulnar-D5 response is affected in isolation and with T1 APR lesions, the MABC response is affected in isolation. On motor NCS, the Ulnar-ADM, the Ulnar-FDI, the Median-APB, and the Radial-EI NCS assess the lower plexus. These four motor NCS assess the C8 and T1 APR to differing degrees—the Radial-EI NCS assesses solely the C8 APR, the Ulnar-ADM and Ulnar-FDI NCS assess the C8 and T1 more equally, and the Median-APB NCS assesses the T1 APR to a greater extent than the C8 APR [7, 17, 18]. On needle EMG, C8-radial and C8-T1 ulnar and median nerve-innervated muscles are utilized.

When involved, the C8-radial axons (Radial-EI motor NCS; extensor indicis and extensor pollicis brevis muscles on needle EMG study) are especially useful in differentiating a lower plexus lesion (involved) from a medial cord lesion (spared).

The Lateral Cord

The lateral cord contains motor axons derived from the C5 through C7 spinal cord segments and sensory axons derived from the C6 and C7 spinal cord segments. The SNAP, CMAP, and muscle domains of the lateral cord are provided (Table 7.2). On sensory NCS testing, the LABC, the Median-D1, the Median-D2, and the Median-D3 NCS assess its fibers 100%, 100%, and 100%, and 80% of the time [7]. In general, with lateral cord lesions, the LABC, Median-D1 and Median-D2 are affected to similar degrees, whereas with upper plexus lesions, the LABC and Median-D1 responses are typically affected to a greater extent than the Median-D2 response [7]. On motor NCS, the Musculocutaneous-Biceps response may be affected (depending on lesion severity), whereas the Axillary-Deltoid response is spared. Needle EMG abnormalities are confined to musculocutaneous nerve and C6,7-median nerve innervated muscles (e.g., pronator teres; flexor carpi radialis). With lateral cord lesions, the C5,6 muscles innervated by the axillary, radial, suprascapular, long thoracic, and dorsal scapular nerves are spared.

The Posterior Cord

The posterior cord contains motor axons derived from the C5 through C8 spinal cord segments and sensory axons derived from the C5 through C7 spinal cord segments. The SNAP, CMAP, and muscle domains of the lateral cord are provided (Table 7.2). On sensory NCS, it is assessed by the S-Radial NCS. On motor NCS, it is assessed by the Axillary-Deltoid and both radial motor NCS (recording extensor digitorum communis and extensor indicis). On needle EMG, muscles innervated by the axillary, radial, and thoracodorsal nerves are helpful.

Posterior cord lesions are differentiated from middle trunk lesions by the Median-D2 and Median-D3 sensory NCS (spared with posterior cord lesions) and by needle EMG of C6,7-median nerve innervated muscles (e.g., pronator teres; flexor carpi radialis), which are spared with posterior cord lesions.

The Medial Cord

The medial cord contains motor and sensory axons derived from the C8 and T1 spinal cord segments. The SNAP, CMAP, and muscle domains of the medial cord are provided (Table 7.2). On sensory NCS, it is assessed by the Ulnar-D5 and MABC NCS. On motor NCS, the Ulnar-ADM, Ulnar-FDI, and Median-APB are useful. On needle EMG, C8,T1-median and ulnar nerve-innervated muscles are helpful.

As previously stated, the C8-radial nerve-innervated muscles (extensor indicis; extensor pollicis brevis) are helpful in differentiating lower plexus lesions (potentially involved) from medial cord lesions (always spared). It is important to understand that sparing of these muscles does not always indicate that the lesion localizes to the medial cord because partial lower plexus lesions may also spare them.

The Preterminal and Terminal Nerves

Sensory NCS are available for all of the terminal nerves except the axillary nerve. Motor NCS are available for all 5 terminal nerves. Many of the preterminal nerves are assessable by motor NCS (e.g., Phrenic-Diaphragm; Suprascapular-Infraspinatus). Because of identical sensory and motor axon composition, a terminal nerve lesion of the brachial plexus cannot be differentiated from a proximally-located upper extremity neuropathy of the same name.

EDX Exercises in Brachial Plexus Localization

Although the EDX study is an extension of the clinical examination, it is nonetheless an independent study. In order to maintain its independence, it must remain unbiased by the clinical features once it begins. The EDX findings, not the clinical findings, generate the EDX study conclusions. Nonetheless, following the EDX conclusion, it is often helpful to the referring provider to relate the EDX conclusions to the clinical features. Again, this is done, when indicated, after the EDX conclusions have already been clearly stated.

To convey the fact that the EDX study is an independent study, these 8 exercises provide very little clinical detail so that the independence of the EDX study is exemplified. Even in the setting of the EDX assessment of individuals with brachial plexus lesions, very little clinical detail is required. In fact, simply knowing which limb is symptomatic is enough to obtain a detailed history and focused examination. The clinical features obtained generate a differential diagnosis and, thus, a starting point for the EDX study. Once initiated, the EDX study continues along in a dynamic fashion. Additional EDX studies are determined by results of the previous EDX studies. The EDX study continues in this manner until the lesion has been fully localized and characterized (pathology, severity, temporal features).

Each of the 8 exercises begins with the information provided by the referring provider and the abbreviated clinical features collected by the EDX provider. The sensory NCS are performed first. The sensory NCS permit axon loss lesion localization (axon loss lesions represent the overwhelming majority of brachial plexopathies). The motor NCS are performed next. These studies localize focal demyelinating lesions and, most importantly, assess lesion severity. Finally, the needle EMG study is performed. It is helpful to confirm and fine tune the NCS conclusions and to define the temporal characteristics of the lesion. The EDX data are presented and discussed as the study unfolds, rather than all at once. This permits a deeper understanding of the dynamic nature of EDX testing (e.g., the need for additional EDX studies and why they are needed).

Regarding the sensory NCS, it is important to realize the DRG from which the sensory axons subserving the sensory NCS are derived. In this manner, just like motor axons, the pathways of the sensory axons through the brachial plexus are determinable. This information is included in the tables and is derived from our original work published in 1995 [7]. Each exercise begins with 3 screening sensory NCS—the median sensory NCS, recording index finger (Median-D2), the ulnar sensory NCS, recording little finger (Ulnar-D5), and the S-Radial sensory NCS, recording from the dorsolateral aspect of the hand (S-Radial)—along with any studies required based on the clinical features collected prior to the start of the EDX study. Whenever the Median-D2 or S-Radial response is abnormal (i.e., the sensory NCS that assess C6 and C7 DRG-derived sensory axons), we add the LABC and the Median-D1 sensory NCS because they only assess the C6 DRG-derived sensory axons and, thus, clarify the potential lesion localization sites. Whenever the Ulnar-D5 response is abnormal (assesses C8 DRG-derived sensory axons), we add the MABC NCS (assesses T1 DRG-derived sensory axons) to better clarify the potential lesion localization sites.

Because the overwhelming majority of brachial plexopathies are related to axon loss and a minority to demyelinating conduction block, only the amplitude values of the responses are presented, all of which are rounded to the nearest whole number. Although the latency and conduction velocity values are helpful for identifying demyelinating conduction slowing, this pathophysiology does not produce negative symptoms (i.e., weakness; numbness) but, instead, only isolated positive symptoms (e.g., episodic tingling). Isolated demyelinating conduction slowing is never observed among individuals with brachial plexopathies. For this reason, and to simplify the collected data for the 8 exercise presented below, the peak latency values (sensory NCS), the distal onset latency values (motor NCS), and the motor NCV values are replaced with an "X" in the data tables. Except with severe axon loss, unless all of the large-diameter, heavily myelinated fibers are disrupted, the latency and conduction velocity values are normal. Thus, in general, with axon loss disorders, the latency and conduction velocity values do not contribute to the EDX study. In the 8 cases discussed below, as expected, the latency and conduction velocity values were normal. Thus, it is easiest to discuss these exercises with the values replaced by an "X." Over a

12-year period, we successfully used this method of presenting NCS data in our popular American Academy of Neurology course: *EDX of the Brachial Plexus*. For NCS, the amplitude value is the most important measurement made. With needle EMG, however, the duration of the MUAP is the most important measurement collected. MUAP duration is much more sensitive to reinnervation via collateral sprouting than is MUAP amplitude. Unless significant collateral sprouting has occurred, the MUAP amplitude is normal, whereas the MUAP duration becomes abnormal with even mild degrees of collateral sprouting, especially when the MUAPs are compared to the contralateral side. The MUAP duration is muscle-dependent and age-dependent. For example, for the upper extremity, the brachioradialis has the shortest duration MUAPs, whereas the triceps and deltoid muscles have the longest. This hierarchy is addressed in some EDX textbooks (Ferrante TB).

When indicated, contralateral NCS were performed. The performance of contralateral studies helps to identify relative abnormalities. We consider a study to be relatively abnormal whenever its amplitude value is more than 50% smaller than the value recorded from the contralateral side. Often, as will be demonstrated by many of these exercises, the lesion is localized during the sensory NCS. When we use the term upper plexus (upper trunk and C5 and C6 roots), middle plexus (middle trunk and C7 root), and lower plexus (lower trunk and C8 and T1 roots), we are referring to the expanded definition of root, which includes the anterior primary ramus and all of the neural structures proximal to it (with the expanded definition, the root element is composed of the anterior primary ramus, the mixed spinal nerve, the primary root, and the rootlets exiting from the spinal cord). Using this approach, an avulsion lesion involving the C5 root would be considered an upper plexus brachial plexopathy.

Because these EDX exercises are included to teach brachial plexus lesion localization using our regional approach, rather than listing all of the individual needle EMG findings, the muscles are simply identified as normal or abnormal. Like other EMG laboratories, we consider a muscle to be abnormal whenever EDX evidence of acute motor axon loss (e.g., fibrillation potentials), chronic motor axon loss (e.g., increased MUAP duration or, less commonly, increased MUAP amplitude), or neurogenic recruitment is observed.

Muscle abbreviations utilized for these exercises are: ADM (abductor digiti minimi), APB (abductor pollicis brevis), ECR (extensor carpi radialis), ECU (extensor carpi ulnaris), ED (extensor digitorum), EI (extensor indicis), EPB (extensor pollicis brevis), FCR (flexor carpi radialis), FDI (first dorsal interosseous), FCU (flexor carpi ulnaris), FDP-4,5 (flexor digitorum profundus to the fourth vand fifth digits), and FPL (flexor pollicis longus).

Brachial Plexus Exercises

Exercise 1

A 58-year-old right hand dominant female is referred for EDX assessment of left upper extremity pain and weakness. These symptoms began 2 months ago. She reports a history of breast cancer, for which she did not receive radiation therapy.

The limited clinical features provided indicate involvement of the right upper extremity. Thus, the 3 screening sensory NCS are performed on the right side. In our EMG laboratories, we begin with 3 sensory NCS—the median sensory NCS, recording index finger (Median-D2), the ulnar sensory NCS, recording little finger (Ulnar-D5), and the S-Radial sensory NCS, recording from the dorsolateral aspect of the hand (Radial).

Nerve Conduction Studies

Case 1		Upper extremity nerve conduction study worksheet Left				Right			
NCS Performed	**DRG**	**LAT**	**AMP**	**CV**	**nAUC**	**LAT**	**AMP**	**CV**	**nAUC**
Sensory									
Median-D2	C6,7	X	26						
Ulnar-D5	C8	X	18						
S-radial	C6,7	X	4						

DRG Dorsal root ganglion/ganglia, *LAT* Latency, *AMP* Amplitude, *CV* Conduction velocity, *nAUC* Negative area under the curve

The sensory NCS are abnormal. The amplitude value of the left superficial radial response is reduced, indicative of axon loss. Because the sensory axons subserving the superficial radial nerve derive from the C6 and C7 DRG, the potential lesion sites include the superficial radial nerve, the radial nerve, the posterior cord, or the upper or middle plexus [7]. The two normal sensory responses support this list of potential lesion localizations, but do not shorten it.

To address these potential localization sites, the LABC and Median-D1 responses are needed. Also, the contralateral S-Radial NCS is needed (for comparison purposes).

Case 1		Upper extremity nerve conduction study worksheet Left				Right			
NCS Performed	**DRG**	**LAT**	**AMP**	**CV**	**nAUC**	**LAT**	**AMP**	**CV**	**nAUC**
Sensory									
Median-D2	C6,7	X	26						
Ulnar-D5	C8	X	18						
S-radial	C6,7	X	4			X	20		

DRG Dorsal root ganglion/ganglia, *LAT* Latency, *AMP* Amplitude, *CV* Conduction velocity, *nAUC* Negative area under the curve

Based on these findings, additional sensory NCS are required. Thus, prior to advancing to the motor NCS, the following sensory NCS are performed:

Case 1		Upper extremity nerve conduction study worksheet Left				Right			
NCS Performed	**DRG**	**LAT**	**AMP**	**CV**	**nAUC**	**LAT**	**AMP**	**CV**	**nAUC**
Sensory									
Median-D2	C6,7	X	26						
Ulnar-D5	C8	X	18						
S-radial	C6,7	X	4			X	20		
LABC	C6	X	NR			X	10		
Median-D1	C6	X	NR			X	16		

DRG Dorsal root ganglion/ganglia, *LAT* Latency, *AMP* Amplitude, *CV* Conduction velocity, *nAUC* Negative area under the curve

The LABC and Median-D1 responses are absent. Their involvement eliminates the superficial radial nerve, the radial nerve, the posterior cord, and the middle plexus as lesion localization sites. Thus, at this point, the lesion is axon loss in nature and involves the upper plexus, at least its C6 DRG derived sensory axons. Whether the C5 DRG-derived sensory axons are affected is unclear because there are no sensory NCS available to assess these axons.

With upper plexus lesions, to the routine motor NCS, we bilaterally add the axillary NCS, recording deltoid (Axillary-Deltoid) and musculocutaneous NCS, recording biceps (Musculocut-Biceps) to assess lesion severity.

Case 1		Upper extremity nerve conduction study worksheet Left				Right			
NCS Performed	**DRG**	**LAT**	**AMP**	**CV**	**nAUC**	**LAT**	**AMP**	**CV**	**nAUC**
Sensory									
Median-D2	C6,7	X	26						
Ulnar-D5	C8	X	18						
S-radial	C6,7	X	4			X	20		
LABC	C6	X	NR			X	10		
Median-D1	C6	X	NR			X	16		
Motor	**Stim Site**								
Median-APB		X	12						
			12	X					
Ulnar-ADM		X	13						
			13	X					
Musculocut-biceps		X	3			X	6		
			3	X					
Axillary-deltoid		X	4			X	9		

DRG Dorsal root ganglion/ganglia, *LAT* Latency, *AMP* Amplitude, *CV* Conduction velocity, *nAUC* Negative area under the curve

The screening motor NCS, as expected, are normal. The amplitude values of the musculocutaneous and axillary motor responses are abnormal and indicate an axon loss lesion. The relationship between the distal motor responses on the two sides indicates that approximately 50% of the musculocutaneous motor axons innervating the biceps muscle are disrupted (1–3/6 = 0.5) and approximately 56% of the axillary motor axons innervating the deltoid muscle are disrupted (1–4/9 = 0.56). it is important to appreciate that reinnervation through collateral sprouting improves the motor response because it reflects the number of muscle fibers innervated, not the number of motor axons composing the nerve. Given that the symptoms started 2 months ago, we use the term "approximately." Had the symptoms started more than 3 months ago, we would replace "approximately" with "at least" to indicate that the degree of motor axon loss might be an underestimate due to the presence of collateral sprouting. This should be supported by the needle EMG as long duration MUAPs.

The Needle EMG Study

- Abnormal muscles: Deltoid, brachioradialis, biceps, pronator teres, FCR
- Normal muscles: Trapezius, serratus anterior, supraspinatus, infraspinatus, triceps, EDC, EIP, FCU, FPL, APB, FDI, paraspinals.

The abnormal muscles are all within the muscle domain of the upper plexus. Sparing of the spinati muscles and the serratus anterior suggest that the lesion involves the upper trunk because the long thoracic nerve exits the plexus from the C5, C6, and C7 anterior primary rami and the suprascapular nerve exits just after the formation of the upper trunk (i.e., it is usually spared with upper trunk disorders). The presence of large amplitude fibrillation potentials and mildly long duration MUAPs indicates recent denervation and some reinnervation, respectively, consistent with a lesion that occurred 2 months ago.

EDX Conclusion

1. Upper Plexopathy

The above is axon loss in nature, involves the sensory and motor axons, and is at least moderate-severe in degree.

Final Comments

- The amplitude values of the sensory NCS are essential for localizing axon loss brachial plexopathies
  - The LABC and Median-D1 sensory NCS are extremely useful for assessing the upper plexus because the sensory axons subserving them derive from the C6 DRG [7]. Thus,

their involvement could not be explained by a middle plexus lesion.
  - Because the sensory axons subserving the Median-D2 sensory NCS are only abnormal in 20% of upper plexus lesions [7], they are not useful for screening this element of the brachial plexus.
- The musculocutaneous and axillary motor responses are helpful for determining the severity of the lesion. This can be calculated for axon loss lesions by comparing the distal motor response amplitude values (or negative AUC values) of the two sides. After enough time has elapsed for reinnervation via collateral sprouting to occur, the calculated value is an underestimate because the calculated value reflects the number of innervated muscle fibers not the number of functioning motor axons. Thus, we study the muscle on needle EMG for evidence of reinnervation via collateral sprouting. For lesions of less than 3 months duration without evidence of reinnervation via collateral sprouting (i.e., absence of long duration MUAPs), we use the term "approximately," whereas with lesions of greater than 3 months with evidence of reinnervation via collateral sprouting (i.e., the presence of long duration MUAPs), we use "at least."
- The because the dorsal scapular and long thoracic nerves exit the plexus from its anterior primary ramus level, they are spared with upper trunk lesions. Because the suprascapular nerve exits from the upper trunk just after its formation, it is frequently spared with upper trunk lesions.
- When involved, the C5,6-axillary nerve innervated muscles (deltoid; teres minor) and the C5,6-radial nerve innervated muscles (e.g., brachioradialis) are helpful for differentiating an upper plexus lesion (involved) from a lateral cord lesion (spared).

Exercise 2

A 41-year-old female is referred for EDX assessment of distal upper extremity sensory and motor abnormalities that followed a fall onto her outstretched left arm 4 weeks earlier.

The distal weakness suggests C8 and T1 fiber involvement, given that it includes the hand, but otherwise, there are no clinical clues. We do know that the left upper extremity is the symptomatic limb. Thus, the screening sensory NCS are performed on that limb first.

		Upper extremity nerve conduction study worksheet							
Case 2		Left				Right			
NCS Performed	**DRG**	**LAT**	**AMP**	**CV**	**nAUC**	**LAT**	**AMP**	**CV**	**nAUC**
Sensory									
Median-D2	C6,7	X	30						
Ulnar-D5	C8	X	NR						
S-radial	C6,7	X	21						

DRG Dorsal root ganglion/ganglia, *LAT* Latency, *AMP* Amplitude, *CV* Conduction velocity, *nAUC* Negative area under the curve

The left Ulnar-D5 sensory response is absent, indicative of an axon loss lesion that is localized to the ulnar nerve, the medial cord, or the C8 fibers of the lower plexus [7]. The other responses are normal and do not affect this list of potential lesion localizations. In our EMG laboratories, whenever the Ulnar-D5 sensory response is abnormal, we add the MABC NCS to better assess the medial cord and lower plexus. When the MABC is unaffected, we add the DUC NCS. We also need to add the contralateral Ulnar-D5.

Case 2		Upper extremity nerve conduction study worksheet Left				Right			
NCS Performed	**DRG**	**LAT**	**AMP**	**CV**	**nAUC**	**LAT**	**AMP**	**CV**	**nAUC**
Sensory									
Median-D2	C6,7	X	30						
Ulnar-D5	C8	X	NR			X	14		
S-radial	C6,7	X	21						
MABC	T1	X	NR			X	12		

DRG Dorsal root ganglion/ganglia, *LAT* Latency, *AMP* Amplitude, *CV* Conduction velocity, *nAUC* Negative area under the curve

The MABC response is absent, indicative of an axon loss process involving the MABC nerve, the medial cord, or the T1 fibers of the lower plexus. Thus, this cannot be an ulnar neuropathy and, for this reason, there is no need to perform the DUC NCS. Also, because the ulnar response is abnormal, this cannot be an MABC lesion. Thus, because the ulnar and the MABC responses are both affected, the lesion must involve the medial cord or the lower plexus (both its C8 and its T1 fibers).

Thus, at this point, there is an axon loss lesion involving the medial cord or the lower plexus. More accurate localization is not possible with the sensory NCS as they do not differentiate between medial cord and lower trunk localizations. This differentiation requires C8-radial motor axon assessment via the motor NCS or the needle EMG study. The C8-radial motor axons traverse the lower plexus and the posterior cord. Thus, their involvement would indicate a lower plexus lesion. However, their sparing does not indicate a medial cord lesion because a partial lower plexus lesion would still be possible. The C8 radial motor axons innervate the extensor indicis muscle. Thus, the Radial-EI NCS is added to the routine motor NCS. If the screening ulnar motor NCS is abnormal, the Ulnar-FDI NCS will be added to better assess lesion severity. Finally, any abnormal motor responses on the symptomatic side will be compared to the contralateral side for severity assessment.

Case 2		Upper extremity nerve conduction study worksheet Left				Right			
NCS Performed	**Stim site**	**LAT**	**AMP**	**CV**	**nAUC**	**LAT**	**AMP**	**CV**	**nAUC**
Sensory									
Median-D2	C6,7	X	30						
Ulnar-D5	C8	X	NR			X	14		
S-radial	C6,7	X	21						
MABC	T1	X	NR			X	12		
Motor									
Median-APB		X	4			X	13		
			4	X					
Ulnar-ADM		X	4			X	12		
			4	X					
Ulnar-FDI		X	5			X	9		
			5	X					
Radial-EI		X	1			X	4		
			1	X					

DRG Dorsal root ganglion/ganglia, *LAT* Latency, *AMP* Amplitude, *CV* Conduction velocity, *nAUC* Negative area under the curve

The left Median-APB, Ulnar-ADM, Ulnar-FDI, and Radial-EI responses are severely reduced in amplitude, consistent with an axon loss process (as already indicated by the sensory NCS) that is severe in degree (as suggested by the absent sensory NCS), and that involves the lower plexus (since the Radial-EI response is affected). The lesion involves 69% of the median motor axons to the APB muscle (1–4/13 = 0.69), 67% of the ulnar motor axons to the ADM muscle (1–0.33 = 0.67), 44% of the motor axons to the FDI muscle (1–5/9 = 0.44), and 75% of the motor axons to the EI muscle (1–1/4 = 0.75).

The Needle EMG Study

- Abnormal muscles: APB, FPL, FCU, FDP-3,4, FDI, ADM, EIP, EPB
- Normal muscles: Deltoid, biceps, triceps, brachioradialis, pronator teres, paraspinals

The needle EMG study shows involvement of muscles in the muscle domain of the lower plexus. The extensor indicis and the extensor pollicis brevis are both involved, consistent with the lower plexus localization identified on motor NCS.

EDX Conclusion

1. Lower plexopathy

The above is axon loss in nature, involves the sensory and motor nerve fibers, and is severe in degree.

Final Comments

- When the sensory NCS localize the lesion to the medial cord or the lower plexus, the C8-radial motor axons, when involved, are helpful in localizing the lesion to the lower plexus because they are never involved with medial cord lesions. Importantly, their lack of involvement does not indicate a medial cord lesion because a partial lower plexus could be responsible.
- The extensor indicis and extensor pollicis brevis are good C8-radial muscles. The extensor indicis is assessable by motor NCS and by needle EMG, whereas the extensor pollicis brevis is usually studied by needle EMG.
- When the Radial-EI response is normal on motor NCS, the EI and EPB should be studied on needle EMG because the needle EMG is more sensitive to axon loss than the motor NCS (especially in the 21- to 35-day window when fibrillation potentials are at their densest).

Exercise 3

A 26-year-old female is referred for EDX assessment of left upper extremity pain and numbness. According to the patient, she has a several-year history of intermittent numbness along the medial aspect of her left forearm and hand. She reports that the tingling can be precipitated by lying in a supine position. She also reports a 10-year history of aching pain along the medial aspect of her left arm and forearm.

The distribution of the pain and tingling along the medial aspect of the arm, forearm, and hand suggest C8 and T1 nerve fiber involvement. To address this presentation, the screening sensory NCS are performed on the left upper extremity.

Nerve Conduction Studies

		Upper extremity nerve conduction study worksheet							
Case 3		Left				Right			
NCS Performed	**DRG**	**LAT**	**AMP**	**CV**	**nAUC**	**LAT**	**AMP**	**CV**	**nAUC**
Sensory									
Median-D2	C6,7	X	51						
Ulnar-D5	C8	X	16						
S-radial	C6,7	X	59						

DRG Dorsal root ganglion/ganglia, *LAT* Latency, *AMP* Amplitude, *CV* Conduction velocity, *nAUC* Negative area under the curve

The screening sensory NCS are normal. However, it is important to assess the relationship of the sensory responses to each other so as not to miss a relative abnormality. Notice that the amplitude value of the median response is roughly 2.5 times the lower limit of normal (the lower limit of normal is 20 microvolts for a patient of this age), that the amplitude value of the ulnar response is 1.25 times the lower limit of normal (the lower limit of normal is 12 microvolts for a patient of this age), and that the amplitude value of the superficial radial response is roughly 3.5 times the lower limit of normal (the lower limit of normal is 17 microvolts for a patient of this age). Thus, the ulnar sensory response is questionably lower than the other two responses. To address this, this NCS should be performed on the contralateral side.

		Upper extremity nerve conduction study worksheet							
Case 3		Left				Right			
NCS Performed	**DRG**	**LAT**	**AMP**	**CV**	**nAUC**	**LAT**	**AMP**	**CV**	**nAUC**
Sensory									
Median-D2	C6,7	X	51						
Ulnar-D5	C8	X	16			X	41		
S-radial	C6,7	X	59						

DRG Dorsal root ganglion/ganglia, *LAT* Latency, *AMP* Amplitude, *CV* Conduction velocity, *nAUC* Negative area under the curve

The contralateral ulnar response is roughly 3.5 times the lower limit of normal, which is in line with the other responses. Moreover, the amplitude value of the contralateral ulnar study is more than twice that of the ipsilateral response, rendering the ipsilateral response relatively abnormal.

The relatively abnormal left ulnar response indicates an axon loss process involving the ulnar nerve, the medial cord, or the C8 fibers of the lower plexus. As discussed in Exercise 2, for localization purposes, the MABC NCS is added. Because this is not one of our routine screening studies, we usually add it bilaterally, especially in the setting of a relatively abnormal ulnar response.

		Upper extremity nerve conduction study worksheet							
Case 3		Left				Right			
NCS Performed	**DRG**	**LAT**	**AMP**	**CV**	**nAUC**	**LAT**	**AMP**	**CV**	**nAUC**
Sensory									
Median-D2	C6,7	X	51						
Ulnar-D5	C8	X	16			X	41		
S-radial	C6,7	X	59						
MABC	T1		NR			X	15		

DRG Dorsal root ganglion/ganglia, *LAT* Latency, *AMP* Amplitude, *CV* Conduction velocity, *nAUC* Negative area under the curve

The absent MABC, when considered in the setting of an abnormal ulnar response, limits the potential lesion localization sites to the medial cord or the lower plexus (both the C8 and T1 fibers must be affected).

It is important to notice the degree of involvement of the two abnormal responses—the ulnar response is relatively abnormal and the MABC response is absent. Although this might represent a lower trunk lesion that happens to be affecting the MABC axons to a much greater extent than the ulnar axons, the other possibility is that the lesion is located in the proximal portion of the lower plexus (i.e., at the anterior primary ramus level, where the C8 and T1 fibers are separate from each other). At this site, they could more readily be affected to varying degrees because the majority of MABC fibers emanate from the T1 DRG and the majority of the ulnar sensory fibers emanate from the C8 DRG [7].

Similar to Exercise 2, the C8-radial motor axons can be useful in differentiating between medial cord and lower plexus lesion localizations. Thus, the Radial-EI motor NCS is added bilaterally to the routine motor NCS. Because the ulnar sensory response was abnormal, both ulnar motor NCS are performed bilaterally.

Case 3		Upper extremity nerve conduction study worksheet Left				Right			
NCS Performed		**LAT**	**AMP**	**CV**	**nAUC**	**LAT**	**AMP**	**CV**	**nAUC**
Motor	**Stim site**								
Median-APB	Wrist	X	2			X	12		
	Elbow		2	X					
Ulnar-ADM	Wrist	X	12			X	14		
	AE		11	X					
Ulnar-FDI	Wrist	X	10			X	15		
	AE		10	X					
Radial-EI	Forearm	X	2			X	4		
	ACF		2	X					

DRG Dorsal root ganglion/ganglia, *LAT* Latency, *AMP* Amplitude, *CV* Conduction velocity, *nAUC* Negative area under the curve

The median motor response is very low in amplitude, indicating a severe axon loss process. The two ulnar motor responses are normal, but clearly lower than the contralateral side. However, they do not meet our criteria for relative abnormal (i.e., less than 50% of the contralateral side). The amplitude value of the radial motor response is abnormal. Its involvement excludes a medial cord localization. Thus, at this point, there is an axon loss process involving the lower plexus.

The degree of median motor response involvement (very severe) when considered in relation to the degree of ulnar sensory nerve fiber involvement (relatively abnormal) argues against a lesion involving a single element because, in general, when an element containing both sensory and motor axons is affected, whenever the motor response from that element is more than 50% reduced, the sensory response from that element is typically absent or very low in amplitude. Thus, although a fascicular process is still possible, the lower trunk is a less likely localization site.

Finally, it is important to recognize that the T1 > C8 pattern on sensory NCS (i.e., absent MABC response; relatively abnormal Ulnar-D5 response) is also present here (i.e., the APB muscle is primarily innervated by motor axons derived from the T1 spinal cord segment). This also argues against a lower trunk localization and, instead, favors an APR-level lesion involving the T1 APR to a greater extent than the C8 APR. this is the typical pattern of NCS abnormalities observed with true neurogenic thoracic outlet syndrome (TN-TOS).

For these reasons, the needle EMG is expanded to better evaluate the lower plexus.

The Needle EMG Study

- Abnormal muscles
  - APB (the most severely affected), FPL, FDI, adductor pollicis, EI, EPB
- Normal muscles
  - Deltoid, brachioradialis, biceps, triceps, pronator teres, FDP-3,4,
- paraspinals.

The extensor indicis and extensor pollicis brevis muscle are involved, confirming a lower plexus localization. Because the APB muscle was the most severely affected and because it predominantly receives motor axons from the T1 spinal cord segment, this pattern of needle EMG abnormalities, like the sensory NCS and the motor NCS, indicates that the severity of T1 nerve fiber involvement exceeds the severity of the C8 nerve fiber involvement.

EDX Study Impression

1. Left Lower Plexopathy (suspect true neurogenic thoracic outlet syndrome)

The above is axon loss in nature and severe in degree. The abnormalities localize to the lower plexus and the pattern of abnormalities suggests more proximal lower plexus involvement at the level of the anterior primary rami. The constellation of EDX abnormalities identified are essentially pathognomonic of true neurogenic thoracic outlet syndrome.

As you know, this disorder is a very slowly progressive one that permits reinnervation to keep pace with denervation. For this reason, it does not respond to conservative therapy and, hence, surgical intervention is the recommended treatment. This is best done by a neurosurgeon specializing in brachial plexus disorders using a supraclavicular approach and leaving the normal first thoracic rib in place. Please contact my office for recommendations.

Final Comments

- Again, when the sensory NCS localize the lesion to the medial cord or lower plexus, the C8-radial motor axons are useful for differentiating these two sites.
- The pattern of T1 > C8 should be appreciated because it is the pattern observed with true neurogenic thoracic outlet syndrome, a disorder usually related to a taut fibrocartilaginous band that extends from the first thoracic rib to the C7 vertebral body (to either a C7 cervical rib or an elongated transverse process) and that displaces the lower plexus upward. The contact site is usually at the APR level of the brachial plexus and, therefore, the traction on the more inferiorly located T1 APR is greater than that on the more superiorly located C8 APR [21, 22].
- The T1 > C8 pattern of EDX abnormalities is typically seen at all levels of the EDX study
  - Sensory NCS: MABC more affected than Ulnar-D5
  - Motor NCS: Median-APB more affected than ulnar motor NCS
  - Needle EMG: APB affected out of proportion to the other muscles of the lower plexus muscle domain
- Because this is a very slowly progressive process, maximum reinnervation has typically already occurred. Thus, surgical intervention is required (i.e., there is no place for conservative treatment with this condition). The normal first thoracic rib is ideally left in place. A supraclavicular approach to section the band is preferred over a transaxillary approach because the latter has been associated with significant surgical complications [22].
- At surgery, this patient was found to have a fibrocartilaginous band extending from her first thoracic rib to a rudimentary C7 rib. The band deflected the T1 APR to a greater extent than the C8 APR, as expected from the EDX findings.

Exercise 4

A 71-year-old male is referred for EDX assessment of a suspected postoperative left ulnar neuropathy. According to the patient, he noted left grip weakness following open heart surgery 3–4 weeks ago. It is associated with numbness along the medial aspect of his left hand.

The distribution of the sensory symptoms implies a lesion along the pathway form the ulnar nerve to the C8 root. This pathway could also account for the grip weakness.

To address this presentation, the screening sensory NCS are performed on the left.

Nerve Conduction Studies

Case 4		Upper extremity nerve conduction study worksheet							
		Left				Right			
NCS Performed	**DRG**	**LAT**	**AMP**	**CV**	**nAUC**	**LAT**	**AMP**	**CV**	**nAUC**
Sensory									
Median-D2	C6,7	X	14						
Ulnar-D5	C8		NR						
S-radial	C6,7	X	18						

DRG Dorsal root ganglion/ganglia, *LAT* Latency, *AMP* Amplitude, *CV* Conduction velocity, *nAUC* Negative area under the curve

The left ulnar response is absent, indicating an axon loss process that is localized to the left ulnar nerve, medial cord, or lower plexus. To better define this list of potential lesion sites, the MABC NCS is added.

Case 4		Upper extremity nerve conduction study worksheet							
		Left				Right			
NCS Performed	**DRG**	**LAT**	**AMP**	**CV**	**nAUC**	**LAT**	**AMP**	**CV**	**nAUC**
Sensory									
Median-D2	C6,7	X	14						
Ulnar-D5	C8		NR						
S-radial	C6,7	X	18						
MABC	T1	X	11						

DRG Dorsal root ganglion/ganglia, *LAT* Latency, *AMP* Amplitude, *CV* Conduction velocity, *nAUC* Negative area under the curve

The MABC sensory response is normal, arguing against a medial cord or lower plexus process involving the T1 fibers. To better localize this process, further NCS are required, including bilateral DUC and contralateral Ulnar-D5 and MABC NCS.

Case 4		Upper extremity nerve conduction study worksheet							
		Left				Right			
NCS Performed	**DRG**	**LAT**	**AMP**	**CV**	**nAUC**	**LAT**	**AMP**	**CV**	**nAUC**
Sensory									
Median-D2	C6,7	X	14						
Ulnar-D5	C8		NR			X	8		
S-radial	C6,7	X	18						
MABC	T1	X	11			X	12		
DUC	C8		NR			X	7		

DRG Dorsal root ganglion/ganglia, *LAT* Latency, *AMP* Amplitude, *CV* Conduction velocity, *nAUC* Negative area under the curve

The left Ulnar-D5 and DUC responses are absent, indicative of an axon loss process that localizes to the ulnar nerve, the medial cord, or the C8 APR. given that both ulnar responses are absent and the MABC response is normal, it is less likely that this represents a partial lower trunk lesion. Involvement of the DUC response indicates that the lesion is proximal to the departure site of this nerve (i.e., it is above the wrist).

At this point, an axon loss process has been identified that involves the ulnar nerve proximal to the wrist, the medial cord, or the C8 fibers of the lower plexus.

Similar to Exercise 2 and Exercise 3, the C8 radial motor axons should be included on the motor NCS (to help differentiate between ulnar nerve/ medial cord and lower plexus localization. Also, the ulnar motor NCS should be performed bilaterally.

Case 4		Upper extremity nerve conduction study worksheet Left				Right			
NCS Performed		**LAT**	**AMP**	**CV**	**nAUC**	**LAT**	**AMP**	**CV**	**nAUC**
Motor	**Stim site**								
Median-APB			7				9		
			7						
Ulnar-ADM			4				10		
			4						
Ulnar-FDI			2				8		
			2						
Radial-EI			1				3		

DRG Dorsal root ganglion/ganglia, *LAT* Latency, *AMP* Amplitude, *CV* Conduction velocity, *nAUC* Negative area under the curve

The median motor response is normal. The ulnar motor responses are severely reduced in amplitude, indicative of an axon loss process involving the ulnar nerve, medial cord, or lower plexus. Sparing of the MABC response argues against a lower trunk process but does not exclude a C8 APR process because the MABC NCS is predominantly subserved by T1 DRG-derived sensory axons.

Because the Radial-EI response is reduced in amplitude, both an ulnar neuropathy and a medial cord are excluded. Thus, the NCS indicate an axon loss process involving the lower plexus, most likely at the C8 APR level.

The needle EMG study of the left upper extremity should be expanded to include additional muscles in the muscle domain of the lower plexus.

The Needle EMG Study

- Abnormal muscles
  - FCU, FDP-3,4, ADM, FDI, FPL, EIP, EPB
- Normal muscles
  - Deltoid, biceps, triceps, pronator teres, APB, paraspinals

The involved muscles all belong to the muscle domain of the lower plexus. Again, the C8-radial muscles are extremely helpful in identifying lower plexus pathology.

EDX Study Impression

1. Lower Plexopathy (median sternotomy brachial plexopathy)

The above is axon loss in nature and severe in degree. The temporal relationship to the median sternotomy and the pattern of EDX abnormalities (i.e., best localizing to the C8 anterior primary ramus) strongly suggest that this represents median sternotomy brachial plexopathy, a disorder associated with the rib retraction required by surgical procedures requiring median sternotomy (median sternotomy causes first thoracic rib-related trauma of the C8 anterior primary ramus). Although the majority of these lesions are predominantly demyelinating conduction block (about two-thirds), this lesion is predominantly axon loss.

Final Comments

- This case exemplifies the importance of adhering to the admonition to always surround the abnormal studies with normal studies. Had the EDX provider mistakenly assumed that the patient had a typical postoperative ulnar neuropathy and only performed standard NCS and needle EMG assessments to verify that impression (i.e., not assessed the C8-radial motor axons), the patient would have been misdiagnosed as having an ulnar neuropathy. Had an unnecessary ulnar transposition been

performed with resultant neurological worsening, a medicolegal issue would be generated (misdiagnosis with harm).
- This particular pattern of NCS findings—involvement of the ulnar sensory and motor nerve fibers with sparing of the MABC sensory and median motor nerve fibers—has long been associated with C8 anterior primary ramus lesion related to median sternotomy. This entity is termed *median sternotomy brachial plexopathy* [5, 6].

Exercise 5

A 56-year-old right hand dominant female is referred for EDX assessment of left upper extremity weakness and numbness. According to the patient, following pacemaker placement, she noted weakness of elbow flexion and pain and numbness along the lateral aspect of the left forearm. Examination shows an infraclavicular scar at the surgical site.

The sensory and motor symptoms following the surgical procedure suggest involvement of the peripheral nervous system and the infraclavicular location of the scar suggest an infraclavicular lesion. Forearm flexion weakness implies musculocutaneous nerve, lateral cord, or upper plexus involvement. The numbness is in the cutaneous distribution of the LABC nerve. Thus, this might represent a musculocutaneous neuropathy or a lateral cord lesion, but is clinically unlikely to represent an upper plexus lesion.

To address this presentation, the screening sensory NCS are performed on the left.

Nerve Conduction Studies

		Upper extremity nerve conduction study worksheet							
Case 5		**Left**				**Right**			
NCS Performed		**LAT**	**AMP**	**CV**	**nAUC**	**LAT**	**AMP**	**CV**	**nAUC**
Sensory	**DRG**								
Median-D2	C6,7	X	14						
Ulnar-D5	C8	X	22						
S-radial	C6,7	X	20						

DRG Dorsal root ganglion/ganglia, *LAT* Latency, *AMP* Amplitude, *CV* Conduction velocity, *nAUC* Negative area under the curve

The Median-D2 response is abnormal. It is reduced in amplitude, indicative of an axon loss process that localizes to the median nerve, lateral cord, or to the C6 or C7 fibers of the upper or middle plexus. The presence of median sensory fibers excludes an isolated musculocutaneous nerve as a consideration, as was postulated by the distribution of sensory and motor symptoms elicited clinically.

As stated previously, whenever the Median-D2 response is reduced in amplitude, the LABC and Median-D1 NCS are added bilaterally. In addition, the Median-D2 and S-Radial NCS should be performed on the contralateral side.

		Upper extremity nerve conduction study worksheet							
Case 5		Left				Right			
NCS Performed		**LAT**	**AMP**	**CV**	**nAUC**	**LAT**	**AMP**	**CV**	**nAUC**
Sensory	**Drg**								
Median-D2	C6,7	X	8				32		
Ulnar-D5	C8	X	22						
S-radial	C6,7	X	20				24		
LABC	C6		5				16		
Median-D1	C6		12				28		

DRG Dorsal root ganglion/ganglia, *LAT* Latency, *AMP* Amplitude, *CV* Conduction velocity, *nAUC* Negative area under the curve

The left LABC and Median-D1 responses are abnormal, indicative of an axon loss process involving the lateral cord or the upper plexus. Given that the sensory axons subserving the Median-D2 NCS only traverse the upper plexus 20% of the time, the lateral cord is favored. In this setting, the Median-D3 NCS may also be helpful, as it assesses the lateral cord 80% of the time and the upper plexus only 10% of the time [7]. In this individual, it was deferred given that this issue would likely be resolved during the motor NCS and the needle EMG study.

In addition to the routine motor NCS on the left, the Axillary-Deltoid and the Musculocutaneous-Biceps motor NCS were added bilaterally.

		Upper extremity nerve conduction study worksheet							
Case 5		Left				Right			
NCS Performed		**LAT**	**AMP**	**CV**	**nAUC**	**LAT**	**AMP**	**CV**	**nAUC**
Motor	**Stim site**								
Median-APB		X	7						
			7	X					
Ulnar-ADM		X	8						
			8	X					
Musculocut-biceps		X	2			X	5		
			2	X					
Axillary-deltoid		X	9.2			X	8.6		

DRG Dorsal root ganglion/ganglia, *LAT* Latency, *AMP* Amplitude, *CV* Conduction velocity, *nAUC* Negative area under the curve

The routine motor NCS are normal, as is the axillary motor response. The musculocutaneous response is moderately to severely reduced. This pattern of motor NCS abnormalities supports a lateral cord localization, as was previously suggested by the sensory NCS.

The needle EMG study is expanded to include muscles belonging to the upper plexus muscle domain that are not a part of the lateral cord muscle domain. These include C5,6 muscles innervated by the suprascapular (supraspinatus; infraspinatus), axillary (deltoid; teres minor), and radial (brachioradialis) nerves.

The Needle EMG Study

- Abnormal muscles
  - Biceps, pronator teres, FCR
- Normal muscles
  - Infraspinatus, deltoid, brachioradialis, FDI, EI, FPL, triceps, paraspinals

The abnormal muscles all belong to the muscle domain of the lateral cord. Sparing of.

the suprascapular, axillary, and radial nerve innervated C5,6 muscles further support this.

localization.

EDX Study Impression

1. Lateral Cord Lesion

The above is axon loss in nature, involves the sensory and motor nerve fibers, and is moderate-severe in degree.

Final Comments

- Unlike upper plexus lesions, with lateral cord lesions, the Median-D1 and the Median-D2 sensory responses tend to be more uniformly affected (they are more uniformly affected with upper plexus lesions). In addition, the radial sensory response is never affected by a lateral cord lesion (it is affected by upper plexus lesions 60% of the time) [7].
- With lateral cord lesions, the musculocutaneous motor response may be affected (depending on severity), but the axillary motor response is always spared. With upper plexus lesions, both of these responses may be affected, depending on lesion severity [7].
- On needle EMG, distinguishing between a lateral cord lesion and an upper plexus lesion is best done by studying C5,6-suprascapular

nerve, C5,6-axillary nerve, and C5,6-radial nerve innervated muscles.

Exercise 6

A 31-year-old right hand dominant male is referred for EDX assessment of progressive left upper extremity weakness. According to the patient, he first noted left upper extremity weakness about 12 years ago. The weakness initially produced a mild finger and wrist drop. Since then, it has slowly worsened and he now can trouble raising his arm over his shoulder level. He also reports left hand numbness. He denies associated bulbar or lower extremity involvement. He denies numbness along the lateral aspect of the arm, proximally.

The wrist and finger drop suggest radial nerve distribution weakness. The shoulder abduction weakness suggests axillary nerve distribution weakness. The distribution of the hand numbness suggests superficial radial nerve involvement. Together, these features suggest posterior cord involvement. We begin the EDX study with screening sensory NCS on that side.

Nerve Conduction Studies.

		Upper extremity nerve conduction study worksheet							
Case 6		Left				Right			
NCS Performed		**LAT**	**AMP**	**CV**	**nAUC**	**LAT**	**AMP**	**CV**	**nAUC**
Sensory	**DRG**								
Median-D2	C6,7		32						
Ulnar-D5	C8		24						
S-radial	C6,7		NR						

DRG Dorsal root ganglion/ganglia, *LAT* Latency, *AMP* Amplitude, *CV* Conduction velocity, *nAUC* Negative area under the curve

The S-Radial response is absent, indicative of an axon loss process involving the S-Radial or radial nerve, the posterior cord, or the upper or middle plexus because the sensory axons subserving the S-Radial predominantly derive from the C6 or the C7 DRG. The normal median response argues against a middle plexus localization because the sensory fibers subserving the Median-D2 response derive from the C7 DRG about 80% of the time [7]. However, middle plexus localization cannot be excluded because the those fibers derive predominantly from the C6 DRG 20% of the time [7]. Further localization requires additional sensory NCS. Thus, as discussed earlier, whenever the screening sensory NCS identify n abnormality involving a sensory NCS whose axons derive from the C6 or C7 DRG, we bilaterally add the LABC and the Median-D1 NCS. In addition, the contralateral S-Radial NCS is added.

		Upper extremity nerve conduction study worksheet							
Case 6		Left				Right			
NCS Performed		**LAT**	**AMP**	**CV**	**nAUC**	**LAT**	**AMP**	**CV**	**nAUC**
Sensory	**DRG**								
Median-D2	C6,7		32						
Ulnar-D5	C8		24						
S-radial	C6,7		NR			X	36		
LABC	C6		26				19		
Median-D1	C6		25						

DRG Dorsal root ganglion/ganglia, *LAT* Latency, *AMP* Amplitude, *CV* Conduction velocity, *nAUC* Negative area under the curve

Because the amplitude value of the Median-D1 response was what would be expected when compared to the Median-D2 response (i.e., more than two-thirds the value of the Median-D2 response), we did not add the contralateral Median-D1 NCS for comparison purposes. We did add the contralateral LABC NCS.

Sparing of the LABC and the Median-D1 sensory responses excludes an upper plexus localization. Thus, the potentials localization sites are the superficial radial or radial nerve or the posterior cord. To hone this list further, the Axillary-Deltoid motor NCS is added. Also, to better define the severity of the lesion, the Radial-ED motor NCS is added (and possibly the Radial-EI NCS). For severity assessment, contralateral comparison studies are also required. Because the upper plexus has been excluded as a possibility, the Musculocutaneous-Biceps motor NCS, previously included when the screening sensory NCS include the upper plexus or the middle plexus as potential lesion localization sites, is not required. This response assesses the musculocutaneous nerve, the lateral cord, and the upper plexus—none of which are lesion localization considerations.

Case 6		Upper extremity nerve conduction study worksheet Left				Right			
NCS Performed		**LAT**	**AMP**	**CV**	**nAUC**	**LAT**	**AMP**	**CV**	**nAUC**
Motor	**Stim site**								
Median-APB		X	18						
			17	X					
Ulnar-ADM		X	10						
			10	X					
Radial-EDC		X	NR						
				X					
Axillary-deltoid		X	NR						

DRG Dorsal root ganglion/ganglia, *LAT* Latency, *AMP* Amplitude, *CV* Conduction velocity, *nAUC* Negative area under the curve

The radial and axillary motor responses are absent. For this reason, the contralateral motor NCS are of no benefit in grading severity (regardless of their value, the lesion involves 100% of the motor axons and is severe). Thus, they were not required and, hence, not performed. The motor response abnormalities are consistent with a posterior cord localization, although a lesion involving both the axillary and the radial nerves near their site where they separate from each other (i.e., at the point where the posterior cord divides to become the axillary nerve and the radial nerve) cannot be excluded.

The needle EMG study, in addition to the screening muscles, is expanded to include additional muscles within the muscle domain of the posterior cord, as well as one C5,6 muscle within the upper plexus domain that is not also in the posterior cord domain (e.g., the infraspinatus).

The Needle EMG Study

- Abnormal muscles
  - Deltoid, teres minor, triceps, brachioradialis, TC, ECR, ED, EI
- Normal muscles
  - Infraspinatus, biceps, pronator teres, FDI, FPL, paraspinals

EDX Study Impression

1. Left Posterior Cord Lesion

The above is axon loss in nature, involves the sensory and motor nerve fibers, and is extremely severe in degree. The relationship between the acute (sparse, low amplitude fibrillation potentials) and the chronic features (many long duration MUAPs) are indicative of a slowly progressive process. As you know, imaging to exclude a structural process may be of further diagnostic utility.

Final Comments

- In the setting of posterior cord lesions, the addition of the LABC and Median-D1 sensory NCS is helpful in excluding a supraclavicular process and thereby decreasing the list of potential lesion localization sites to the posterior cord or the radial or superficial radial nerve.
- Following the sensory NCS, the motor NCS are helpful in differentiating a posterior cord lesion from one restricted to either the radial nerve or the axillary nerve.
- On needle EMG examination, muscles should be added to differentiate a posterior cord lesion from an upper plexus lesion (e.g., C5,6

long thoracic, dorsal scapular, or suprascapular nerve innervated muscles, of which the infraspinatus is the easiest to assess). In addition, muscles belonging to the axillary and radial nerve muscle domains are included to differentiate a posterior cord from one involving just one of its branches.

- Posterior cord lesions are differentiated from middle plexus lesions by assessing C7 motor axons that traverse the lateral cord (e.g., those innervating the pronator teres and FCR muscles).

Exercise 7

A 32-year-old right hand dominant female was referred for EDX assessment of left hand weakness and atrophy. According to the patient, she first noted left hand weakness about 10 years ago. Since that time, it has slowly worsened but has not progressed proximally. More recently, she noted left axillary pain. The latter radiates distally to the hand.

Clinically, the axillary pain suggests that the underlying etiology of the left hand weakness and atrophy is located proximally, possibly in the axillary region. The distribution of the weakness (hand intrinsic muscle weakness) suggests C8 and T1 nerve fiber involvement. The clinical features—the location of the pain and the distribution of the weakness—suggest possible medial cord or lower plexus involvement.

To address this presentation, screening sensory NCS of the left upper extremity are performed first.

Nerve Conduction Studies

		Upper extremity nerve conduction study worksheet							
Case 7		Left				Right			
NCS Performed		**LAT**	**AMP**	**CV**	**nAUC**	**LAT**	**AMP**	**CV**	**nAUC**
Sensory	**DRG**								
Median-D2	C6,7	X	38						
Ulnar-D5	C8	X	4						
S-radial	C6,7	X	33						

DRG Dorsal root ganglion/ganglia, *LAT* Latency, *AMP* Amplitude, *CV* Conduction velocity, *nAUC* Negative area under the curve

The low amplitude value of the Ulnar-D5 response indicates an axon loss process involving the ulnar nerve, the medial cord, or the C8 fibers of the lower plexus. To shorten this list of potential lesion localization sites, the MABC NCS is added bilaterally. Should it be normal, the DUC NCS will be added bilaterally. For comparison purposes, the ulnar response is performed on the contralateral side.

		Upper extremity nerve conduction study worksheet							
Case 7		Left				Right			
NCS Performed		**LAT**	**AMP**	**CV**	**nAUC**	**LAT**	**AMP**	**CV**	**nAUC**
Sensory	**DRG**								
Median-D2	C6,7	X	38						
Ulnar-D5	C8	X	4				28		
S-radial	C6,7	X	33						
MABC	T1		NR				17		

DRG Dorsal root ganglion/ganglia, *LAT* Latency, *AMP* Amplitude, *CV* Conduction velocity, *nAUC* Negative area under the curve

The absent MABC response eliminates the ulnar nerve from the list of possible lesion localization sites. Because the sensory response is nearly absent, we would expect the ulnar motor response to be at least mildly involved.

To address this, the screening motor NCS are expanded to include the Radial-EI motor NCS bilaterally. Although radial motor response involvement localizes the process to the lower plexus, radial motor response sparing does not localize the lesion to the medial cord because a partial lower plexus lesion could also spare it (i.e., the radial motor response contributes to lesion localization when it is abnormal, but not when it is normal). The Ulnar-FDI motor NCS is added bilaterally (to better define lesion severity). To better define lesion severity, those routine motor responses that are abnormal, will be compared to the contralateral side.

		Upper extremity nerve conduction study worksheet							
Case 7		Left				Right			
NCS Performed		**LAT**	**AMP**	**CV**	**nAUC**	**LAT**	**AMP**	**CV**	**nAUC**
Motor	**Stim site**								
Median-APB		X	4			X	10		
			4	X					
Ulnar-ADM		X	5			X	11		
			5	X					
Ulnar-FDI		X	8			X	14		
			8	X					
Radial-EI		X	5			X	5		
			5	X					

DRG Dorsal root ganglion/ganglia, *LAT* Latency, *AMP* Amplitude, *CV* Conduction velocity, *nAUC* Negative area under the curve

The amplitude values of the left Median-APB response and the left Ulnar-ADM response are reduced, consistent with an axon loss process involving the medial cord or the lower plexus. Although asymmetric. The two Ulnar-FDI responses are normal because the amplitude value of the response is above the lower limit of normal (i.e., not an absolute abnormal) and more than 50% of the contralateral response value (i.e., not a relative abnormal). Still, the asymmetry implies axon loss and, thus, the needle EMG study of this muscle is expected to be abnormal.

Again, sparing of the Radial-EIP response does not exclude a lower plexus localization (it may be a partial lower plexus lesion sparing the C8-radial nerve fibers) or rule in a medial cord localization.

The routine needle EMG study can now be performed, with special attention to C8 radial nerve innervated muscles (EI; EPB) and the FDI (to look for axon loss).

The Needle EMG Study

- Abnormal muscles: FCU, FDI, ADM, FPL, APB, FPL
- Normal muscles: Deltoid, triceps, biceps, pronator teres, EI, EPB, paraspinals

This pattern of abnormal muscles is most consistent with a medial cord lesion (i.e., involvement of C8 and T1 median and ulnar nerve innervated muscles, with sparing of C8 radial nerve innervated muscles). Of course, a partial lower trunk lesion cannot be excluded with certainty.

EDX Study Impression

1. Probable Medial Cord Lesion

The EDX study identifies a brachial plexopathy that is axon loss in nature and that involves the sensory and motor nerve fibers. The distribution of the EDX abnormalities is most consistent with a medial cord localization, although a partial lower plexus lesion could produce a similar pattern and, hence, cannot be excluded.

Final Comments

Differentiation between lower plexus and medial cord lesions is best accomplished by studying the C8-radial motor axons. Although lesions involving the lower plexus may affect them, lesions involving the medial cord never do. Thus, although their involvement excludes a medial cord localization, the converse statement—that C8-radial muscle sparing localizes the lesion to the medial cord—is inaccurate.

Exercise 8

A 17-year-old male violinist is referred for EDX assessment of left upper extremity numbness and weakness. According to the patient, he first noted muscle wasting involving the left thenar eminence about 1 year ago. At that time, he also noted numbness along the lateral aspect of his left forearm and thumb. On examination by the referring physician, there was also biceps and brachioradialis weakness. Based on the distribution of the weakness and the numbness, a tentative diagnosis of left C6 radiculopathy had been provided by the referring physician.

Clinically, the sensory loss involves C6-derived axons, so the list of possible lesions sites includes the lateral cord and the upper plexus, whereas the weakness involves C5- or C6-derived motor axons (biceps; brachioradialis) and C8,T1-derived motor axons (thenar eminence muscles). No single PNS element could account for this distribution. Although it is possible that the thenar eminence atrophy is congenital, the patient is certain that it was not present prior to 1 year ago.

On examination, it would be helpful to separately assess the dorsal (superficial radial nerve, radial nerve, posterior cord distribution) and ventral (median nerve, lateral cord distribution) aspects of the thumb to determine if a single region or both regions (upper plexus distribution) are involved. This was done, but the information is not being provided because we have enough information to move forward with the EDX study.

The screening sensory NCS are performed on the symptomatic (left) limb.

Nerve Conduction Studies

		Upper extremity nerve conduction study worksheet							
Case 8		Left				Right			
NCS Performed		**LAT**	**AMP**	**CV**	**nAUC**	**LAT**	**AMP**	**CV**	**nAUC**
Sensory	**DRG**								
Median-D2	C6,7	X	7						
Ulnar-D5	C8	X	14						
S-radial	C6,7	X	21						

DRG Dorsal root ganglion/ganglia, *LAT* Latency, *AMP* Amplitude, *CV* Conduction velocity, *nAUC* Negative area under the curve

The amplitude response value of the Median-D2 response indicates an axon loss lesion involving the median nerve, the lateral cord, or the upper or middle plexus. The normal radial response argues against a supraclavicular localization but, because the sensory fibers subserving the Median-D2 and S-Radial sensory NCS could theoretically emanate from either the C6 DRG or the C7 DRG (i.e., one could be affected in isolation), a supraclavicular site cannot be excluded.

As always, because the median screening response is abnormal, the LABC and median-D1 sensory NCS are added bilaterally. The contralateral Median-D2 is also added. Although the radial and ulnar responses are normal, in a 17-year-old the amplitude values could have been much higher. Thus, they are also added. In addition, we need to assess the C8 fibers because of the thenar eminence muscle weakness and atrophy.

		Upper extremity nerve conduction study worksheet							
Case 8		Left				Right			
NCS Performed		**LAT**	**AMP**	**CV**	**nAUC**	**LAT**	**AMP**	**CV**	**nAUC**
Sensory	**DRG**								
Median-D2	C6,7	X	7			X	24		
Ulnar-D5	C8	X	14			X	17		
S-radial	C6,7	X	21			X	19		
LABC	C6	X	4			X	17		
Median-D1	C6	X	6			X	18		

DRG Dorsal root ganglion/ganglia, *LAT* Latency, *AMP* Amplitude, *CV* Conduction velocity, *nAUC* Negative area under the curve

The left LABC and Median-D1 responses are reduced in amplitude, arguing for a lateral cord or upper plexus localization. Sparing of the left radial response does not differentiate between these two possibilities as it could be spared with both if the sensory axons subserving it predominantly emanate from the C7 DRG.

To address this list of possibilities, the Musculocutaneous-Biceps and Axillary-Deltoid motor NCS are added bilaterally and the contralateral Median-APB motor NCS is added to address the thenar muscle atrophy.

		Upper extremity nerve conduction study worksheet							
Case 8		Left				Right			
NCS Performed		**LAT**	**AMP**	**CV**	**nAUC**	**LAT**	**AMP**	**CV**	**nAUC**
Motor	**Stim site**								
Median-APB	Wrist	X	2			X	8		
	Elbow		2	X			8	X	
Ulnar-ADM	Wrist	X	8			X	9		
	Elbow		8	X			9	X	
Musculocutaneous-BC	Axilla	X	4			X	8		
	SCF		4	X			8	X	
Axillary-deltoid	SCF	X	14			X	12		

DRG Dorsal root ganglion/ganglia, *LAT* Latency, *AMP* Amplitude, *CV* Conduction velocity, *nAUC* Negative area under the curve

The amplitude value of the median motor response is reduced, indicating an axon loss process involving the median nerve, the medial cord, or the lower plexus. However, the medial cord and lower plexus localizations are excluded by the normal Ulnar-D5 sensory response, leaving only the median nerve as an explanation. The low amplitude Musculocutaneous-Biceps response indicates an axon loss process involving the musculocutaneous nerve, the lateral cord, or the upper plexus. Sparing of the Axillary-Deltoid response argues against an upper plexus localization.

Thus, the sensory NCS argues for a lateral cord lesion (but cannot exclude upper plexus with certainty) and the motor NCS argue for a lateral cord and median nerve lesion (but cannot exclude upper plexus with certainty. Given that we are seeking a single focus that could account for all of the abnormalities, and given that the lateral cord and the terminal median nerve are adjacent structures, a lateral cord lesion with extension into the terminal median nerve is suggested. Thus, on needle EMG, we will need to look at the lateral cord and median nerve muscle domains closely (as well as the upper plexus muscle domain given that the needle EMG study is more sensitive to motor axon loss than are the motor NCS).

The Needle EMG Study

- Abnormal muscles
  - Biceps, brachialis, pronator teres, FCR, FPL, APB
- Normal muscles
  - Infraspinatus, deltoid, triceps, brachioradialis, EI, FDI, paraspinals

The needle EMG shows abnormalities in the distribution of the lateral cord (biceps; brachialis; pronator teres) and the terminal median nerve (APB, FPL, pronator teres, FCR). Note that the brachioradialis is normal (it was reported to be weak by the referring physician).

EDX Study Impression

1. Probable Lateral Cord Brachial Plexopathy with extension into the Median Terminal Nerve

The above is axon loss and best localizes to the lateral cord with extension into the terminal median nerve. Based on the motor responses, the lesion is severe in degree. An MRI study of the brachial plexus may be of further diagnostic utility. Evidence of brachioradialis involvement was not noted.

Final Comments

- Magnetic resonance imaging of the brachial plexus disclosed a mass involving the lateral cord that, as predicted by the EDX study, extended into the terminal median nerve. At surgery, the lesion extended from the proximal aspect of the lateral cord (proximal to the departure site of the musculocutaneous nerve) to the proximal aspect of the terminal median nerve. Pathology showed the lesion to be a perineurioma.
- The strength of the brachioradialis muscle is not easily assessed. Even when the forearm is oriented in the neutral position (i.e., forearm pronation so that the thumb is superior), the biceps and brachialis are the predominant forearm flexors. Moreover, in this case, the biceps and brachialis muscles are both affected.
- The author assesses the brachioradialis muscle by having the patient first position both forearms in their neutral position and flexed against the examiner's forearm, which is held perpendicular to the patient's forearms. The examiner then uses his other hand to palpate the contracting brachioradialis muscles of the two sides for differences in bulk and consistency. In this individually, the brachioradialis muscles of the two sides had identical features.

References

1. Stewart JD. Focal peripheral neuropathies. 2nd ed. New York: Raven Press; 1993. p. 506.
2. Wilbourn AJ. Brachial plexus disorders. In: Dyck PJ, Thomas PK, editors. Peripheral neuropathy, vol. 2. 3rd ed. Philadelphia: WB Saunders; 1993. p. 911–50.
3. Ferrante MA. Brachial plexopathies: classification, causes, and consequences. Muscle Nerve. 2004;30:547–68.
4. Ferrante MA. Comprehensive electromyography: with clinical correlations and case studies. New York: Cambridge University Press; 2018.
5. Ferrante MA, Tsao BE. Brachial plexopathies. In: Katirji B, Kaminski HJ, Ruff RL, editors. Neuromuscular disorders in clinical practice, vol. 2. 2nd ed. New York: Springer; 2014. p. 1029–62.
6. Ferrante MA. Brachial plexopathies. Continuum. 2014;20:1323–42.
7. Ferrante MA, Wilbourn AJ. The utility of various sensory nerve conduction responses in assessing brachial plexopathies. Muscle Nerve. 1995;18:879–89.
8. Bonnel F. Microscopic anatomy of the adult human brachial plexus: an anatomical and histological basis for microsurgery. Microsurgery. 1984;5:107–17.
9. Slingluff CL Jr, Terzis JK, Edgerton MT. The quantitative microanatomy of the brachial plexus in man: reconstructive relevance. In: Terzis JK, editor. Microreconstruction of nerve injuries. Philadelphia: WB Saunders; 1987. p. 285–324.
10. Wolock B, Millesi H: Brachial plexus: applied anatomy and operative exposure. In Gelberman RH, editor. Operative nerve repair and reconstruction, volume 2. Philadelphia: Lippincott; 1991; p 1255–1272.
11. Wilbourn AJ. Brachial plexus lesions. In: Dyck PJ, Thomas PK, editors. Peripheral neuropathy. 4th ed. Philadelphia: Elsevier Saunders; 2005. p. 1339–73.
12. Swash M. Diagnosis of brachial root and plexus lesions. J Neurol. 1986;233:131–5.
13. Leffert RD. Brachial plexus injuries. London: Churchill Livingstone; 1985.
14. Hollinshead WH. Anatomy for surgeons, vol 3: the back and limbs. 3rd. ed. Philadelphia: Harper & Row; 1982.
15. Ferrante MA. The management of peripheral nerve trauma. Curr Treat Options Neurol. 2018 Jun 1;20(7):25. https://doi.org/10.1007/s11940-018-0507-4).
16. Brunelli GA, Brunelli GR. A fourth type of brachial plexus injury: middle lesion (C7). Ital J Orthop Traumatol. 1992;18:389–93.
17. Maggiano H, Levin KH, Wilbourn AJ. Relationship between the medial antebrachial cutaneous sensory and median motor responses in brachial plexopathies (abstract). Muscle Nerve. 1993;16:1113–4.
18. Nishida T, Price SJ, Minieka MM. Medial antebrachial cutaneous nerve conduction in true neurogenic thoracic outlet syndrome. Electromyogr Clin Neurophysiol. 1993;33:285–8.
19. Walsh JF. The anatomy of the brachial plexus. Am J Med Sci. 1877;74:387–98.
20. Gilliatt RW. Thoracic outlet syndromes. In: Dyck PJ, Thomas PK, Lambert EH, Bunge R, editors. Peripheral neuropathy. 2nd ed. Philadelphia: Saunders; 1984. p. 1409–24.
21. Tsao BE, Ferrante MA, Wilbourn AJ, Shields RW Jr. Electrodiagnostic features of true neurogenic thoracic outlet syndrome. Muscle Nerve. 2014;49:724–7. https://doi.org/10.1002/mus.24066.
22. Ferrante MA, Ferrante ND. The thoracic outlet syndromes: part 1. Overview of the thoracic outlet syndromes and review of true neurogenic thoracic outlet. Muscle Nerve. 2017;55:782–93. https://doi.org/10.1002/mus.25536.

8 Radiculopathies

Karen A. Karwa and John A. Morren

Etiology

There are several causes of radiculopathy, however, the vast majority of radiculopathies are compressive in etiology. Typically, in patients younger than 40–50 years of age, nerve root compression occurs from disc protrusion. Whereas, in patients older than 40–50 years of age, nerve root compression is due to bony impingement from spondylosis. Compressive radiculopathy is more commonly seen in cervical and lumbosacral regions. Lumbar spinal stenosis most commonly affects L4-5 followed by L3-4, L5-S1 and L1-2 in descending order [1]. The likelihood of nerve root compression by disc rupture at the lumbosacral levels is increased by extrathecal dural and foraminal ligaments that anchor nerve roots and reduce plasticity [2, 3]. Radiculopathy in the thoracic region due to disc protrusion is uncommon (this region benefits from less range of movements, especially given the effects of ribs) and is more likely to be secondary to local infection such as herpes zoster, diabetes mellitus, or spinal tumors. Below is a more extensive list of the causes of radiculopathies.

<u>Causes of Radiculopathy:</u>

- Compression: Disc herniation, degenerative spine disease/spondylosis [4, 5]
- Vascular: Vasculitis (e.g. in diabetes mellitus), epidural/subdural hematomas, dural fistulae/arteriovenous malformations, spinal epidural cavernous hemangiomas [3, 5]
- Infections: e.g. Tuberculosis, mycoplasma, herpes zoster virus (HZV), herpes simplex virus (HSV), cytomegalovirus (CMV), Epstein-Barr virus (EBV), Lyme, syphilis, HIV [6–10]
- Iatrogenic: including complication of spinal anesthesia [11], spinal cord stimulator placement [12]
- Trauma: e.g. Root avulsion, fracture of vertebral body [13]
- Toxic: e.g. Procainamide polyradiculoneuropathy [14]
- Autoimmune: e.g. Chronic Inflammatory Demyelinating Polyradiculoneuropathy (CIDP) [15]
- Metabolic: e.g. Diabetic polyradiculopathy, adrenal insufficiency [16]
- Inflammatory: e.g. Sarcoidosis [17–19]
- Mass (non-neoplastic): e.g. Epidural abscess, spinal cysts [20–22]
- Neoplastic: Epidural/vertebral metastases, leptomeningeal metastases, malignant angiotrophic lymphoma; benign such as meningioma, ependymoma, schwanommas, [23–25]

The original version of this chapter was revised. A correction to this chapter can be found at https://doi.org/10.1007/978-3-030-74997-2_14

K. A. Karwa (✉)
Neurology of the Rockies, Englewood, Colorado, USA

J. A. Morren
Neuromuscular Center, Neurological Institute, Cleveland Clinic, and Cleveland Clinic Lerner College of Medicine of Case Western Reserve University, Cleveland, OH, USA
e-mail: morrenj@ccf.org

N. Galvez-Jimenez et al. (eds.), *Electrodiagnostic Medicine*,
https://doi.org/10.1007/978-3-030-74997-2_8

- Radiation
- Neurodegenerative: Amyotrophic lateral sclerosis (involvement may extend beyond anterior horn cell proper), juvenile amyotrophy [26]

Anatomy

Neural foramina are formed between each pair of vertebral bodies and are bounded superiorly and inferiorly by pedicles, anteriorly by intervertebral disc and vertebral body, and posteriorly by facet joint.(See Fig. 8.1) [3]. Through the neural foramina pass the spinal nerve roots, recurrent meningeal nerves and radicular blood vessels. The blood supply to the nerve roots arises from a capillary network derived from radicular arteries [3]. There are 31 pairs of spinal roots: 8 cervical, 12 thoracic, 5 lumbar, 5 sacral, 1 coccygeal. The number designation of the exiting cervical spinal root corresponds with the number of the vertebral body below it, for example the C3 nerve root exits the spinal canal at C2-3 neural foraminal level. The cervical spinal column is comprised of 7 vertebral bodies, as a result at the C7-T1 intervertebral level, the exiting nerve root is numbered C8. Thus all thoracic, lumbar and sacral nerve roots exit below the vertebral body of the same number [3]. For example the T1 nerve root exits at the T1-2 vertebral level, and the L4 nerve root exits at L4-5 vertebral level. At lumbosacral levels, all lumbar and sacral spinal nerve roots are constituted at the T12-L1 vertebral level, where the spinal cord ends as the conus medullaris. The roots then course down the canal as the cauda equina, until they exit at their respective neural foramina. Depending on the nature and location of intraspinal compression, roots may be injured at any disk level, from the L1-2 level to the level of their exit through the neural foramen. For example, the L5 root can be compressed by a central disk protrusion at the L2-3 or L3-4 level, a posterolateral disk protrusion at the L4-5 level, or foraminal stenosis at the L5-S1 level. (Figs. 8.2 and 8.3) [3, 27].

The cell bodies of the motor nerve roots are located in the anterior horn of the spinal cord (anterior horn cells), and are therefore within the spinal canal, whereas the sensory dorsal root ganglion (DRG) is typically located outside the spinal canal proper. The DRG is in a protected position within the neural foramen. This location is of significance as nerve conduction studies demonstrate preservation of sensory nerve action potentials (SNAP) in radiculopathies. However, there are cadaveric and radiographic (including magnetic resonance imaging studies) that demonstrate about 11%-38% of L5 DRG and 3% of L3 and L4 DRG are intraspinal canal in loca-

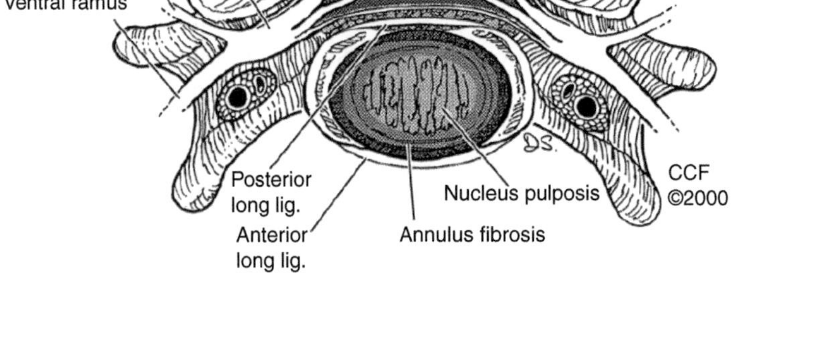

Fig. 8.1 Diagram of cross section of the spine at the cervical level [3]

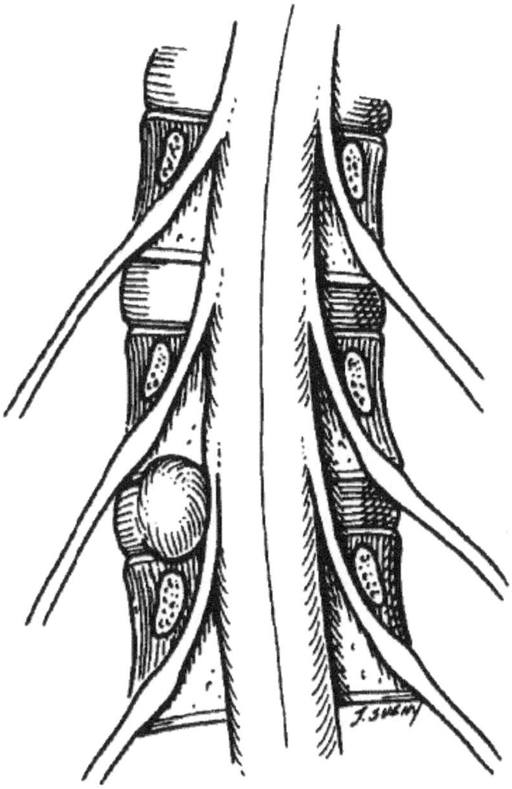

Fig. 8.2 Posterolateral disc herniation compresses the nerve root descending to exit the intervertebral foramen one level below corresponding vertebrae (i.e L4 -5 disc herniation compresses L5 nerve root) [27]

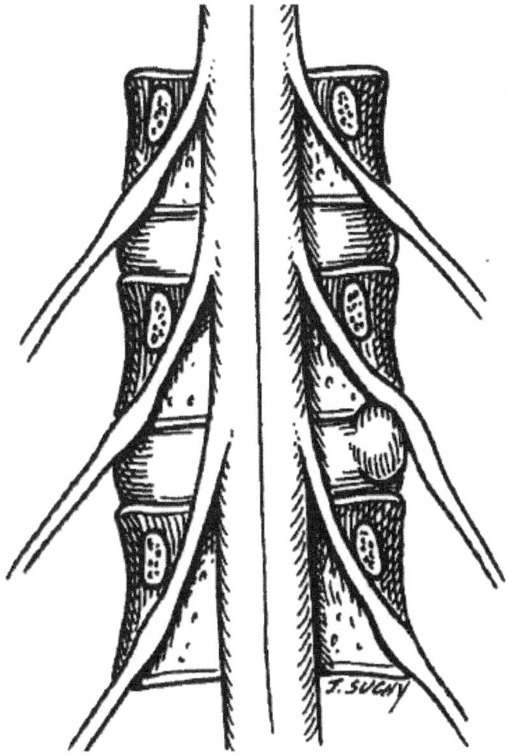

Fig. 8.3 Far lateral disc herniation compresses the nerve root exiting foramen through foramen at that vertebral level (ie. L4-5 disc compressing the L4 nerve root) [27]

tion [28, 29]. In addition, the C5 and C6 DRG also have a tendency to reside in intraspinal locations [30]. Intraspinal location of DRG can result in degeneration of sensory nerves and loss of SNAP on nerve conduction studies which can present diagnostic dilemmas in the case of radiculopathies.

Mild injury to the nerve root may result in focal demyelination leading to conduction block or conduction velocity slowing along nerve root fibers. Axon loss at the root level results in wallerian degeneration along the entire course of affected nerve fibers [3].

Clinical Features

Radiculopathies present clinically as pain and/or paresthesia originating from the spine and generally following the distribution of the nerve root (i.e. the dermatomal distribution). They are also associated with sensory loss and weakness following the distribution of the nerve root. Due to significant dermatomal overlap dense numbness is uncommon and is more classically seen in a peripheral nerve lesion rather than radiculopathy. Similarly, weakness can be seen in muscles supplied by the same nerve root, however, it is very unusual for a radiculopathy to result in complete muscle paralysis due to myotomal overlap. Conduction block and axon loss only produce symptoms and neurologic deficits if a sufficient number of nerve fibers are affected. Conduction velocity slowing alone is insufficient to produce significant weakness or sensory loss, although sensory modalities requiring timed volleys of impulse transmission along their pathways, such as vibration and proprioception, can be altered [3]. Deep tendon reflexes may be absent depending on the nerve root involved in the muscle tendon reflex [31]. Involvement of a single nerve root is termed monoradiculopathy, whereas multiple, usually contiguous nerve root level involvement is termed polyradiculopathy.

Cervical Radiculopathies

The clinical diagnosis of cervical radiculopathy is supported by neck or shoulder pain radiating into the arm. Cervical radiculopathies involving the C7 nerve root is most common, while pure T1 radiculopathy occurs the least commonly [32]. Provocative tests such as Spurling's test (neck compression maneuver or foraminal compression test) and relief tests such as *shoulder abduction relief sign* have been used at the bedside to assist with diagnosis of cervical radiculopathy. One study reviewed various provocative and relief signs and reported that for roots C6-8 neck compression maneuvers had a specificity of 100% for radicular pain and 92-100% for neurological and radiological signs, respectively. For shoulder abduction relief sign, the specificity was 100% for neurological signs and 80% for radiological signs. The sensitivity of these tests for radicular symptoms, neurological signs and radiological signs varied from 40–60% [33].

There are classical clinical attributes in solitary cervical root lesions which are detailed below:

<u>C5 Radiculopathy:</u> Typically presents with neck or shoulder pain, with numbness generally following axillary nerve distribution. Weakness is classically seen in C5 innervated muscles—shoulder abduction, external rotation, elbow flexion, forearm supination. There can be loss of biceps and brachioradialis reflex.

<u>C6 Radiculopathy:</u> Typically presents with pain in neck, shoulder, lateral upper arm, lateral forearm, thumb and lateral hand; numbness typically seen in lateral forearm, thumb and index fingers. Weakness is classically seen in C6 innervated muscles—shoulder abduction, external rotation, elbow flexion, forearm supination and pronation. There can be loss of biceps and brachioradialis reflex. C6 radiculopathies have the most variable presentation with half of the cases presenting similar to C5 and other half similar to C7 radiculopathies [32].

<u>C7 Radiculopathy:</u> Typically presents with pain in neck, shoulder, middle finger and hand; numbness typically seen in index, middle finger, palm. Weakness is classically seen in C7 innervated muscles—elbow and wrist extension, forearm pronation.

An important part of the clinical diagnosis of C7 radiculopathy rests on the finding of a diminished triceps deep tendon reflex, but several studies have shown that the reflex is abnormal in less than 70% of patients [32, 34].

<u>C8 Radiculopathy:</u> Typically presents with pain in shoulder, medial forearm, fourth and fifth digits, medial hand; numbness typically seen in medial forearm, fourth and fifth digits, medial hand. Weakness is classically seen in C8 innervated muscles—finger and wrist extension, distal finger flexion, finger abduction and adduction. There can be loss of triceps reflex.

<u>T1 radiculopathy:</u> Typically presents with pain in medial arm, medial forearm, axillary chest wall; numbness typically seen in medial forearm, fourth and fifth digits, medial hand. Weakness is classically seen in T1 innervated muscles—thumb abduction, distal thumb flexion, finger abduction and adduction. T1 radiculopathy is the most uncommon isolated root lesion affecting the arm. Although all C8 muscles of the hand are said to have some T1 contributions, the abductor pollicis brevis muscle seems to be the only muscle with predominantly T1 innervation [32, 35].

Thoracic Radiculopathies

The classic presentation of thoracic radiculopathies involve pain and paresthesias radiating from the posterior thorax in the dermatomal distribution of the involved nerve root. Sensory loss may be present only in a portion of the involved dermatome. Muscle weakness is often subtle and can be demonstrated by having patient cough or attempt a sit up which may result in a bulging intercostal or abdominal muscle [5].

Lumbosacral Radiculopathies

Lumbosacral radiculopathies typically present as pain and/or paresthesias radiating from lower back into the lower limbs. Symptoms are often worsened by Valsalva maneuvers, straight leg raising test and reverse straight leg raising test. However, straight leg raising test and reverse straight leg raising are not quite specific and may be seen in lumbosacral plexopathies, femoral neuropathies and diseases of hip joint [5]. Lumbar disc herniation leading to electromyographically-determined motor radiculopathy occurs at L4-5, L5-S1 and L3-4 levels 55%,43% and 2% of the time respectively [3, 36].

L1 radiculopathy: Extremely uncommon. Typically presents with pain and/or paresthesias and/or loss of sensation in inguinal region. No corresponding muscle weakness in the lower limb, or loss of reflexes [5].

L2 Radiculopathy: Very uncommon. Typically presents with pain and/or paresthesias and/or loss of sensation in anterolateral thigh with weakness of hip flexors [5].

L3 Radiculopathy: More likely to occur than L1 or L2 however, less common than L4-S1 levels. Typically presents with pain and/or paresthesias and/or loss of sensation in medial thigh or knee with weakness of hip flexors, quadriceps, and adductors. The knee jerk may be reduced or absent [5].

L4 Radiculopathy: Disc herniation is fairly common at this level. Typically presents with pain and/or paresthesias and/or loss of sensation in the medial leg with weakness of quadriceps, hip adductors, occasionally tibialis anterior. The knee jerk is often reduced or absent [5].

L5 Radiculopathy: Typically presents with pain and/or paresthesias and/or loss of sensation in lateral lower leg and great toe with weakness including that of the tibialis anterior, extensor hallucis, ankle invertors and evertors, and gluteus medius. There is no specific deep tendon reflex abnormality [5].

S1 Radiculopathy: Typically presents with pain and/or paresthesias and/or loss of sensation in the sole/plantar aspect, lateral aspect of the foot and lateral three toes with weakness of gastrocnemius, soleus and gluteus maximus. The ankle reflex may be absent or reduced [5]. The biceps femoris short head, long head and medial gastrocnemius are near exclusively innervated by the S1 root although some studies do suggest significant L5 innervation [3, 37–39].

S2-4 Radiculopathy: Typically occurs as a polyradiculopathy. Typically presents with pain and/or paresthesias and/or loss of sensation in the perineal and medial buttocks and is associated with urinary and fecal incontinence. There can be absence of anal wink and bulbocavernosus reflexes [5].

Differential Diagnosis of Cervical Radiculopathy

1. Neuralgic Amyotrophy: This can often present similar to an acute cervical radiculopathy. Classically patient presents with debilitating pain in shoulder or scapula that is followed by progressive weakness. The motor component can involve spinal accessory, suprascapular, long thoracic, axillary, and musculocutaneous nerves. Most patient recover although atrophy and muscle weakness may persist. This condition can be hard to differentiate from a C5-6 radiculopathy [4, 40].
2. Rotator cuff tear: Typically results in weakness of shoulder abductor, external rotation and can be associated with suprascapular mononeuropathy [41].
3. Amyotrophic lateral sclerosis: May initially present as a radiculopathy (although radicular pain typically absent) especially if predominant C8-T1 muscle involvement (the weakness and atrophy may produce the so-called "split-hand pattern").
4. Multifocal motor neuropathy: Early on, when an isolated nerve trunk is involved it may also mimic involvement of an isolated nerve root [4].
5. Neurogenic thoracic outlet syndrome: Classically involves T1> > C8 nerve root with severe axon loss in the abductor pollicis brevis muscle and medial antebrachial SNAP [42].

6. Median sternotomy brachial plexopathy: Typically occurs in the setting of coronary artery bypass graft and cardiac valve repair surgeries (operations requiring sternotomy) with severe axon loss in C8> > T1 nerve root [42].
7. Ulnar mononeuropathy: Can present similar to C8-T1 radiculopathy. However, weakness is limited to ulnar innervated muscles with sparing of median and radial innervated C8-T1 muscles [43].

Differential Diagnosis of Lumbosacral Radiculopathies

1. Ilioinguinal and genitofemoral neuropathy: Can present similar to L1 radiculopathy [44]
2. Lateral femoral cutaneous neuropathy: Can present similar to L2 radiculopathy, however classically a pure sensory neuropathy with no associated weakness [44].
3. Femoral neuropathy: Can present similar to L2/L3/L4 radiculopathy. However, classically only femoral innervated muscles are weak with essentially preserved strength in hip abductors/adductors [44].
4. Common peroneal (fibular) neuropathy: Can present similar to L5 radiculopathy, however, there is preservation of ankle inversion which is typically weak in a L5 radiculopathy [44].
5. Sciatic neuropathy: Can present similar to multilevel lumbosacralradiculopathy, but glutei muscles are spared in sciatic neuropathy [44].
6. Tibial neuropathy: Can present similar to S1 radiculopathy, but hamstrings and glutei muscles are spared in tibial neuropathy [44].

Electrodiagnostic Evaluation

Nerve Conduction Studies

Nerve conduction studies are an essential part of the work up of patients with suspected radiculopathies. Due to the intraspinal location of the DRG, the sensory nerve responses are classically preserved. The SNAP amplitude may be affected if the DRG is involved in the pathologic process such as with a variant intraspinal location of DRG. In patients with radiculopathy, nerve conduction studies are typically normal (unless lesion is severe/has marked motor axon loss) and electrodiagnosis is primarily established by needle electrode examination (NEE) [31]. There can be abnormalities in routine motor nerve conduction studies especially in C8-T1 and L5-S1 with significant axon loss. Late responses include F-waves and H-reflex. The absence of motor F-wave, in the presence of normal motor nerve conduction is suggestive of recent/acute demyelination, classically seen in acute demyelinating neuropathies however, this finding may also be seen in an isolated motor radiculopathy. Abnormalities in F-waves are not specific and can be seen in several disorders and alone is insufficient to make an electrodiagnosis of radiculopathy. An evidence-based review demonstrated the peroneal (fibular) and tibial motor F-waves have a low sensitivity in diagnosis of lumbosacral radiculopathy [45]. Although the H-reflex is the electrodiagnostic equivalent of the ankle deep tendon reflex, in normal individuals there may be a discordance between presence of the ankle reflex and ability to elicit the H reflex [46]. The tibial H-reflex is routinely used in clinical practice and is a very sensitive test for tibial S1 sensory pathway including intraspinal course of S1 nerve root [3]. In the H-reflex electrical stimulus travels orthodromically along 1a afferents to the spinal cord activating the motor neuron in the same segment and resulting in a peripheral motor response [47, 48]. The H-reflex is absent or low in 80% patients with surgically proven S1 radiculopathy [49].

Theoretically, somatosensory evoked potentials (SEPs) should be a valuable tool in the assessment of conduction abnormalities along sensory fibers at the root level. Electrical stimuli are delivered on the skin surface to a mixed sensory and motor nerve trunk, a sensory nerve trunk, or the skin in a specific dermatomal distribution. Responses are recorded over the spine and scalp, and latencies are measured to assess the conduction time along large-diameter sensory fibers across various segments of the peripheral and central conduction pathways primarily subserving proprioception and vibratory sense [3]. Unfortunately, a number of limitations diminish the value of this technique including variable amplitude measurements in normal individuals; activation of nerve fibers belonging to more than one root segment, time consuming procedure and subject to technical artifacts [50]. Given these limitations, SEPs obtained from nerve trunk stimulation have been shown to add little diagnostic value [51, 52].

Tables 8.1 and 8.2 demonstrate "screening" nerve conduction studies that can be performed to evaluate cervical and lumbosacral radiculopathies, respectively.

Table 8.1 Nerve conduction studies evaluating for cervical radiculopathy

Nerve	Recording Site	Nerve Root
Median sensory	Index/digit 2	C6-7
Median sensory	Digit 3	C7
Ulnar sensory	Digit 5	C8
Radial sensory	Snuffbox	C5-C6
Lateral antebrachial cutaneous	Lateral forearm	C5-6
Medial antebrachial cutaneous	Medial forearm	T1
Median motor	Abductor pollicis brevis	T1
Ulnar motor	Abductor digiti minimi	C8-T1
Radial motor	Extensor digitorum (communis)	C7-8
Musculocutaneous motor	Biceps	C5-6
Axillary	Deltoid	C5-6

Table 8.2 Nerve conduction studies to evaluate for lumbosacral radiculopathy

Nerve	Recording Site	Nerve Root
Sural sensory	Ankle	S1
Superficial peroneal (fibular) sensory	Ankle	L5
Saphenous sensory	Ankle	L4
Peroneal (fibular) motor	Extensor digitorum brevis	L5 (-S1)
Tibial motor	Abductor Hallucis	S1
Peroneal (fibular) motor	Tibialis anterior	(L4-)L5
Femoral motor	Rectus Femoris	L3-4
H-reflex	Soleus	S1

The Needle Electrode Examination

NEE is the most specific and sensitive electrodiagnostic test for the identification of axon loss radiculopathy. NEE can identify one or more of the following abnormalities: increased insertional activity (usually in the form of unsustained positive sharp waves just after needle movement); further evidence of active/ongoing motor axon loss (typically in the form of fibrillation potentials); reduced ("neurogenic") recruitment pattern of motor unit firing; and features of chronic motor unit action potential (MUAP) reinnervation, such as increased duration, increased amplitude, and polyphasia [3]. The NEE can help localize nerve root involvement by identifying motor axon loss changes in at least two muscles that share the same nerve root however, involve separate peripheral nerve distributions. When a single nerve root is localized, muscles of surrounding myotomes must be examined to rule out additional nerve root involvement. Corresponding paraspinal muscle evaluation should be routinely performed as it is very helpful in ruling out generalized polyneuropathy or plexopathy (also the first muscles to be affected early in the process). NEE can also determine degree of active/ongoing and chronic motor axon loss, thereby establishing the chronicity of the process. In patients with nonspecific arm or leg paresthesias, screening of several muscles can be performed to help identify an underlying radiculopathy. Tables 8.3 and 8.4 outline the "screening" NEE for radiculopathy [3].

Anatomic, clinical, and electromyographic myotomal charts are used to correlate the pattern of EMG abnormalities in a limb with a specific root level involvement. Anatomical and clinical charts although useful, are not entirely applicable to the NEE. Muscles are chosen for the NEE because of specific attributes of root innervation and accessibility.

NEE can easily isolate muscles that are difficult to examine clinically and with assistance of myotomal chart, play a key role in root localization. Thus, electromyographically derived myotomal charts are quite useful in the electrodiagnosis of radiculopathy [3, 32, 49, 53]. Tables 8.5 and 8.6 demonstrate myotomal innervation patterns in upper and lower extremities respectively [54].

Table 8.3 Screening muscles to evaluate cervical radiculopathy* [3]

Muscle	Nerve Root	Nerve Trunk
First dorsal Interosseus	C8(−T1)	Ulnar
Abductor pollicis brevis	(C8-)T1	Median
Flexor Pollicis longus	C8(−T1)	Anterior Interosseus (median)
Extensor Indicis Proprius	C8	Posterior Interosseus (radial)
Pronator Teres	C6-7	Median
Triceps	C6-7(-C8)	Radial
Biceps	C5-6	Musculocutaneous
Deltoid	C5-6	Axillary
C7 Paraspinal	Overlap	

Table 8.4 Screening muscles to evaluate lumbosacral radiculopathy* [3]

Muscle	Nerve Root	Nerve Trunk
Abductor Hallucis	S1	Tibial
Medial gastrocnemius	S1	Tibial
Biceps Femoris, short head	S1	Peroneal (fibular) division of sciatic
Extensor digitorum brevis	L5 (S1)	Peroneal (fibular) (deep branch)
Tibialis anterior	(L4) L5	Peroneal (fibular) (deep branch)
Tibialis posterior (or flexor Digitorum longus)	L5	Tibial
Gluteus Medius	L5 (S1)	Superior gluteal
Rectus Femoris	(L2)L3-4	Femoral
S1 Paraspinal	Overlap	

Table 8.5 Myotomal Innervatation Upper Extremity* [54]

ANTERIOR PRIMARY RAMI	C5	C6	C7	C8	T1
PROXIMAL NERVES					
Rhomboid major/minor (dorsal scapular)	■				
Supraspinatus (suprascapular)	■	▓			
Infraspinatus (suprascapular)	■	▓			
Deltoid (axillary)	■	▓			
Biceps brachii (musculocutaneous)	■	■			
Brachialis (musculocutaneous)	■	■			
RADIAL NERVE					
Triceps		■	■		
Anconeus		▓	■		
Brachioradialis	▓	■			
Extensor Carpi Radialis		▓	■		
Extensor Pollicis Brevis			░	■	
Extensor Indicis Proprius			░	■	
MEDIAN NERVE					
Pronator Teres		■	■		
Flexor Carpi Radialis		▓	■		
Flexor Pollicis Longus				■	▓
Pronator Quadratus				■	▓
Abductor Pollicis Brevis				▓	■
ULNAR NERVE					
Flexor Carpi ulnaris				■	░
Flexor digitorum Profundus Dig 4,5				■	░
Abductor Digiti Minimi				■	▓
Adductor Pollics				■	▓
First Dorsal Interosseus				■	▓

Table 8.6 Myotomal Innervation Lower extremity [54]

ANTERIOR PRIMARY RAMI	L2	L3	L4	L5	S1	S2
PROXIMAL NERVES						
Iliacus (lumbar plexus-femoral)	■	■	▒			
Adductor Longus (obturator)	▒	■	■			
Vastus Lateralis (femoral)	▒	■	■			
Rectus Femoris (femoral)	▒	■	■			
Tensor Fascia Lata (superior gluteal)			░	■	▒	
Gluteus Medius (superior gluteal)			░	■	▒	
Gluteus Maximus (inferior gluteal)				▒	■	░
SCIATIC NERVE						
Semitendinosus/Semimembranosus (tibialdivision of sciatic)			░	■	▒	
Biceps Femoris, shorthead (peroneal (fibular) division of sciatic)			░	▒	■	
Biceps Femoris long head (tibial division of sciatic)				▒	■	
PERONEAL (FIBULAR) NERVE						
Tibialis Anterior			▒	■		
Extensor Hallucis				■	▒	
Peroneus Longus				■	▒	
Extensor Digitorum Brevis				■	▒	
TIBIAL NERVE						
Tibialis Posterior				■	▒	
Flexor Digitorum Longus				■	▒	
Gastrocnemius, lateral					▒	■
Gastrocnemius, medial					■	▒
Soleus					■	▒
Abductor Hallucis					■	▒
Abductor Digiti Quinti Pedis					■	▒

■ Usually dominant contribution
▒ Sometimes significant contribution
░ Minor/equivocal contribution

Determining the Age of a Radiculopathy

There are characteristic electrophysiological changes that occur within the muscle in the setting of conduction block and axon loss injury which help identify the age of a radiculopathy. Table 8.7 summarizes the typical changes in axon loss radiculopathy.

A. Acute Axonal radiculopathy: Motor unit potentials are of normal configuration and size, the presence of abnormal insertional or spontaneous activity in the form of trains of brief sharp spikes or positive waves indicates recent motor axon loss. Increased insertional activity alone suggests that the process may be only several weeks old. The presence of additional spontaneous activity in the form of fibrillation potentials indicates a process at least ~3 weeks of age (may be earlier in proximal limb and paraspinal muscles).

B. Acute Demyelinating Radiculopathy: There is evidence of a prominent conduction block lesion at the root level as the cause for weakness. In these cases, CMAP (with stimulation point distal to the root-level conduction block) is of normal amplitude and NEE of the muscle demonstrates reduced recruitment pattern, normal motor unit configuration/morphology and the absence of positive sharp wave and fibrillation potentials (which may be collectively referred to as "denervation potentials"). The corresponding late responses (F-wave and/or H-reflex responses) may be prolonged

Table 8.7 Findings in Needle Electrode Examination at progressive stages of axon loss radiculopathy * [3]

	Reduced Recruitment	Insertion	PSP	Fib	Poly/Var	Neuro	CRD
<3 week	++	+/++	+	–	–	–	–
3-6 week	++	++	++	+++	–	–	–
6-26 week	++	+	+/–	++	+++	–	–
Chronic/active	++	–	+/–	+	++	++	–
Chronic/remote	+/++	–	–	–	–	+++	+

Abbreviations: *Fib* fibrillation potentials in myotomal limb muscles; *Insertion* abnormal insertional activity in myotomal muscles; *CRD* complex repetitive discharges; *Neuro* neurogenic motor unit potential changes (increased duration and amplitude); *Poly/Var* polyphasic motor unit potential changes/motor unit potential variation/variability; *PSP* paraspinal muscle fibrillation potentials; –negligible/equivocal amount; +, mild amount; ++, moderate amount; +++, greatest amount [3]

or absent. Ttogether, these findings suggests conduction block. If this pattern is seen in multiple muscles of a specific myotome, a diagnosis of radiculopathy can be made. This strategy is not reliable for the diagnosis of conduction block if the onset of weakness is less than ~4 weeks before the electrodiagnostic study, because an acute axon loss lesion may share these features, including not clearly manifesting denervation potentials for ~3 or more weeks after onset of symptoms [3].

C. Chronic-active Radiculopathy: NEE demonstrates neurogenic MUAP with chronic reinnervation changes along with considerabledenervation potentials. In root distributions where the myotome includes muscles in distal and proximal regions of a limb, the presence of a chronic and ongoing axon loss process can be even more clearly defined when fibrillation potentials are seen in distal and proximal muscles in the root distribution. In lesions where fibrillation potentials are seen in distal muscles only, the presence of an ongoing axon loss process is less certain. Some inactive but severe axon loss processes never fully reinnervate, especially in muscles farthest from the injury site, leaving some muscle fibers denervated indefinitely.
D. Chronic-remote Radiculopathy: NEE demonstrates neurogenic MUAP with chronic reinnervation changes, in the absence of denervation potentials. These changes in motor unit action potentials are permanent, reflecting the histopathologic changes in the reinnervated muscle, and remain unchanged unless the motor unit is injured again. After a significant motor axon loss process has occurred, MUAPs never return to their preinjury morphology.

Determining the Severity of a Radiculopathy

The severity of an axon loss is based on the degree of motor unit loss in the specific root distribution. This is determined by a subjective/semi-objective measurement of the degree of reduced recruitment of motor unit potentials. Of note, reduced recruitment (without definite MUAP morphological changes) is not necessarily caused by axon loss unless the CMAP elicited from the same muscle is also reduced in amplitude (although, less commonly, this may also result from distal conduction blocks). Thus, defining the severity of an axon loss radiculopathy requires evaluation of the CMAPs in the myotome in question (when possible) and the degree of reduced recruitment of MUAPs. Quantifying the degree of denervation potentials does not correlate as well with the degree of axon loss [3].

Electrodiagnostic Pitfalls and Limitations

The value of electrodiagnostic studies in establishing a diagnosis of radiculopathy is highly variable and depends on patient selection, nerve root involved and study used for electrodiagnostic testing [3, 55–57].

Limitations of Nerve Conduction Studies in Diagnosis of Radiculopathy

There are several limitations to the use of nerve conduction studies in the diagnosis of radiculopathy. Nerve conduction studies are more useful to exclude other clinical conditions mimicking radiculopathies.

1. In most radiculopathies, typically there is damage only to a portion of nerve root fibers, thus there may not be significant axon loss to result in abnormalities in (motor) nerve conduction studies.
2. Early in the course of a radiculopathy patients present with pain/paresthesia.

   Sensory radiculopathy can only rarely be reliably localized segmentally by electrodiagnostic techniques. Pain is primarily mediated through C-type sensory fibers that are too small to be studied by routine electrodiagnostic techniques, and because the peripheral processes of sensory root fibers remain intact with intraspinal lesions, SNAPs typical remain normal. The intraspinal location of most lesions makes it impossible to perform direct nerve conduction studies on the nerve root proximal to the damaged segment, precluding the diagnosis of conduction block or focal conduction velocity slowing along the damaged segment.
3. Sensory NCS performed along peripheral nerve trunks are characteristically normal in radiculopathy. When DRG reside in an intraspinal location they become vulnerable to compression/injury by disk protrusion and spondylosis (or other intraspinal canal pathological process). L5 radiculopathy can uncommonly be associated with loss of the superficial peroneal (fibular) SNAP [58]. However, an intraspinal location of DRG alone does not result in abnormal SNAP, for example S1 radiculopathy is almost never associated with sural SNAP amplitude loss. Although S1 DRG are even more commonly intraspinal than L5 DRG, their intraspinal location is caudal to the L5-S1 disk space where most compressive S1 radiculopathies occur. When nerve root damage occurs distal to the neural foramen, SNAP amplitude is affected [3, 58, 59].
4. Motor nerve conduction are often normal in radiculopathies as typically a loss of close to 50% of motor axons in a nerve trunk is required to reliably establish a significant reduction in the compound muscle action potential (CMAP) amplitude compared with the same response on the uninvolved side [60].
5. To identify an abnormality of CMAP amplitude in a motor radiculopathy, the muscle belly from which the CMAP is generated must be in the myotomal distribution of the injured root. Illustratively, this is as follows: A severe C8 radiculopathy is expected to produce some change in the ulnar CMAP amplitude, recording from either the abductor digiti minimi or the first dorsal interosseus. In the C5 myotome, the musculocutaneous and axillary nerve trunks can be stimulated to assess CMAPs from the biceps and deltoid muscles, respectively. However, muscles in the C6 and C7 myotomal distributions are not well spatially isolated from muscles of other myotomes, and therefore CMAPs derived from them are generally less reliable [3].

Limitations of Needle Examination in Diagnosis of Radiculopathy

Although needle examination plays a key role in the diagnosis of radiculopathy, there are several limitations that may pose diagnostic challenges.

1. Most muscles are innervated by more than one myotome making it challenging to isolate a single root involvement. For example, L2, L3, and L4 root lesions cannot be reliably distinguished from each other because if the overlap of innervation of the anterior (and medial) thigh muscles.
2. The problem in reliable localization is compounded if there is absence of proximal and distal muscles to examine for example C5-6 and L2-4 radiculopathies.
3. Reinnervation occurs in proximal muscles before distal muscles, in chronic radiculopathies there may be residual denervation only in distal muscles making it challenging to differentiate from distal neuropathy especially in older individuals when sensory responses can be absent.
4. Electrodiagnostic localization of a specific root lesion does not specify the vertebral level of damage/injury in lumbosacral radiculopathies.
5. NEE can be normal in acute lesions and mild demyelinating radiculopathy. In acute demyelinating radiculopathy abnormalities are

only seen if associated with prominent conduction block.

6. NEE cannot identify a pure sensory radiculopathy.
7. Fascicular sparing can result patchy involvement of muscles within the same myotome and often requires sampling of several muscles to increase yield of study.
8. Paraspinal muscle denervation potentials are not specific to radiculopathies and can also be seen in processes affecting anterior horn cells and in muscle disorders, such as necrotizing myopathy.
9. Paraspinal muscle involvement cannot precisely localize the segmental level of root damage because the segmental innervation of paraspinal muscles can overlap by as much as four to six segments [61].
10. Clear evidence of paraspinal denervation with cervical and lumbosacral radiculopathies is seen only in approximately 50% of cases due to overlapping segmental innervation of paraspinal muscles and the tendency for muscles close to the site of the nerve lesion to reinnervate sooner and more completely than muscles at greater distance from the point where nerve regeneration must begin [3, 32, 49].
11. In paraspinal muscles close to a prior laminectomy/similar spinal surgery site, denervation potentials may persist indefinitely because of iatrogenic denervation [3].

For cervical radiculopathy, a systematic evidence-based literature review concluded that needle EMG examination provided confirmatory evidence of cervical root pathology in 30% to 72% of patients presenting with appropriate symptoms or signs. Needle EMG abnormalities were highly correlated with weakness. Good agreement between imaging studies and needle EMG was seen in 65% to 85% of cases [62]. For lumbosacral radiculopathy, an evidence-based review concluded that needle EMG of the limb is probably effective in clinical diagnosis (class II evidence) [45].

One study retrospectively analyzed 47 patients with a clinical history compatible with either cervical or lumbosacral radiculopathy who were evaluated with an EMG and a spine MRI. Among these patients, 55% had an EMG abnormality and 57% had an MRI abnormality that correlated with the clinically estimated level of radiculopathy.

The two studies agreed in 60% of patients, with normal in 11 and abnormal in 17; however, only one study was abnormal in a significant minority (40%), suggesting that the two studies were complementary diagnostic modalities. The agreement was higher in patients with abnormal findings on neurologic examination [63].

Case Studies

Case 1: A 48 year-old right-handed woman was referred for an EMG/NCS to evaluate for a possible lumbosacral radiculopathy. Patient typically exercises regularly at the gym. Approximately 4 weeks ago she was lifting weights when she experienced sudden onset back pain radiating down into her right leg. On neurological examination she appears to have positive straight leg raising test on lifting her right leg up to 45 degrees. On formal muscle strength testing she had normal strength in her left leg, her right leg appeared to be strong proximally, ankle and toe dorsiflexion, foot inversion and eversion was approximately 4+/5 as per Medical Research Council (MRC) grading scale. She had difficulty standing on heels with relative preservation of standing on toes. Sensory exam reveals subtle decreased sensation over dorsum of right foot to pinprick and all deep tendon reflexes are preserved.

Approach to electrodiagnostic evaluation: In this case, history and physical examination is classic for of a lumbosacral radiculopathy involving the right L5 nerve root. Also on the differential is a proximal lesion of the sciatic nerve or lower lumbosacral plexus. In order to reach electrodiagnosis of a lumbosacral radiculopathy, one must (typically) obtain normal sensory nerve responses with L5 and S1 nerve root thus ruling out a sciatic mononeuropathy and plexopathy. Needle examination must sample muscles from several nerve roots, in addition, it is important to sample L5-S1 muscles that are supplied by different nerves. The summary of her electrodiagnostic study findings is presented in Table 8.8.

Table 8.8 Case electrodiagnostic data

Sensory nerve conductions

Nerve stimulated	Stimulation site	Recording site	Amplitude (μV)		Peak Lat (ms)		Normal values		Temperature (°C)
			L	R	L	R	Amp (μV)	Peak Lat (msec)	
Sural	Posterior leg	Lateral malleolus		8.45		3.3	>4	<4	31.2
Superficial peroneal (fibular)	Lateral leg	Dorsum of foot		6.20		3.6	>4	<4	31.5

Motor nerve conductions

Nerve stimulated	Stimulation site	Recording site	Amplitude (mV)		Onset Lat (ms)		Cond Vel (m/s)		Distance (mm)		Normal values			F-wave Lat (ms)		Temperature (°C)
			L	R	L	R	L	R	L	R	Amp (mV)	Distal Lat (msec)	Cond Vel (m/s)	L	R	
Peroneal (fibular)	Ankle Pop fossa	EDB		5.26 4.54		4.00 13.00		N/A 48.9		70 440	>4	<6	> 40			31.7
Tibial	Ankle Pop fossa	AH		11.44 8.30		4.00 13.00		N/A 48.9		80 440	>5	<5.9	> 40			30.8
Peroneal (fibular)	Fib Head Pop fossa	TA		4.50 4.02		2.60 4.30		N/A 58.8		80 100	>3	<4.1	> 40			31.0
Tibial	Ankle	AH										<66			57.5	31.2
Tibial	H-reflex M response	Soleus	1.50 7.26	1.60 7.16	32.5 5.0	33.80 6.00					>1 >7	<35 <7				31.5

Needle EMG

Muscle	Insertion	Spontaneous activity				Motor unit action potentials				
	Activity	Fibs	PSW	Fasc	Other	Rec pattern	Duration	Amp	Polys	Descript
L tibialis anterior	Normal	0	0	0		Normal	Normal	Normal	None	NC
R. lumbar 1 PSP	Normal	0	0	0						
R sacral 1 PSP	Normal	2+	0	0		Normal	Normal	Normal	None	NC
R gluteus medius	Normal	0	2+	0		Rapid, Reduced 2-	Normal	Normal	None	NC
R gluteus maximus	Normal	0	0	0		Normal	Normal	Normal	None	NC
R rectus femoris	Normal	0	0	0		Normal	Normal	Normal	None	NC
R semitendinosus	Normal	0	2 +	0		Rapid, Reduced 2-	Normal	Normal	None	NC
R biceps femoris, short head	Normal	0	0	0		Normal	Normal	Normal	None	NC
R tibialis anterior	Normal	2+	0	0	Rapid,	Rapid, Reduced 3-	Normal	Normal	None	NC
R extensor hallucis longus	Normal	1+	0	0		Rapid, Reduced 2-	Few 1+	Normal	None	NC
R medial gastrocnemius	Normal	0	0	0		Normal	Normal	Normal	None	NC
R flexor digitorum longus	Normal	0	0	0		Rapid, Reduced 3-	Few 1+	Normal	None	NC

Abbreviations: *μV* microvolt; *mV* millivolt; *msec* milliseconds; *m/s* meter/second; *mm* millimeter; *L* left; *R* right; *mV* millivolt; *Lat* Latency; *Cond Vel* Conduction Velocity; *Sup Peroneal (fibular)* Superficial Peroneal (fibular); *Pop* Popliteal; *EDB* Extensor Digitorum Brevis; *AH* Abductor Hallucis; *TA* Tibialis Anterior; *Fib* fibrillation potentials; *PSW* positive sharp waves; *Fasc* fasciculations; *Rec Pattern* Recruitment pattern; *Amp* Amplitude; *Polys* polyphasic motor unit potential changes; *PSP* paraspinal muscle; *NC* no comment; Descript description; fibrillation potentials: *1+* mild amount; *2+* moderate amount; *3+* great amount

Interpretation of electrodiagnostic studies:

1. Right sural and superficial sensory nerve conduction studies are within normal limits which would rule out a generalized large fiber polyneuropathy or a lumbosacral plexopathy (or multiple mononeuropathies).
2. Motor nerve conduction studies including right peroneal (fibular) recording from extensor digitorum brevis (EDB) and tibialis anterior (TA) muscles and tibial nerve recording from abductor hallucis (AH) muscle are within normal limits. Tibial H-reflex is without definite abnormality bilaterally.
3. Extensive needle examination performed in right lower extremity with additional study in left lower extremity reveals significant active/ongoing motor axon loss changes in the form of fibrillation and positive sharp wave potentials and/or neurogenic recruitment pattern in several muscles including right gluteus medius, semitendinosus, tibialis anterior, extensor hallucis and S1 paraspinal muscles. MUAP morphology is essentially normal in the muscle sampled throughout. Of note, although the S1 paraspinal muscle reveals fibrillations, all of the muscles with associated denervation potentials are predominantly L5 innervated muscles and one must keep in mind that there is significant overlap in innervation of paraspinal muscles. Abnormalities in paraspinal muscles have greater value in localizing lesion at or proximal to the root rather than specific root involvement.

Taken together these findings are supportive of a subacute intraspinal canal lesion involving the right L5 nerve root, axon loss in type and at least moderate in degree electrically.

Case 2: A 66 year-old right-handed man presents for an EMG referral with a long-standing history of neck pain who, over the past 3 months, has been experiencing pain, tingling, numbness travelling from right elbow into digits III, IV, V. On neurological examination patient appears to have diffuse dysesthetic sensory perception distortion along the right forearm and hand, but no classic dermatomal sensory loss pattern. He appears to have mild decreased strength (4+/5 MRC grading) in right hand muscles specifically finger flexors, extensors, thumb abductors. Examination is somewhat limited due to pain.

Approach to electrodiagnostic evaluation: In this case, the history may suggest a possible right ulnar mononeuropathy at the elbow, however, on exam patient appears to have diffuse hand muscle weakness including median and radial innervated hand muscles. Electrodiagnostic studies should be performed to primarily differentiate between right ulnar mononeuropathy, right (lower trunk) brachial plexopathy and right C7-T1 radiculopathy. The summary of his electrodiagnostic study findings is presented in Table 8.9.

Interpretation of electrodiagnostic studies:

1. Sensory nerve conduction studies including right median (digit II) and bilateral ulnar (digit V), dorsal ulnar cutaneous and medial antebrachial cutaneous nerves are within normal limits which would rule out a brachial plexopathy, or multiple mononeuropathies.
2. Motor nerve conduction studies reveal normal right median recording from abductor pollicis brevis (APB) muscle and bilateral ulnar motor nerves recording from first dorsal interosseous (FDI) as well as Abductor digiti minimi (ADM) muscles including proximal stimulations up to Erb's point. Bilateral ulnar F-wave distal latencies are within normal limits. No evidence of conduction block or other demyelination features along bilateral ulnar motor nerves.
3. On extensive needle examination performed in right upper extremity with additional studies in left upper extremity, there appears to be neurogenic (motor axon loss-related) changes of different ages/chronicities in the muscles studied. For example, there appears to be mixed active/ongoing on chronic motor axon loss changes involving right FDI, APB, flexor digitorum profundus (to digits 4,5), and flexor carpi ulnaris, with predominantly chronic motor axon loss changes involving right triceps, pronator teres, ADM, flexor pollicis longus, extensor indicis (proprius) and extensor digitorum (communis) muscles.

Taken together these findings are most consistent with chronic intraspinal canal lesions involving the right C7-T1 nerve roots/segments, axon loss in type, overall moderate-to-severe in

Table 8.9 Case electrodiagnostic data

Sensory nerve conductions

Nerve stimulated	Stimulation site	Recording site	Amplitude (μV)		Peak Lat (ms)		Normal values		Temperature (°C)
			L	R	L	R	Amp (μV)	Peak Lat (msec)	
Median	Wrist	Digit II		24.66		3.0	>10	<3.8	33.0
Ulnar	Wrist	Digit V	20.21	22.95	3.0	2.7	>5	<3.2	33.1
Radial	Forearm	Snuffbox		21.73		2.2	>10	<2.8	33.7
Ulnar	Wrist	Dorsal hand	10.26	8.45	2.8	2.6	>5	<3.2	33.6
Medial antebrachial cutaneous	Proximal Elbow	Forearm	7.18	7.23	2.6	2.6	>5	<3.2	34.2

Motor nerve conductions

Nerve stimulated	Stimulation site	Recording site	Amplitude (mV)		Onset Lat (ms)		Cond Vel (m/s)		Distance (mm)		Normal values			F-wave Lat (ms)		Temperature (°C)
			L	R	L	R	L	R	L	R	Amp (mV)	Distal Lat (msec)	Cond Vel (m/s)	L	R	
Median	Wrist	APB		11.48		3.1		N/A		50	>5	<4.0	>50			34.0
	Elbow			10.72		8.3		55.8		290						
Ulnar	Wrist	FDI	9.27	9.50	3.00	3.00	N/A	N/A	210	210	>7	<4.5	>50			33.7
	Dist elbow		9.05	9.31	6.80	6.90	55.3	53.8	310	310						
	Prox elbow		8.00	8.42	9.00	8.80	51.7	53.4								
Ulnar	Wrist	ADM	9.92	9.80	2.25	2.00	N/A	N/A	50	50	>7	<3.1	>50			34.2
	Dist elbow		9.03	9.11	5.80	5.65	59.2	57.5	210	210						
	Prox elbow		8.81	8.90	8.15	8.00	52.5	51.7	310	310						
	Axilla		8.57	8.61	10.95	10.60	51.7	52.3	450670	450						
	Erb's point		8.05	8.10	14.00	13.75	57.0	57.0		670						
Ulnar	Wrist	ADM										<34		29.65	29.90	33.6

(continured)

Table 8.9 (continued)

Needle EMG										
	Insertion	Spontaneous activity				Motor unit activity				
Muscle	Activity	Fibs	PSW	Fasc	Other	Rec pattern	Duration	Amp	Polys	Descript
L triceps	Normal	0	0	0		Normal	Normal	Normal	None	NC
L flexor pollicis longus	Normal	0	0	0		Normal	Normal	Normal	None	NC
L first dorsal interosseus	Normal	0	0	0		Normal	Normal	Normal	None	NC
R cervical 7 PSP	Normal	0	0	0		Normal	Normal	Normal	None	NC
R deltoid	Normal	0	0	0		Normal	Normal	Normal	None	NC
R biceps	Normal	0	0	0		Normal	Normal	Normal	None	NC
R triceps	Normal	0	0 +	0		Rapid, Reduced 2-	Many 2+	Many 1+	Many 1+	NC
R extensor digitorum communis	Normal	0	0	0		Rapid, Reduced 3-	Many 2+	Many 2+	None	NC
R extensor indicus proprius	Normal	0	0 +	0 +		Rapid, Reduced 2-	Many 1+	Few 1+	Some 1+	NC
R pronator teres	Normal	0	0+	0		Rapid, Reduced 2-	Some 1+	Few 1+	None	NC
R flexor pollicis longus	Normal	0	0+	0		Rapid, Reduced 2-	Some 1+	Some 1+	None	NC
R flexor carpi ulnaris	Normal	1+	0	1+		Rapid, Reduced 3-	Most1+	Most 1+	None	NC
R flexor digitorum profundus 4,5	Normal	1+	2+	0		Rapid, Reduced 3-	Many 1+	Some 1+	None	NC
R abductor pollicis brevis	Normal	0	2+	0		Rapid, Reduced 2-	Some 1+	Some 1+	None	NC
R abductor digiti minimi	Normal	0	0	0+		Rapid, Reduced 2-	Many 1+	Some 1+	None	NC
R first dorsal interosseus	Normal	0	1+	1+		Rapid, Reduced 3-	Many 2+	Many 2+	Some 1+	NC
R thoracic 1 PSP	Normal	0	0	0		Normal	Normal	Normal	None	pain-limited

Abbreviations: *μV* microvolt; *mV* millivolt; *msec* milliseconds; *m/s* meter/second; *mm* millimeter; *L* left; *R* right; *mV* millivolt; *Lat* Latency; *Cond Vel* Conduction Velocity; *APB* Abductor pollicis brevis muscle; *FDI* First Dorsal Interosseus muscle; *ADM* Abductor Digiti minimi; *Fib* fibrillation potentials; *PSW* positive sharp waves; *Fasc* fasciculations; *Rec Pattern*. Recruitment pattern; *Amp* Amplitude; *Polys* polyphasic motor unit potential changes; *PSP* paraspinal muscle; *NC* no comment; Descript description; fibrillation potentials: *1+* mild amount; *2+* moderate amount; *3+* great amount degree electrically, and with a superimposed subacute component mostly in the C8-T1 distributions.

References

1. Binder DK, Schmidt MH, Weinstein PR. Lumbar spinal stenosis. Semin Neurol. 2002 Jun;22(2):157–66.
2. Spencer DL, Irwin GS, Miller JA. Anatomy and significance of fixation of the lumbosacral nerve roots in sciatica. Spine. 1983 Sep;8(6):672–9.
3. Levin KH. Approach to the patient with suspected radiculopathy. Neurol Clin. 2012 May 1;30(2):581–604.
4. Levin KH. Cervical radiculopathy. In: Neuromuscular disorders in clinical practice. 2nd ed. New York: Springer; 2014. p. 981–1000.
5. Raynor E, Baruchow S, Nardin R, Kleiner-Fisman G. Lumbosacral and thoracic radiculopathies. In: Neuromuscular disorders in Clinical Practice. 2nd ed. New York: Springer; 2014. p. 1001–28.
6. Thomas JE, Howard FM. Segmental zoster paresis--a disease profile. Neurology. 1972 May;22(5):459–66.
7. So YT, Olney RK. Acute lumbosacral polyradiculopathy in acquired immunodeficiency syndrome: experience in 23 patients. Ann Neurol. 1994 Jan;35(1):53–8.
8. Logigian EL. Peripheral nervous system Lyme borreliosis. Semin Neurol. 1997 Mar;17(1):25–30.
9. Masjuan J, Corral I, Fernåndez-Ruiz LC. Mycobacterial acute lumbosacral polyradiculopathy as the initial manifestation of AIDS. J Acquir Immune Defic Syndr Hum Retrovirology Off Publ Int Retrovirology Assoc. 1997 Jun 1;15(2):175.
10. Corral I, Quereda C, Casado JL, Cobo J, Navas E, Pérez-Elías MJ, et al. Acute polyradiculopathies in HIV-infected patients. J Neurol. 1997 Aug;244(8):499–504.
11. Yuen EC, Layzer RB, Weitz SR, Olney RK. Neurologic complications of lumbar epidural anesthesia and analgesia. Neurology. 1995 Oct;45(10):1795–801.
12. Mammis A, Bonsignore C, Mogilner AY. Thoracic radiculopathy following spinal cord stimulator placement: case series. Neuromodulation Technol Neural Interface. 2013 Sep 1;16(5):443–8.
13. Liveson JA. Thoracic radiculopathy related to collapsed thoracic vertebral bodies. J Neurol Neurosurg Psychiatry. 1984 Apr;47(4):404–6.
14. Sahenk Z, Mendell J, Rossio J, Hurtubise P. Polyradiculopathy accompanying procainamide-induced lupus erythrematosus: evidence for drug-induced enhanced sensitization to peripheral nerve myelin. Ann Neurol. 1977;1:378–84.
15. Goldstein JM, Parks BJ, Mayer PL, Kim JH, Sze G, Miller RG. Nerve root hypertrophy as the cause of lumbar stenosis in chronic inflammatory demyelinating polyradiculoneuropathy. Muscle Nerve. 1996 Jul;19(7):892–6.
16. Bastron JA, Thomas JE. Diabetic polyradiculopathy: clinical and electromyographic findings in 105 patients. Mayo Clin Proc. 1981 Dec;56(12):725–32.
17. Atkinson R, Ghelman B, Tsairis P, Warren RF, Jacobs B, Lavyne M. Sarcoidosis presenting as cervical radiculopathy: a case report and literature review. Spine. 1982 Oct;7(5):412–6.
18. Vargas DL, Stern BJ. Neurosarcoidosis: diagnosis and management. Semin Respir Crit Care Med. 2010 Aug;31(4):419–27.
19. Koffman B, Junck L, Elias SB, Feit HW, Levine SR. Polyradiculopathy in sarcoidosis. Muscle Nerve. 1999 May;22(5):608–13.
20. Schutta H. Spinal tumors. In: Joynt RG, editor. Clinical neurology. Philadelphia: Lippincott Williams & Wilkins; 1994. p. 1–126.
21. Hlavin ML, Kaminski HJ, Fenstermaker RA, White RJ. Intracranial suppuration: a modern decade of postoperative subdural empyema and epidural abscess. Neurosurgery. 1994;34(6):974–80. discussion 980-981
22. Schutta H. Diseases of the dura mater. In: Joynt RG, editor. Clinical neurology. Philadelphia: Lippincott Williams & Wilkins; 1993. p. 67–91.
23. Black P. Spinal metastasis: current status and recommended guidelines for management. Neurosurgery. 1979 Dec;5(6):726–46.
24. Taylor JW, Schiff D. Metastatic epidural spinal cord compression. Semin Neurol. 2010 Jul;30(3):245–53.
25. Engelhard HH, Villano JL, Porter KR, Stewart AK, Barua M, Barker FG, et al. Clinical presentation, histology, and treatment in 430 patients with primary tumors of the spinal cord, spinal meninges, or cauda equina. J Neurosurg Spine. 2010 Jul;13(1):67–77.
26. Hirayama K, Tomonaga M, Kitano K, Yamada T, Kojima S, Arai K. Focal cervical poliopathy causing juvenile muscular atrophy of distal upper extremity: a pathological study. J Neurol Neurosurg Psychiatry. 1987 Mar;50(3):285–90.
27. Hardy R, Plank N. Clinical diagnosis of herniated lumbar disc. In: Lumbar Disc Disease. New York: Raven Press; 1982. p. 17–28.
28. Hamanishi C, Tanaka S. Dorsal root ganglia in the lumbosacral region observed from the axial views of MRI. Spine. 1993 Oct;18(13):1753–6.
29. Kikuchi S, Sato K, Konno S, Hasue M. Anatomic and radiographic study of dorsal root ganglia. Spine. 1994 Jan 1;19(1):6–11.
30. Yabuki S, Kikuchi S. Positions of dorsal root ganglia in the cervical spine. An anatomic and clinical study. Spine. 1996 Jul 1;21(13):1513–7.
31. Preston D, Shapiro B. Radiculopathy. In: Electromyography and neuromuscular disorders: clinical-electrophysiological correlates. 3rd ed. China: Elsevier Saunders; 2013. p. 448–67.
32. Levin KH, Maggiano HJ, Wilbourn AJ. Cervical radiculopathies: comparison of surgical and EMG localization of single-root lesions. Neurology. 1996 Apr;46(4):1022–5.
33. Viikari-Juntura E, Porras M, Laasonen EM. Validity of clinical tests in the diagnosis of root compression in cervical disc disease. Spine. 1989 Mar;14(3):253–7.
34. Yoss RE, Corbin KB, Maccarty CS, Love JG. Significance of symptoms and signs in local-

ization of involved root in cervical disk protrusion. Neurology. 1957 Oct;7(10):673–83.
35. Levin KH. Neurologic manifestations of compressive radiculopathy of the first thoracic root. Neurology. 1999 Sep 22;53(5):1149–51.
36. Knutsson B. Comparative value of electromyographic, myelographic and clinical-neurological examinations in diagnosis of lumbar root compression syndrome. Acta Orthop Scand Suppl. 1961;49:1–135.
37. Liguori R, Krarup C, Trojaborg W. Determination of the segmental sensory and motor innervation of the lumbosacral spinal nerves. An electrophysiological study. Brain J Neurol. 1992 Jun;115(Pt 3):915–34.
38. Thage O. The myotomes L2-S2 in man. Acta Neurol Scand. 1965;41(Suppl 13):241–3.
39. Young A, Getty J, Jackson A, Kirwan E, Sullivan M, Parry CW. Variations in the pattern of muscle innervation by the L5 and S1 nerve roots. Spine. 1983 Sep;8(6):616–24.
40. Feinberg JH, Radecki J. Parsonage-Turner Syndrome. HSS J. 2010 Sep;6(2):199–205.
41. Bachasson D, Singh A, Shah S, Lane JG, Ward SR. The role of the peripheral and central nervous Systems in Rotator Cuff Disease. J Shoulder Elb Surg Am Shoulder Elb Surg Al. 2015 Aug;24(8):1322–35.
42. Levin KH, Wilbourn AJ, Maggiano HJ. Cervical rib and median sternotomy-related brachial plexopathies: a reassessment. Neurology. 1998 May;50(5):1407–13.
43. Preston DC. Compressive and entrapment neuropathies of the upper extremity. In: Neuromuscular disorders in clinical practice. 2nd ed. New York: Springer; 2014. p. 871–902.
44. Katirji B. Compressive and entrapment neuropathies of the lower extremity. In: Neuromuscular disorders in clinical practice. 2nd ed. New York: Springer; 2014. p. 903–52.
45. Cho SC, Ferrante MA, Levin KH, Harmon RL, So YT. Utility of electrodiagnostic testing in evaluating patients with lumbosacral radiculopathy: an evidence-based review. Muscle Nerve. 2010 Aug;42(2):276–82.
46. Katirji B, Weissman JD. The ankle jerk and the tibial H-reflex: a clinical and electrophysiological correlation. Electromyogr Clin Neurophysiol. 1994 Sep;34(6):331–4.
47. Burke D, Gandevia SC, McKeon B. Monosynaptic and oligosynaptic contributions to human ankle jerk and H-reflex. J Neurophysiol. 1984 Sep;52(3):435–48.
48. Fisher M. H reflexes and F waves: physiology and clinical indications. Muscle Nerve. 1992;15:1223–33.
49. Tsao BE, Levin KH, Bodner RA. Comparison of surgical and electrodiagnostic findings in single root lumbosacral radiculopathies. Muscle Nerve. 2003 Jan;27(1):60–4.
50. Wilbourne A, Aminoff M. Radiculopathies. In: Brown W, Bolton C, editors. Clinical electromyography. 2nd ed. Boston: Butterworth- Heinemann; 1993. p. 177–209.
51. Yiannikas C, Shahani BT, Young RR. Short-latency somatosensory-evoked potentials from radial, median, ulnar, and peroneal nerve stimulation in the assessment of cervical spondylosis: comparison with conventional electromyography. Arch Neurol. 1986 Dec 1;43(12):1264–71.
52. Aminoff M, Goodin D. Electrophysiological evaluation of lumbosacral radiculopathy; electromyography, late responses and somatosensory evoked potentials. Neurology. 1985;35:1514–8.
53. Phillips LH, Park TS. Electrophysiologic mapping of the segmental anatomy of the muscles of the lower extremity. Muscle Nerve. 1991 Dec;14(12):1213–8.
54. Wilbourn AJ, Aminoff MJ. AAEM Minimonograph 32: the electrodiagnostic examination in patients with radiculopathies. Muscle Nerve. 1998 Dec 1;21(12):1612–31.
55. Johnson E, Melvin J. Value of electromyography in lumbar radiculopathy. Arch Phys Med Rehabil. 1971;52:239–43.
56. LaJoie W. Nerve root compression: correlation of electromyographic, myelographic, and surgical findings. Arch Phys Med Rehabil. 1972;53:390–2.
57. Tullberg T, Svanborg E, Isacsson J. A preoperative and postoperative study of the accuracy and value of electrodiagnosis in patients with lumbosacral disc herniation. Spine. 1993;18:837–42.
58. Levin KH. L5 radiculopathy with reduced superficial peroneal sensory responses: intraspinal and extraspinal causes. Muscle Nerve. 1998 Jan;21(1):3–7.
59. Wiltse LL, Guyer RD, Spencer CW, Glenn WV, Porter IS. Alar transverse process impingement of the L5 spinal nerve: the far-out syndrome. Spine. 1984 Feb;9(1):31–41.
60. Berger AR, Sharma K, Lipton RB. Comparison of motor conduction abnormalities in lumbosacral radiculopathy and axonal polyneuropathy. Muscle Nerve. 1999 Aug;22(8):1053–7.
61. Gough JG, Koepke GH. Electromyographic determination of motor root levels in erector spinae muscles. Arch Phys Med Rehabil. 1966 Jan;47(1):9–11.
62. American Association of Electrodiagnostic Medicine, So YT. Guidelines in electrodiagnostic medicine. Practice parameter for needle electromyographic evaluation of patients with suspected cervical radiculopathy. Muscle Nerve Suppl. 1999;(8):S209–21.
63. Nardin RA, Patel MR, Gudas TF, Rutkove SB, Raynor EM. Electromyography and magnetic resonance imaging in the evaluation of radiculopathy. Muscle Nerve. 1999 Feb;22(2):151–5.

Recommended Reading

Levin KH. Approach to the patient with suspected radiculopathy. Neurol Clin. 2012 May 1;30(2):581–604.

Levin KH. Cervical radiculopathy. In: Neuromuscular disorders in clinical practice. 2nd ed. New York: Springer; 2014. p. 981–1000.

Raynor E, Baruchow S, Nardin R, Kleiner-Fisman G. Lumbosacral and thoracic radiculopathies. In: Neuromuscular disorders in clinical practice. 2nd ed. New York: Springer; 2014. p. 1001–28.

Preston D, Shapiro B. Radiculopathy. In: Electromyography and neuromuscular disorders: clinical electrophysiological correlates. 3rd ed. China: Elsevier Saunders; 2013. p. 448–67.

9 Motor Neuron Diseases

Michelle M. Dompenciel

Etiology

Motor neuron diseases (MND) are very challenging to diagnose, and it is imperative that the correct diagnosis is reached early after the onset of symptoms, because of the poor prognosis associated with the disease. Amyotrophic Lateral Sclerosis (ALS) is the most frequent form of MND. It causes gradual dysfunction of the upper motor neurons (UMN) and lower motor neurons (LMN). The median survival of ALS is about 2–3 years after onset of symptoms, typically related to respiratory muscle weakness/failure. However, because the disease is variable, there are a few exceptions, with some patients living past the typical estimated life expectancy.

UMN symptoms comprise spasticity, weakness, and pathologic hyperreflexia, and the expression of symptoms varies between patients depending on which motor neurons are affected. LMN signs include fasciculations, cramps, muscle atrophy and weakness. ALS patients are typically diagnosed in late middle age (average age of about 55 years at diagnosis), but more cases have been diagnosed as being genetic/familial affecting much younger adult patients as well. ALS is typically more common in men than in women, but this is rapidly changing as the incidence can equal between men and women with increasing age. Genetic influence plays an important role as more gene mutations are found, some linked with environmental risk factors causing degeneration of the motor neurons. ALS cases were initially described and studied by Jean-Martin Charcot in 1869 as a pure motor neuron disease with a very distinct pathology, and the term amyotrophic lateral sclerosis was later introduced in his 1874 research paper. Nowadays, ALS is considered a multi-systemic disease that can be at times associated with non-motor symptoms, causing dysfunction of the fronto-temporal lobes, cerebellar circuits (as may sometimes be seen in Madras MND), autonomic nervous system, basal ganglia [1], dorsal columns, and even cases described as related to idiopathic sensory neuropathy [2]. Rare forms of ALS that can be inherited in endemic areas and which can present with ALS-Parkinsonism-Dementia complex have also been reported. Madras motor neuron disease (MMND) is another rare subtype of motor neuron disease presenting typically in the young, having weakness and wasting of limb muscles, together with multiple lower cranial nerve palsies and sensorineural hearing loss. Infrequently, there may be cerebellar involvement, with cerebellar atrophy described in at least 1 case [3].

A small percentage of ALS patients may manifest with frontotemporal dementia (FTD) with cognitive deficits, personality changes, and

M. M. Dompenciel (✉)
Department of Neurology, Cleveland Clinic, Weston, FL, USA
e-mail: dompenm@ccf.org

N. Galvez-Jimenez et al. (eds.), *Electrodiagnostic Medicine*,
https://doi.org/10.1007/978-3-030-74997-2_9

behavioral changes (up to 50% of ALS patients with at least some of these features). Even though the majority of cases of ALS are sporadic, now it is considered a genetically heterogeneous disorder with a complex genetic etiology [4]. The most frequently mutated disease genes discovered are: *C9ORF72*, *SOD1* (the first gene mutation identified for ALS), *NEK1* (sporadic and familial cases), *TDP-43* (mostly dominant forms of inheritance cases), and *FUS* (mostly dominant inheritance pattern). *C9ORF72* DNA expansion gene accounts for more ALS cases with a genetic influence (seen in up to ~40%), including a predisposition to developing FTD, and to a lesser extent seen in sporadic cases (up to ~7%). More genes have been discovered that are associated with the development of ALS, and having an understanding of their role in the disease will affect future therapeutic avenues. Nevertheless, there are limitations with genetic testing in patients with suspected family history of ALS, mostly because of variable expression and incomplete penetrance of the genes [4]. ALS has been linked to excessive stimulation of glutaminergic NMDA (activation of glutamate receptors causing elevation of neuronal intracellular calcium, leading ultimately to cell death) and AMPA (*alpha-amino-3-hydroxy-5-methyl-4-isoxazolepropionate*) receptors, impaired axonal transport, increased oxidative stress, glial cell dysfunction, reactive astrocytes, among other hypotheses, ultimately leading to motor neuron degeneration [5].

Primary Lateral Sclerosis (PLS) selectively affects the UMN with a clinical presentation of spasticity, pathologic hyperreflexia, weakness, and even pseudobulbar affect [6]. It affects about 1–3% of patients diagnosed with MND, with also a slight male predominance. Symptoms can take years to progress; most commonly exhibiting progressive paraplegia, spastic bulbar weakness, or hemiplegia [7]. Overlaps with other diseases have also been documented [8]. The Pringle criteria suggests that the diagnosis is based on clinical findings, appropriate laboratory testing (infectious, metabolic, or toxic), EDX results not meeting El Escorial criteria, and at least 3 years of observation. This is to ensure that the correct diagnosis is made, as it can be easily mistaken with other diseases/mimics. Lack of LMN involvement on EDX, structural lesions on imaging, or family history of hereditary forms of spastic paraplegia, will make the diagnosis of PLS more convincing. Typically, the prognosis of PLS is better when compared to classic ALS. The etiology is considered mostly similar to ALS with a potential combination of genetic and environmental factors.

Progressive Muscular Atrophy (PMA) is another subtype of MND presenting with purely LMN symptoms of: fasciculations, cramps, reduced/absent reflexes, flaccid muscle weakness, and atrophy. It also carries a better prognosis than ALS. Appropriate diagnostic testing and close clinical observation are needed because some patients with initial physical examination suggestive of PMA could progress to develop UMN signs, hence eventually meeting El Escorial criteria for ALS. EDX evaluation is important to differentiate between PMA and multifocal motor neuropathy with conduction block (MMNCB), which is another disorder mostly affecting the motor fibers with sparing of the sensory fibers. MMNCB is an immune-mediated demyelinating motor neuropathy, and it is imperative for it to be excluded during EDX testing and laboratory investigation (associated with GM1 ganglioside antibody). This is especially important since most MMNCB, patients show improvement with immune-modulating therapies (particularly IV immunoglobulin).

Progressive Bulbar Palsy (PBP) presents with selective damage of the motor nerves supplying the bulbar muscles, affecting speech and swallowing, and may affect the facial muscles as well. Most cases are sporadic and some familial ones have been described. Diagnosis is usually delayed because the initial symptoms are mistaken as gastrointestinal or ENT-related conditions. Patients can present with tongue muscle atrophy with fasciculations, drooling, spastic speech, and brisk facial reflexes. It can remain limited to the bulbar muscles, but in some cases, it may be the initial presentation of the ALS type of MND. Close clinical observation and EDX information over time are integral parts of securing the diagnosis. A small study published in 2016 suggested early changes on imaging that could potentially assist in the future when distinguishing among the different MND variants. The study proposed early disease changes seen in diffusion tensor imaging

(DTI) and magnetic resonance spectroscopic (MRS) studies in patients with bulbar-onset and limb-onset ALS. Extra-motor involvement by the corpus callosum is a feature seen in bulbar-onset patients, when compared to limb-onset ALS, and can suggest poor outcome in such patients [9].

Anatomy

The upper motor neurons (pyramidal tracts) originate in the brain's primary motor cortex, and those tracts carry voluntary motor activity from the cortex to the lower motor neurons. These tracts will descend in the spinal cord to synapse with the lower motor neurons at each spinal nerve root level. Each of those axons will innervate several fibers of a skeletal muscle. The major UMN/pyramidal pathway is the corticospinal tracts, which travel down the anterior horn to connect with interneurons and exit the spinal cord to convey voluntary muscle control to the extremities and trunk. The other pyramidal pathway is the corticobulbar tract, which connects to the cranial nerve motor nuclei, like the nucleus ambiguus (supplying motor fibers of the vagus and glossopharyngeal nerves), and motor fibers of the trigeminal, facial, and accessory nerves. Damage to the nucleus ambiguus will affect speech and swallowing because of its control on the pharynx, larynx, and soft palate muscles. Once the nerve exits the spinal cord or brainstem (in the case of cranial nerve motor nuclei) it becomes a lower motor neuron. Electrodiagnostic evaluation (EDX) will specifically assess the function of the lower motor neurons. ALS affects both the upper and lower motor neurons (see Figs. 9.1 and 9.2), and remains a clinical diagnosis. EDX will assist in detecting lower motor neuron dysfunction, with upper motor neuron involvement primarily assessed during physical examination.

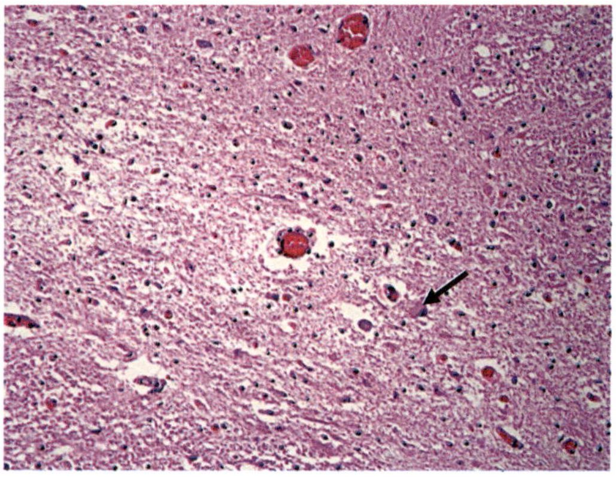

Fig. 9.1 Hematoxylin and eosin stained slide showing loss of neurons in the anterior horn cell region with reactive astrocytes (arrow represents a motor neuron). Courtesy of Dr. Richard Prayson/Section Head of Neuropathology at Cleveland Clinic

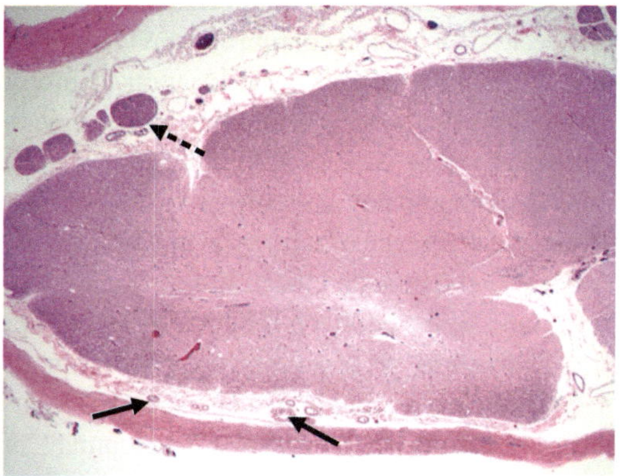

Fig. 9.2 Hematoxylin and eosin stained slide of the cervical spinal cord with atrophy of the anterior spinal rootlets (solid arrows) when compared to the posterior rootlets (dashed arrow). Courtesy of Dr. Richard Prayson/Section Head of Neuropathology at Cleveland Clinic

From a histopathological point of view, astrocytes are vital in supporting and repairing the nervous tissue, and when they become reactive, they promote motor neuron autophagy. It has been stipulated that motor neuron degeneration has been linked to a reactive state of astrocytes, at times triggered by environmental factors like traumatic central nervous system injuries; however, not fully understood. Hence, increased risk for ALS has also been associated with history of traumatic brain injuries [10]. Typically, ALS starts with symptoms affecting one body segment, and depending on the location and degree of spinal cord motor neuron loss, progressive weakness will ultimately involve adjacent myotomes. The disease will continue to spread to other extremities, or bulbar muscles, producing weakness and respiratory complications, leading to death. Prompt diagnosis is paramount in order to offer available treatment to slow the disease progression. Two FDA-approved medications are available for the treatment of ALS: Riluzole and Edaravone. Riluzole may modulate and inhibit glutamate neurotransmission, decreasing glutamate-related excitotoxicity. Edaravone has been associated with decreasing oxidative stress. Free radicals/oxidative stress have been linked to motor nerve cell death, increasing the risk of ALS development.

Clinical Features

Motor neuron diseases can be very difficult to diagnose because they can share clinical features, at its earliest presentation, with other diseases/mimics. At onset, the majority of ALS patients will have subtle features of weakness in either an upper or lower extremity. Symptoms then evolve to muscle atrophy, and continue to spread to other myotomes. Depending on the location of motor neuron involvement, it can clinically mimic a mononeuropathy such as at the ulnar nerve, or a lumbar radiculopathy presenting with foot drop. The clinical absence of sensory symptoms should indicate to the clinician that a motor neuron process could be the etiology. If bulbar motor nerves are involved at presentation, then the patients may have spastic and/or flaccid speech, dysarthria, dysphagia, leading to the development of tongue atrophy with fasciculations and drooling. Most of these cases are initially extensively evaluated by other specialists looking for other causes of dysphagia and dysarthria.

The revised El Escorial criteria (see Table 9.1) were published to assist in the correct diagnosis of ALS. Based on the guidelines, there has to be clinical evidence of disease progression, and absence of alternative causes. Signs of upper and lower motor neuron involvement must be present, which may include that supported by electrophysiological evaluation. Neuroimaging is always recommended to exclude mimics. The revised El Escorial criteria classify cases as: suspected, possible, probable, or definite ALS. Appropriate laboratory evaluations are needed to rule-out other etiologies when the diagnosis is in question. At times, repeating EDX testing is required to discern disease progression. This can be considered in cases where the initial symptoms are bulbar, and the patient starts to develop new symptoms spreading to other limbs. Clinical examinations should be performed at least every 6 months for progression. Four regions have been established to describe the involvement/spread of clinical symptoms: bulbar, cervical, thoracic, and lumbosacral. The diagnosis becomes more evident when the features spread within the same region, or involve other regions. Moreover, if there is sensory, sphincter, or autonomic dysfunction, then alternative diagnoses should be considered. A detailed neurological examination, family history, past medical history, medications/toxin exposure history, and onset/evolution of symptoms review need to be carefully taken into consideration when diagnosing MND. More importantly, electrophysiological studies are always recommended to confirm a lower motor neuron process, and are essentially equivalent to clinical LMN findings. Primary Lateral Sclerosis (PLS) often presents as progressive leg weakness, cramps, and stiffness. The disease course is prolonged, and has a better prognosis than ALS. On examination, patients will develop pathologic hyperreflexia and marked spasticity. Some patients can develop cognitive changes and pseudobulbar affect and dysarthric speech. At least 3 years are required for clinical observation, looking for progression or development of features suggestive of LMN involvement, according to The Pringle criteria. EDX evaluation must show lack of a LMN process. Progressive Muscular Atrophy (PMA) also has a prolonged course of symptom development. On physical examination, the patients will show: reduced or absent reflexes, fasciculations, muscle weakness, and ultimately muscle atrophy. Limited forms of the disease have also been described, like flail arm or leg syndromes. The clinician needs to perform close observation over time, looking for UMN signs or features that meet El Escorial criteria, to exclude the possibility of disease progression to classic ALS. Progressive Bulbar Palsy (PBP) presents with early symptoms of speech, drooling, and swallowing dysfunction. Patients can develop tongue and facial weakness with atrophy and fasciculations. Generally, the symptoms remain lim-

Table 9.1 World Federation of Neurology El Escorial criteria for ALS

LMN signs	UMN signs	Regions	Clinically definite	Clinically probable	Clinically possible	Clinically suspected
– Weakness – Atrophy – Fasciculations	– Spasticity – Pathologic hyperreflexia – Extensor plantar response – Pseudobulbar features	-**Bulbar (craniobulbar)** -**Cervical** -**Thoracic** -**Lumbosacral**	**UMN and LMN features:** →bulbar and at least 2 other spinal regions OR →3 spinal regions →absence of other possible etiologies	**UMN and LMN features:** → 2 regions →some UMN signs must be rostral to (above) LMN signs → "Clinically probable, laboratory-supported ALS": UMN signs in 1 or more regions coupled with LMN signs by EMG in at least 2 regions →absence of other possible etiologies	→UMN and LMN signs in 1 region OR →UMN signs in 2 or more regions OR →UMN and LMN signs in 2 regions without UMN signs rostral to the LMN signs →absence of other possible etiologies	→LMN *or* UMN signs only in 1 or more regions →absence of other possible etiologies

Based on the revised El Escorial criteria ("Clinically Suspected" category carried forward from the original criteria). On electromyography, cervical and lumbar region requires involvement of at least 2 muscles innervated by different nerve roots. Bulbar and thoracic region requires involvement of at least 1 muscle per region. *ALS* Amyotrophic lateral sclerosis; *UMN* upper motor neuron; *LMN* lower motor neuron; *EMG* electromyography ited to the bulbar muscles, but in some cases, it can be the initial presentation of ALS.

Clinically, if there is evidence of widespread LMN process (at least 2 or more regions), then ALS should be suspected, provided that the appropriate diagnostic testing (neuroimaging, laboratory, or genetic testing if warranted) was performed to exclude other possible etiologies. Cognitive testing should also be considered to assess ALS variants like FTD-ALS. More forms of ALS are being described leading to the belief that it is a multi-systemic disease. It has to be recognized that ALS can be associated, in some cases, with mild sensory, autonomic, and cerebellar, among other symptoms.

Differential Diagnosis

Motor neuron diseases have a myriad of symptoms that can be confused with many other diseases at onset [11]. Using the revised El Escorial criteria can assist in the proper clinical evaluation of ALS and its mimics. All of these patients should undergo EDX evaluation, laboratory testing, and neuroimaging studies to exclude other disease possibilities. Requesting imaging studies is very important because a structural lesion can present with both UMN and LMN features. Some examples of structural lesions are: cervical compressive myelopathy/myeloradiculopathy, brainstem or spinal cord tumors, also tandem UMN lesions with LMN lesions from plexopathy, or polyradiculopathy, among others. However, some of these examples may have sensory loss clinical features, and should alert the clinician against the case for ALS. Laboratory studies are recommended to exclude metabolic, toxic (organic pesticides, lead, mercury, arsenic, among others), infectious, or nutritional causes. Vitamin B12 deficiency, thyroid dysfunction, copper deficiency, hyperparathyroidism, heavy metals toxicity, vitamin E deficiency, Lyme disease, HIV myelopathy, and tropical spastic paraparesis (human T-lymphotropic virus type 1 infection), are some other examples. Some of them can present with largely UMN symptoms, like HIV myelopathy and tropical spastic paraparesis. EDX testing can only complement the physical examination, and should not be used in isolation to diagnose ALS. As previously mentioned, EDX evaluation will specifically assess the function of the lower (not upper) motor neurons. One caveat of EDX testing can be seen in multiple sclerosis patients when the plaque involvement is near/at root exit zones, and the patient also has a more typical central nervous system lesion(s). Clinically, the patient will express UMN and LMN involvement, mimicking a motor neuron disease process. Although rare, it may present on EDX testing as a pure LMN process, like a polyradiculopathy. Clinical examination, onset of symptoms review, and neuroimaging will certainly aid in differentiating between the two entities. Post-polio syndrome should be easy to assess, because of prior history of infection and slow muscle weakness and atrophy progression over many years.

Often patients present to the neurologist with muscle twitching or fasciculations, having great concern about the implications of this isolated symptom. In these cases, fasciculation potentials are often detected on EDX evaluation in the absence of any other significant changes. Close clinical observation over time would typically confirm benign fasciculation syndrome, rather than a more sinister motor neuron process. In particular, lack of unequivocal weakness or progressive muscle atrophy suggests a benign disorder like this.

Certain muscle diseases may mimic a disorder of motor neuron dysfunction. This raises the importance of appropriate laboratory including electrodiagnostic testing, and in some cases muscle biopsy to confirm a diagnosis. Inclusion body myositis (IBM) is an idiopathic inflammatory disorder that can present with asymmetric limb weakness (typically, deep finger flexors and quadriceps muscles), with some difficulties in swallowing due to bulbar muscle involvement. IBM can share some EDX features with ALS, hence ideally a muscle biopsy should be performed in suspected cases for diagnosis confirmation. Oculopharyngeal muscular dystrophy is another muscle disease that can present with progressive muscle weakness of the throat, facial, ocular, and eyelid muscles. It can mimic bulbar-onset ALS, specifically when the extraocular muscle symptoms are very subtle at onset. In this case, genetic testing will help in the evaluation. Isolated neck extensor myopathy is one of the etiologies of dropped head syndrome that will show signs of electrical "irritability" on needle electromyography testing in the cervical paraspinal muscles, and can be confused with MND at onset. However, it is usually limited and does not spread to other myotomes, such as in ALS. Diseases of the neuromuscular junction may present with LMN features. Myasthenia gravis may present with bulbar symptoms, and at onset can be mistaken for bulbar-onset ALS. To assist in differentiation, blood evaluation [e.g. for acetylcholine receptor and MuSK (muscle-specific kinase) antibodies], and repetitive nerve stimulation on electrodiagnostic testing (or single fiber EMG), can be performed to establish the diagnosis of myasthenia gravis. One should not rely only on symptom improvement with cholinesterase inhibitors to differentiate between them, because some MND patients may express transient symptom improvement with these medications.

Immune-mediated processes should always be investigated further because some could be potentially treatable. Multifocal motor neuropathy with conduction block (MMNCB) presents with a lower motor neuron dysfunction, and needs to be excluded from the progressive muscular atrophy MND variant. MMNCB is a purely motor demyelinating neuropathy that is slowly progressive, and also begins distally as in many ALS cases. Clinically, they can be differentiated by more multifocal individual motor nerves being affected in MMNCB, rather than progressively involving adjacent myotomal distributions as in ALS/MND. Anti-GM1 antibody presence, and motor conduction block (between distal and proximal motor segments) on EDX evaluation, are typical of MMNCB patients. The distinction between these two processes must be made clear because a trial of intravenous immunoglobulin therapy should be considered in MMNCB patients. Stiff person syndrome patients will develop painful cramps and spasticity, thus clinically mimicking a UMN disease. Typically, it affects the truncal muscles, but there are other variants that are segmental or limited to a limb. Blood evaluation for glutamic acid decarboxylase (GAD) antibodies, and paraneoplastic testing, should be performed to exclude underlying malignancy.

Hereditary spastic paraparesis, spinal muscular atrophy, Kennedy's disease (spinal and bulbar muscular atrophy), and hexosaminidase A deficiency (Tay-Sachs disease), are examples of hereditary diseases that may present with some features of MND clinically or electrodiagnostically. Hereditary spastic paraparesis can present with UMN disorder, whereas spinal muscular atrophy will present as slowly progressive muscle weakness because of anterior horn cell/LMN involvement. Kennedy's disease patients will manifest with muscle cramps, tongue weakness/fasciculations, speech disturbance, and limb weakness. There is dysfunction of the motor neurons at the brainstem and spinal cord, which can be confused with classic ALS, but these patients will also show endocrine dysregulation, and genetic testing will confirm the diagnosis. Hexosaminidase A deficiency/adult or late-onset patients can express speech and swallowing problems, but prominent psychiatric and cognitive deficits can differentiate it from bulbar-onset ALS.

Paraneoplastic processes can also manifest with clinical features of MND. Lymphoma can present with lower extremity LMN features. Radiation therapy can manifest with muscle weakness and atrophy, even many years after radiation exposure, and clinically exhibits a pure LMN process. EDX evaluation will be important in this case because myokymic discharges are very commonly seen in radiation-induced processes, particularly plexopathy.

Electrodiagnostic Evaluation

Nerve Conduction Studies

Nerve conduction studies and needle electromyography play an important role in the diagnostic process of motor neuron diseases, but essentially can only evaluate the presence of lower motor neuron dysfunction. Therefore, ALS is a clinical diagnosis, supported by the presence of UMN dysfunction (signs disclosed on neurological exam) and LMN dysfunction (exam and/or EDX findings). EDX evaluation will also serve to exclude potentially treatable alternative etiologies, including a demyelinating motor/motor-predominant polyneuropathy. Careful testing of several motor nerves should be performed to increase the probability of finding a motor conduction block or focal/segmental demyelination. At times, proximal nerve stimulation can be considered, or contralateral studies, to look for pertinent features including motor conduction block. In addition, if the late-responses are abnormal and the motor studies are normal, contralateral or proximal motor nerve studies are recommended.

Upper and lower extremities must be assessed on nerve conduction studies (NCS). Features of motor axonal loss are classic findings of LMN involvement in ALS. Decreased compound muscle action potentials (CMAP), with relatively normal distal latencies and conduction velocities are typical findings seen with motor axonal loss. If there is involvement of the largest and fastest conducting axons, then there could be mild slowing of the conduction velocities; however, not to the degree seen in a demyelinating process. Only the fastest conducting fibers are measured on conduction velocities and latency testing on NCS. If there is marked motor axonal loss, the CMAP will drop, but the distal latencies and conduction velocities should remain essentially normal (or almost normal), because there will be a few of the fastest conducting fibers still left unaffected. These fibers can only drop to ~75% of the lower limit of normal conduction velocity because these myelinated fibers cannot conduct slower than this range. Distal latencies can be prolonged, but will not be greater than ~130% of the upper limit of normal. Applying these concepts to the evaluation of MND is important to exclude a demyelinating neuropathy. When there is a complete motor conduction block, there is a drop of more than 50% of the CMAP amplitude or area, when comparing the distal and proximal stimulation sites (with or without associated temporal dispersion). This tends to become marked when the nerve is studied utilizing a long distance between stimulation sites. Sensory nerve conduction studies should be normal in MND/ALS, except in those cases where there is a superimposed process like a mononeuropathy or polyneuropathy, in which case relevant investigations should be performed looking for other etiologies.

Routine motor studies should be performed on the following nerves: median (recording at abductor pollicis brevis; stimulating at the wrist and antecubital fossa), ulnar (recording at the abductor digiti minimi; stimulating at the wrist and at below-elbow and above-elbow sites), peroneal (fibular) (recording at extensor digitorum brevis; stimulating at the ankle, below the fibular neck, and lateral popliteal fossa), and tibial (recording at abductor hallucis; stimulating at the ankle and popliteal fossa). Consider peroneal (fibular) motor studies recording at the tibialis anterior muscle if the peroneal (fibular) motor study recording at the extensor digitorum brevis muscle is abnormal. If the CMAP amplitudes are low at the median/abductor pollicis brevis or ulnar/abductor digiti minimi, a brief post-exercise stimulation should be performed to evaluate the presence of a presynaptic disorder of neuromuscular junction transmission. The ulnar/first dorsal interosseous muscle response is also recommended, especially as it pertains to the demonstration of a "split-hand pattern" which may be seen in ALS.

Sensory nerve action potential (SNAP) studies should include the following nerves: median (stimulating at the wrist; recording at second digit), ulnar (stimulating at the wrist; recording at fifth digit), radial (stimulating at the forearm; recording at base of the thumb), superficial peroneal (fibular) (stimulating at the lateral leg; recording at the ankle), and sural (stimulating at the posterior portion of the calf; recording at the posterior ankle). Late responses are important and should include: F-waves (median, ulnar, peroneal (fibular), and tibial nerves), and tibial H-reflexes. Any abnormality should be compared to the contralateral side. More proximal motor nerve stimulation could be considered looking for conduction block, but may be limited due to location and supramaximal stimulation pitfalls at the axilla or Erb's point. Late responses could also be minimally abnormal in MND/ALS, mostly reflecting the reduced number of motor neurons available for the response, but are not typically expected to be absent or significantly delayed, as may be seen in a severe polyradiculopathy.

Needle Electrode Examination

Needle electromyographic assessment must be comprehensive and must show evidence of widespread denervation and re-innervation, specifically in the majority of the four regions discussed previously, and in at least two muscles of different spinal nerve root innervation within each limb region.

Table 9.2 Recommended muscle selections for needle electrode examination- motor neuron disease protocol

Upper extremity	Lower extremity	Craniobulbar	Paraspinal muscles
→first dorsal interosseous →abductor digiti minimi →abductor pollicis brevis →flexor pollicis longus (if question of inclusion body myositis) →extensor indicis proprius →pronator teres →biceps brachii →triceps →deltoid	→tibialis anterior →medial gastrocnemius →tibialis posterior or flexor digitorum longus →rectus femoris or vastus lateralis →gluteus medius	→tongue **Consider:** →sternocleidomastoid →masseter →facial muscles	→cervical **→thoracic (must be performed- typically, mid or low thoracic levels)** →lumbosacral

Abnormal spontaneous activity (fibrillation, positive sharp wave, and/or fasciculation potentials) are usually very prominent in a motor neuron disease process. However, fasciculation potentials alone are not sufficient to be considered as evidence of active/ongoing denervation, as they can be seen in other diseases, or may be a benign finding in some cases. Nonetheless, in MND, fasciculation potentials tend to be large with multiple turns and/or phases comprising a complex "bizarre-appearing" morphology. Noteworthy is the added pathological/diagnostic significance that is conferred by fasciculation potentials when there is superimposition of chronic motor axon loss changes in the same muscle (added diagnostic yield from the Awaji criteria, compared to the revised El Escorial criteria). Complex repetitive discharges (CRDs) can be seen in chronic lower motor neuron processes, but are not a particularly common feature in MND. Abnormal needle EMG findings must show involvement of different myotomes, with careful evaluation of possible sparing of individual nerves that could suggest another process, such as MMNCB.

Careful evaluation of motor unit action potentials (MUAPs) are key in the assessment of a lower motor neuron process. Features of chronic axon loss will be manifested by MUAP configurational changes- high amplitude, long duration, and may include increased polyphasia. There is often evidence of motor unit instability, as typically evidenced by "moment-to-moment amplitude variation". Decreased recruitment would also reflect the loss of motor units. Recruitment analysis will be essential when differentiating a lower motor neuron process from a myopathic process (including one with overalapping denervation/neurogenic) features. With LMN lesions, recruitment is reduced (including the rapid firing frequency of affected MUAPs), but in myopathies there is typically "early" recruitment (of MUAPs which are polyphasic, but short in duration and low in amplitude).

The recommended protocol for needle electromyography should include at least two limbs (distal and proximal muscles of different spinal nerve root innervation), thoracic paraspinal muscles (typically at the mid and low thoracic levels), and may also include craniobulbar muscles (important when excluding the possibility of superimposed cervical or lumbosacral polyradiculopathy). Active/ongoing denervation findings in the thoracic paraspinal muscles are commonly seen in most patients with MND/ALS, and several segments should be examined to increase diagnostic yield. Please refer to Table 9.2 for our recommended protocol of muscle selection for needle electrode examination in motor neuron disease cases.

Electrodiagnostic Pitfalls and Limitations

Sensory nerve action potentials are essential when demonstrating that there is definite electrodiagnostic evidence of a motor neuron process. As mentioned previously, SNAPs are expected to be normal in lower motor neuron disease. However, if the patient has a superimposed mononeuropathy, or polyneuropathy (or plexopathy), then the results can seem confounding because of reduced SNAPs. In this case, history, physical examination, and additional testing may assist in the differential diagnostic investigation. Motor nerve studies must be evaluated with caution, because the examiner has to specifically exclude MMNCB. If there is any indication of selective motor nerves being affected, with sparing of other individual motor nerves, MMNCB (or multifocal motor neuropathy) has to be considered. Since a complete motor conduction block has been established as greater than 50% drop in CMAP amplitude or area between distal and proximal nerve stimulation sites, there needs to be vigilance to prevent spurious responses with similar changes. Accordingly, if supramaximal nerve stimulation was not achieved (or if there are technical factors related to large body habitus), then responses may exhibit a motor conduction block pattern, leading to misdiagnosis. For example, a patient can be misdiagnosed as having a demyelinating polyneuropathy, when the underlying pathological entity is actually motor neuron disease. This can result from improper testing of nerve conduction responses, and the inability to acquire the SNAPs correctly, and consequently documenting an abnormal or absent response which should otherwise be present. Therefore, proficiency in nerve conduction studies is of paramount importance.

Again, at times it is recommended to repeat electrodiagnostic testing after several months to confirm progression of disease over time and to ascertain the diagnosis. Moreover, cervical and lumbosacral polyradiculopathies can manifest with the same nerve conduction features of a lower motor neuron disease, mostly because the SNAPs are normal (lesions are proximal to the dorsal root ganglia). However, in these patients, sensory symptoms and signs are typically present, contrasting with MND patients.

Late responses are not expected to be significantly abnormal in most cases of MND/ALS. This finding can be seen in the late or end stages of the disease, as more motor neurons become affected and can't contribute to the late response. As more of the largest and fastest the constituent fibers are affected, the F-wave latencies are expected to be progressively prolonged. Significant abnormalities of the late responses are commonly seen in a polyradiculopathy, and this feature could assist the electromyographer when making the distinction between this entity and MND, but it is generally not considered sufficient, especially as an isolated finding.

Needle electromyography also has some limitations during the evaluation of a lower motor neuron disease process. Accordingly, the assessment has to be comprehensive and should involve sufficient coverage of the majority of regions (craniobulbar, cervical, thoracic, and lumbosacral). There should be the aforementioned electrical evidence of active/ongoing and chronic axon loss (i.e. overlapping features of denervation and reinnervation), spanning different nerve roots/myotomes, which cannot be reasonably explained by any other etiologies. Thoracic paraspinal muscles are of paramount importance when differentiating motor neuron disease from a polyradiculopathy, as typically they will be abnormal in MND. In contrast, a polyradiculopathy is commonly seen at the cervical and lumbar regions, and is much less likely at the thoracic region. Moreover, some fasciculations can be seen during the needle EMG of patients with a polyradiculopathy (or any other neurogenic process), and need careful interpretation. Fasciculations alone cannot be considered as evidence of active/ongoing denervation. However, in conjunction with chronic motor axon loss changes, they may have similar significance per the Awaji criteria.

Other caveats in the interpretation of needle electromyography include patient's tolerance for testing (intolerance usually manifested by suboptimal activation of MUAPs), and their ability to complete the full extensive protocol. Intolerance issues (e.g. from pain-related effects) could lead to incomplete estimation of MUAP recruitment, because of suboptimal MUAP activation. Additionally, incomplete muscle relaxation hampers reliable spontaneous activity assessment. This is commonly seen during craniobulbar muscle needle EMG, especially with impaired relaxation typically encountered when examining the tongue muscle.

Adequate discussion, including clarification of expectations should occur before requesting electrodiagnostic study to ensure that the patient understands the testing procedure, especially as the MND protocol is very extensive.

Some chronic muscle diseases can be very challenging to differentiate from a motor neuron disorder, particularly if there are superimposed chronic denervation-type changes (as can be commonly seen in inclusion body myositis). On needle electromyography, they may exhibit chronic neurogenic changes with or without abundant spontaneous activity abnormalities (fibrillation potentials/positive wave potentials) which may be seen in both active/ongoing denervation and myopathy with inflammatory/necrotizing features. Therefore, these disorders can sometimes mimic a motor neuron process. As mentioned previously, the MUAP recruitment pattern can be used to differentiate between the two, as well as history and physical examination, and other laboratory testing (e.g. creatine kinase level). This is why electrodiagnostic testing alone cannot be used to diagnose a motor neuron disease, and can only be a component (albeit an important one) of the comprehensive evaluation. Amyotrophic lateral sclerosis remains a clinical diagnosis, supported by electrodiagnostic testing, neuroimaging, laboratory studies, and history/physical examination findings. On this basis, it may be prudent that the interpretation section of the EDX study does not claim that the pertinent results are "diagnostic" for MND/ALS, but rather are compatible/consistent with this diagnosis in the appropriate clinical context.

Case Study

A 68 year-old right-handed Caucasian woman, with a past medical history of hypertension, was referred for progressive left foot drop for about 4 months. The weakness started very distally at the toes, then slowly progressed proximally to involve the ankle. There was no lower back pain, limb numbness or paresthesia, symptoms of bowel/bladder dysfunction, or prior history of falls or trauma. She saw a neurosurgeon who advised her that there was no surgical intervention needed for the essentially unremarkable lumbar spine findings on MRI. There was no involvement of the right lower extremity, or the upper extremities. There were no symptoms of craniobulbar or respiratory muscle weakness. At another facility, she was recently diagnosed with a severe, subacute on chronic mixed axonal-demyelinating peripheral polyneuropathy, based on electrodiagnostic testing, and intravenous immunoglobulin therapy had been commenced. There is no family history of neurodegenerative diseases.

On initial neurological examination: mental status, cranial nerves, and spine/straight leg raise test were normal/negative. Both upper extremities and the right lower extremity were normal in motor and sensory examination. The left lower extremity had mild-to-moderate diffuse muscle atrophy, mostly distal to the knee with motor strength graded at 3- to 4−/5 (MRC scale), throughout the left L2-S1 myotomes. No fasciculations, no tongue atrophy, dystonic posturing, tremors, dysmetria or spasticity were noted. Reflexes were 2+ throughout, even in the context of the weakness noted in the left lower limb. Plantar responses were mute bilaterally, and there was no clonus. Sensory examination was normal to all modalities tested.

Since the history, neurological examination, and recent electrodiagnostic testing were rather contradicting, we decided to order additional testing. A lumbar puncture was performed showing normal: cell count, protein, glucose, albumin, IgG index/synthesis rate, myelin basic protein, culture, and smear. In addition, she tested negative for CSF Lyme antibodies, VDRL, and oligoclonal bands. On blood testing she had normal/negative: 24-hour urine heavy metal panel, comprehensive ganglioside panel, GAD antibody, vitamin B-12, comprehensive metabolic panel, Lyme IgG/IgM, CBC, ESR, and CRP. Neuroimaging showed multilevel degenerative changes in the cervical spine, and very minimal disc degeneration in the lumbar spine without evidence of significant central canal or neuroforaminal stenosis. There was evidence of widespread chronic ischemic white matter changes on the brain MRI, but no acute findings were seen.

On the follow-up appointment 6 months later, there was now more progressive leg weakness, involving the right lower extremity, and hands. She had subjective symptoms of mild swallowing dysfunction, without breathing difficulties. Sensory examination remained normal. Reflexes were now pathologically brisk, and mild spasticity was noted in the lower extremities. Considering normal testing, including CSF protein level, the patient agreed to have the electrodiagnostic testing repeated. Please refer to Table 9.3 for EDX study results.

Table 9.3 Case electrodiagnostic data

Sensory Nerve Conduction

Nerve	Stimulus	Recording	B-P Amp (μV)		LatNPk (ms)		CV (m/s)		Dist (mm)		Norm B-P Amp	Norm LatNPk	Norm CV	Temp (°C)	
			L	R	L	R	L	R	L	R				L	R
Sural	Lower Leg	Lat Malleolus	12.17		3.88		n/a		140		>3 uV	<4.6 ms	>40 m/s	31.9	
Superficial Per	Lower Leg	Ankle	6.25		3.64		n/a		100		>3 uV	<4.6 ms	>40 m/s	31.8	
Median	Wrist	Index	13.49		3.70		n/a		130		>10 uV	<3.8 ms	>50 m/s	32.8	
Ulnar	Wrist	5th Dig	16.02		2.80		n/a		110		>5 uV	<3.2 ms	>50 m/s	32.6	

Motor Nerve Conduction

Nerve	Recording	Stimulus	B-P Amp (μV)		LatOn (ms)		CV (m/s)		Dist (mm)		Norm B-P Amp	Norm Distal LatOn	Norm CV	Temp (°C)	
			L	R	L	R	L	R	L	R				L	R
Peroneal (fibular)/ EDB	EDB	Ankle	**2.40**		4.60		n/a		70		>2.5 mV	<6 ms	>40 m/s	32.3	
		Pop **Foss - Knee**	**2.00**		13.75		45.4		415					32.4	
Tibial/AH	AH	Ankle	4.01		4.05		n/a		80		>4 mV	<6 ms	>40 m/s	32.7	
		Pop **Foss - Knee**	**3.77**		13.20		44.8		410					32.8	
Peroneal (fibular)/ TA	TA	Below Fib Head	**2.67**		2.45		n/a				>3 mV	<4.5 ms	>40 m/s	33.1	
Median	APB	Wrist	5.32		3.90		n/a		50		>5 mV	<4 ms	>50 m/s	33.0	
		Elbow	**4.92**		9.10		57.7		300					33.0	
Ulnar/ADM	ADM	Wrist	9.26		2.96		n/a		50		>7 mV	<3.1 ms	>50 m/s	33.2	
		Below Elbow	8.68		6.90		58.2		230					32.9	
		Above Elbow	8.41		8.90		55.5		330					33.1	
Ulnar/1stDI	1stDI	Wrist	7.28		3.05		n/a				>7 mV	<4.5 ms	>50 m/s	33.3	

F-Wave Side-To-Side Comparison Table

Nerve	Stimulus	Recording	F-Waves Lat (ms)	
			L	R
Tibial/AH	Ankle	AH	56.70	
Ulnar/ADM	Wrist	ADM	29.00	

H-Reflex Summary Table

Nerve	Stimulus	Recording	Side	M-Wave		H-Wave	
				Lat (ms)	Amp (mV)	Lat (ms)	Amp (mV)
	Pop Fossa	Soleus	Left	5.5ms	9.6mV	33.7ms	1.7

Needle EMG Summary

Side	Muscle	Ins Act	Fib	PW	Fasc	Other	Number	Recruit	Dur	Dur	Amp	Amp	Poly	Poly	Descript	Descript	Descript
L	1st Dorsal Inter	Norm	1+	1+	0+		2-	Rapid	Many	1+	Many	1+		Norm	NC	NC	NC
	Abduc.Pol.Brevis	Norm	1+	0	1+		3-	Rapid	All	1+	All	1+	Some	1+	ATR	NC	NC
	Abduc.Digiti.Minimi	Norm	0	0+	0		2-	Rapid	Many	1+	Some	1+		Norm	NC	NC	NC
	Flex.Pollicis Longus	Norm	0	0+	0		1-	Mod-R	Some	1+	Some	1+		Norm	NC	NC	NC
	Extn. Indicis Pro	Norm	0+	0	0+		1-	Rapid	Many	1+	Many	1+		Norm	NC	NC	NC
	Pronator Teres	Norm	0	0+	0+		1-	Mod-R	Few	1+	Few	1+		Norm	NC	NC	NC
	Biceps Brachii	Norm	0	0	0+		Norm	Full		Norm		Norm		Norm	NC	NC	NC
	Triceps-Lat	Norm	0	0	0		1-	Mod		Norm		Norm		Norm	NC	NC	NC
	Deltoid, Middle	Norm	1+	0	0+		1-	Mod-R	Few	1+		Norm	Few	1+	NC	NC	NC
	SCM	Norm	0	0+	0		1-	Mod-R	Few	1+	Few	1+		Norm	NC	NC	NC
	Cervical PSP (Low)	Norm	1+	0	1+			NE							NC	NC	NC
	Abductor Hallucis	Norm	0	0	0+	MTP	3-	Mod-R	Many	1+	Many	1+		Norm	NC	NC	NC
	Extn. Digitorum Brv	Norm	0+	0	0+		3-	Mod-V	Most	1+	Many	1+		Norm	NC	NC	NC
	Flex. Digitrum Longus						2-	Mod-R	Many	1+	Some	1+		Norm	NRLX	NC	NC
	Tibialis Anterior	Norm	2+	1+	1+		3-	Rapid	Most	1+	Many	1+	Some	1+	MMAV	NC	NC
	Gastroc. Medial H	Norm	0	1+	0+		2-	Mod-R	Many	1+	Some	1+	Few	1+	NC	NC	NC
	Rectus Famoris	Norm	0+	0	0		1-	Mod-R	Few	1+	Few	1+		Norm	NC	NC	NC
	Vastus Lateralis	Norm	1+	0	0		2-	Mod-R	Many	1+	Many	1+		Norm	NC	NC	NC
	Gluteus Medius	Norm	0	1+	0		2-	Mod-R	Many	1+	Many	1+	Few	1+	NC	NC	NC
	Lumbar PSP (Low)	Norm	0	0+	0			NE							NC	NC	NC
	Tongue	Norm	1+	0	1+		1-	Mod-R	Few	1+	Few	1+		Norm	NC	NC	NC
	Thoracic PSP (Mid)						2-	Mod-R	Many	1+	Few	1+	Some	1+	NRLX		
	Thoracic PSP (Low)	Norm	1+	0	1+		1-	Mod-R	Few	1+	Few	1+		Norms	NC	NC	NC

Abbreviations: *ATR* atrophy; *MMAV* moment-to-moment amplitude variation; *MTP* myotonic potential; *NE* recruitment pattern not examined (muscle examined at rest only) *NRLX* not relaxed; *SCM* sternocleidomastoid; *EDB* Extensor digitorum brevis; *AH* Abductor hallucis; *TA* Tibialis anterior; *APB* Abductor pollicis brevis; *ADM* Abductor digiti minimi; *1st DI* First dorsal interosseous; *PSP* Paraspinals

Considering the nerve conduction findings, especially the preserved SNAPs, we decided to perform a more extensive needle electromyography evaluation, conforming to the lab's MND protocol. Widespread chronic MUAP neurogenic changes (including increased duration and amplitude, with or without polyphasic units), with evidence of active/ongoing denervation (fibrillation and positive sharp wave potentials) in addition to scattered fasciculation potentials were seen in the muscles of the left upper and lower extremities, as well as the thoracic and craniobulbar regions. No myopathic units were seen. The findings spanned multiple nerve roots/myotomes (also implicating progression from the initial areas described as involved), correlating with the most recent worsening of clinical features disclosed at the follow-up office visit. Collectively, the results were consistent with a generalized active/ongoing on chronic motor axon loss process (conspicuously sparing sensory responses) compatible with an evolving widespread disorder of anterior horn cells/motor neurons.

These results cannot be explained by the neuroimaging, or laboratory/spinal tap results obtained. In this case, it became apparent that the diagnosis of MND/ALS was strongly supported by the latest EDX study, and that the initial study produced erroneous results and interpretation. Electrodiagnostic testing should be repeated for cases in which the clinical presentation is not consistent the EDX results provided. A repeat EDX study may also serve to more objectively demonstrate progression of disease. It is imperative to have the appropriate expertise when performing these studies. In this case, pertinent alternative etiologies were excluded by comprehensive testing.

ALS patients should ideally be further evaluated and managed at ALS multidisciplinary clinics, consistent with recommended best practice guidelines. Such specialized ALS clinics typically provide timely access to several services/resources including assistive devices/adaptive equipment, non-invasive ventilation, feeding tubes, and referral to other medical specialists (e.g. pulmonary, physical/occupational therapy, nutritionist), as well as referral to a medical social worker. Although the diagnosis of ALS may be initially difficult to elucidate, prompt diagnosis can allow the patient to have an opportunity to receive treatment/supportive care that could increase quality of life, even if the improvement in longevity is not very marked.

References

1. Xu J, et al. Abnormal cortical-basal ganglia network in amyotrophic lateral sclerosis: a voxel-wise network efficiency analysis. Behav Brain Res. 2017;333:123–8.
2. Isaacs JD, Dean AF, Shaw CE, Al-Chalabi A, Mills KR, Nigel LP. Amyotrophic lateral sclerosis with sensory neuropathy: part of a multisystem disorder? J Neurol Neurosurg Psychiatry. 2007;78(7):750–3.
3. Ling L, Xiaodong C, Jia L, Zhuang K, Jing L, Zizhen H, Ruomi G, Zhengqi L. A madras motor neuron disease patient with cerebellar atrophy: a new clinical feature. Front Neurosci. 2018;12:722.
4. Volk AE, Weishaupt JH, Andersen PM, Ludolph AC, Kubisch C. Current knowledge and recent insights into the genetic basis of amyotrophic lateral sclerosis. Med Genet. 2018;30(2):252–8.
5. Pehar M, Harlan BA, Killoy KM, Vargas MR. Role and therapeutic potential of astrocytes in amyotrophic lateral sclerosis. Curr Pharm Des. 2017;23(33):5010–21.
6. Tartaglia MC, Rowe A, Findlater K, et al. Differentiation between primary lateral sclerosis and amyotrophic lateral sclerosis: examination of symptoms and signs at disease onset and during follow-up. Arch Neurol. 2007;64(2):232–6.
7. Zhai P, Pagan F, Statland J, Butman JA, Floeter MK. Primary lateral sclerosis: a heterogeneous disorder composed of different subtypes? Neurology. 2003;60(8):1258–65.
8. Statland JM, Barohn RJ, Dimachkie MM, Floeter MK, Mitsumoto H. Neurol Clin. 2015;33(4):749–60.
9. Vora M, Kumar S, Sharma S, et al. Advanced magnetic resonance neuroimaging in bulbar and limb onset early amyotrophic lateral sclerosis. J Neurosci Rural Pract. 2016;7(1):102–8.
10. Tripathi P, Rodriguez-Muela N, Klim JR, et al. Stem Cell Reports. 2017;9(2):667–80.
11. Ghasemi M. Amyotrophic lateral sclerosis mimic syndromes. Iran J Neurol. 2016;15(2):85–91.

10 Disorders of the Neuromuscular Junction

Raghav Govindarajan and Elanagan Nagarajan

Anatomy and Physiology of the Neuromuscular Junction

A synapse is a functional junction between two excitable cells. The neuron which transmits information is the presynaptic neuron, and the one which receives the information is the postsynaptic neuron (in the case of the NMJ, this is the muscle fiber). Between the pre- and postsynaptic membranes, there is a definite anatomical gap called the synaptic cleft [2–5].

The axon of the presynaptic neuron loses its myelin sheath as it reaches the muscle fiber and is branched at the nerve terminal, where it ends as a knob-like structure. This structure contains mitochondria which is rich in adenosine triphosphate (ATP) along with coated and uncoated vesicles. The mitochondrial ATP is used as an energy source for the synthesis of acetylcholine which is stored in the vesicles. These vesicles are not uniformly distributed along the synaptic cleft but are clustered at a region called the active zone [2–5].

R. Govindarajan (✉) · E. Nagarajan
Department of Neurology, Neurology Clinics, ALS and MDA Clinic, EMG/Neurophysiology Lab, Clinical Outcomes for Department of Neurology, University of Missouri, Columbia, MO, USA

Department of Neurology, University of Missouri, Columbia, MO, USA
e-mail: govindarajanr@health.missouri.edu; nagarajane@health.missouri.edu

The skeletal muscle fiber membrane at the end plate is thickened and invaginates into the muscle fiber forming a depression. This depression is known as "synaptic trough or gutter." This synaptic gutter has both chemical and electrical characteristic features that are different from the rest of the muscle membrane and also serves as a location for most of the acetylcholine receptors in the postsynaptic membrane.

The synaptic cleft is filled with an electron-dense material called "ground substance", made up of acetylcholinesterase enzyme (AChE). This AChE degrades the acetylcholine into acetate and choline [5]. The detailed anatomy of the NMJ is shown in Fig. 10.1a.

The series of sequential events needed for the generation and propagation of the action potential leading to muscle contraction is summarized in Fig. 10.1b [2–5].

When an impulse reaches the presynaptic terminal, a delay of 0.5 msec occurs before a response is elicited in the postsynaptic membrane. This time delay is called synaptic delay, and this occurs because the aforementioned sequence of events has to occur [2–5].

The integrity of the AChR at the postsynaptic membrane and its function are determined by the presence of several other proteins in the muscle end plate region. Agrin is a large proteoglycan secreted by the nerve terminal which interacts with muscle-specific tyrosine kinase (MuSK) through its coreceptor, low-density lipoprotein receptor-related

N. Galvez-Jimenez et al. (eds.), *Electrodiagnostic Medicine*,
https://doi.org/10.1007/978-3-030-74997-2_10

protein 4 (LRP4). The resultant MuSK-LRP4 complex results in the activation and clustering of AChRs at the neuromuscular junction.

Myasthenia Gravis

Myasthenia gravis (MG) is a prototypical human autoimmune disorder in which the neuromuscular transmission is impaired due to the presence of antibodies against structural components in the muscle membrane. This results in fluctuating muscle weakness and fatigability. The identification of different antibodies and the relatively easy availability of antibody assays have shown a significant improvement in the diagnosis and tailored therapy. The current management options include symptomatic treatment, immunomodulation/immunosuppression therapy, and thymectomy in a selected subgroup of the MG population.

Epidemiology

Based on the available epidemiological data, there is a significant variation in the incidence and prevalence of MG due to ethnic diversity and geographic region. It was reported that the worldwide prevalence is 40–180 per 100,000 people with an annual incidence of 4–12 per 100,000 people [6]. Recent studies have suggested that the incidence is higher, especially in the elderly and this is due to the more widespread availability of antibody testing, and the better understanding of clinical presentation [7]. Juvenile myasthenia gravis is most commonly seen in patients of East Asian origin and half of the cases have an onset before the age of 15 and is restricted to ocular muscle only [8]. Women are more prone to have MG before the age of 50 years old, which is typical of many autoimmune disorders when compared to male [9]. Late-onset MG which is above

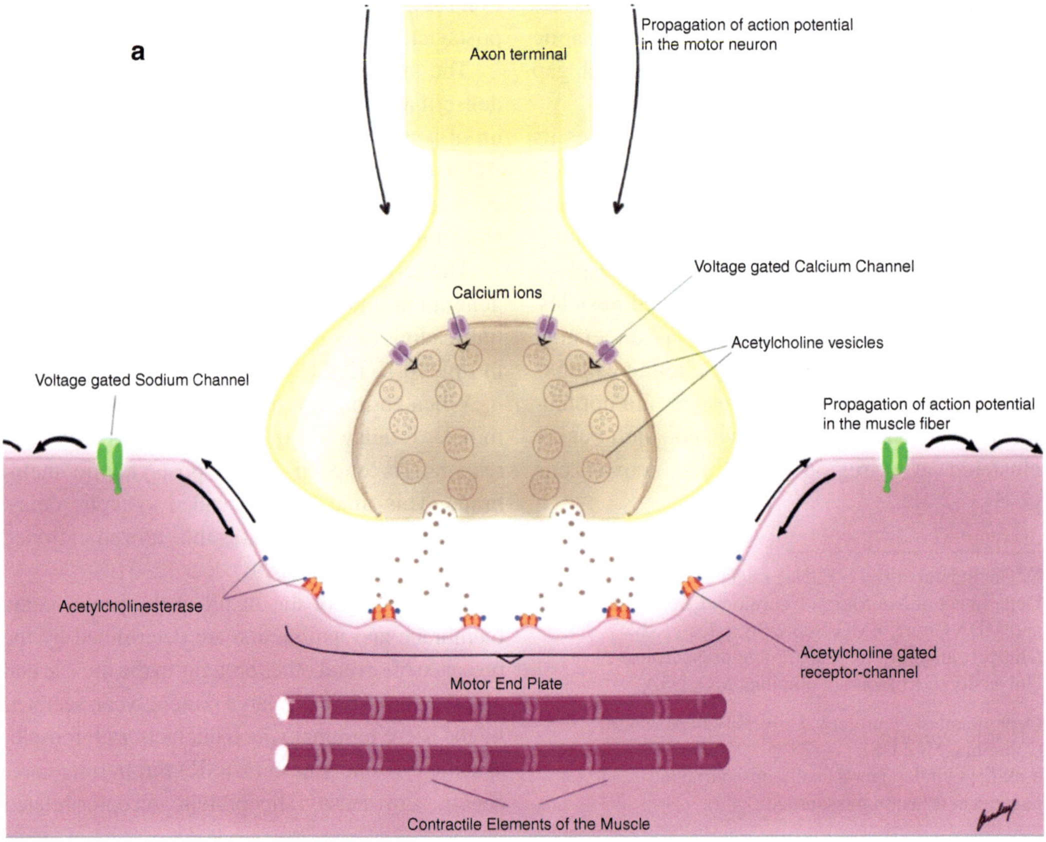

Fig. 10.1 (**a**) The Neuromuscular Junction anatomy and schematic. (**b**) Sequential Physiological Changes During Neuromuscular Junction Transmission

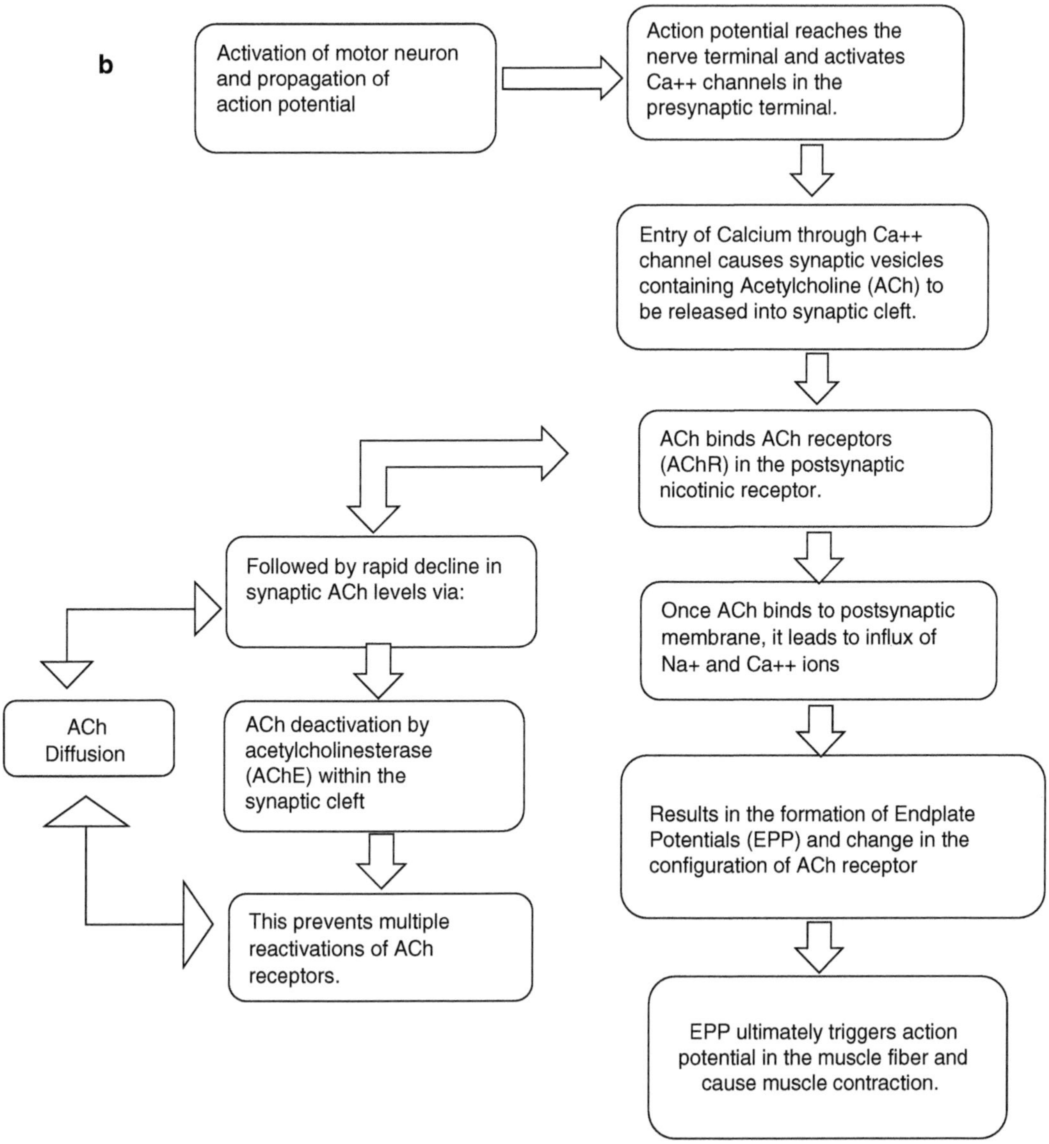

Fig. 10.1 (continued)

50 year old is more commonly seen in males when compared to females [9].

Clinical Presentation

Muscle weakness is the major hallmark in the diagnosis of MG. Accentuation in weakness at the end of the day and exercise-induced weakness is strongly suggestive of MG. Younger individuals often present with unspecified fatigue as a major complaint, whereas the elderly population usually presents with eye and bulbar symptoms [10–12]. The weakness is generally more common in ocular muscles, but it can also be seen in the extraocular eye muscles, other craniobulbar, limb and axial/truncal muscles. Roughly around 60% of patient's presents with ptosis or diplopia or both and in 20% of patients, symptoms remain essentially restricted to the ocular distribution [10, 11, 13]. The weakness of extraocular muscle is almost always asymmetrical whereas limb muscles are generally symmetrically involved with proximal muscles usually being involved more than the distal muscles [13].

Subtypes of Myasthenia Gravis

MG can be classified into different subtypes based upon the presence of antibodies (and the specific antibody) against the structural proteins in the postsynaptic membrane. There may be some noteworthy differences in the clinical features and treatment responses between the subtypes.

Mysthenia Gravis (MG) Associated with Acetylcholine Receptor Antibodies (ACHR) Antibodies

Figure 10.2 below summarizes the key clinical and pathological characteristics of AChR antibody positive MG.

Mysthenia Gravis (MG) Associated with Muscle-Specific Tyrosine Kinase (MuSK) and LDL Receptor Related Protein 4 (LRP4) Receptor Antibodies

Figure 10.3 below summarizes the key clinical and pathological characteristics of MuSK and LRP4 antibody positive MG.

Seronegative Myasthenia Gravis

In this subgroup, patients have clinical features consistent with MG, however, their AChR, MuSK, or LRP4 antibodies levels are found to be undetectable which is probably due to a low affinity or low concentration (below threshold) on routine assays [14, 15]. These antibodies may be detectable through the cell-based assay which is not routinely done in most laboratories [16]. Roughly around 20–50% of patients with seronegative MG were found to have low-affinity antibodies [14, 15]. Cases have also been reported with antibodies against agrin and cortactin, but the pathological role in the disease process remains unclear [17, 18]. The diagnosis becomes more difficult when there is total absence of antibodies. In such a population, the possibility of other myasthenic syndromes, muscle, and non-muscle disorders needs to be considered as well [11].

Ocular Myasthenia Gravis

The weakness remains restricted to ocular muscles in this population. This group of patients has the highest risk of developing generalized MG within 2 years of symptom onset. Approximately half of the patients with ocular myasthenia gravis have a positive acetylcholine receptor antibody, and rarely the presence of MUSK antibodies are also reported [19].

CASE

A 23-year-old woman who has a known history of epilepsy presented with a complaint of excessive daytime fatigue and tiredness. On further questioning, she had a frequent head drop without any loss of awareness and was diagnosed with psychogenic non-epileptic spells. Since then she had a progressive worsening with an increase in the frequency of head drop along with breathing difficulty at rest and worse with activity. Her symptoms were worse in the evening and also associated with dysphagia. Neurological examination was significant for mild neck extensor muscle weakness and fatigable weakness in the upper extremities. EDX including repetitive nerve stimulation (RNS) studies showed 40% decrement in the abductor digiti minimi, and needle examination was notable for fibrillation potentials and myopathic-appearing motor units in the paraspinal and proximal upper limb muscles. Single fiber EMG of the orbicularis oculus showed abnormal jitter. She was started on pyridostigmine for symptomatic control which paradoxically made her symptom worse. Anti-MuSK antibodies were found to be positive and the

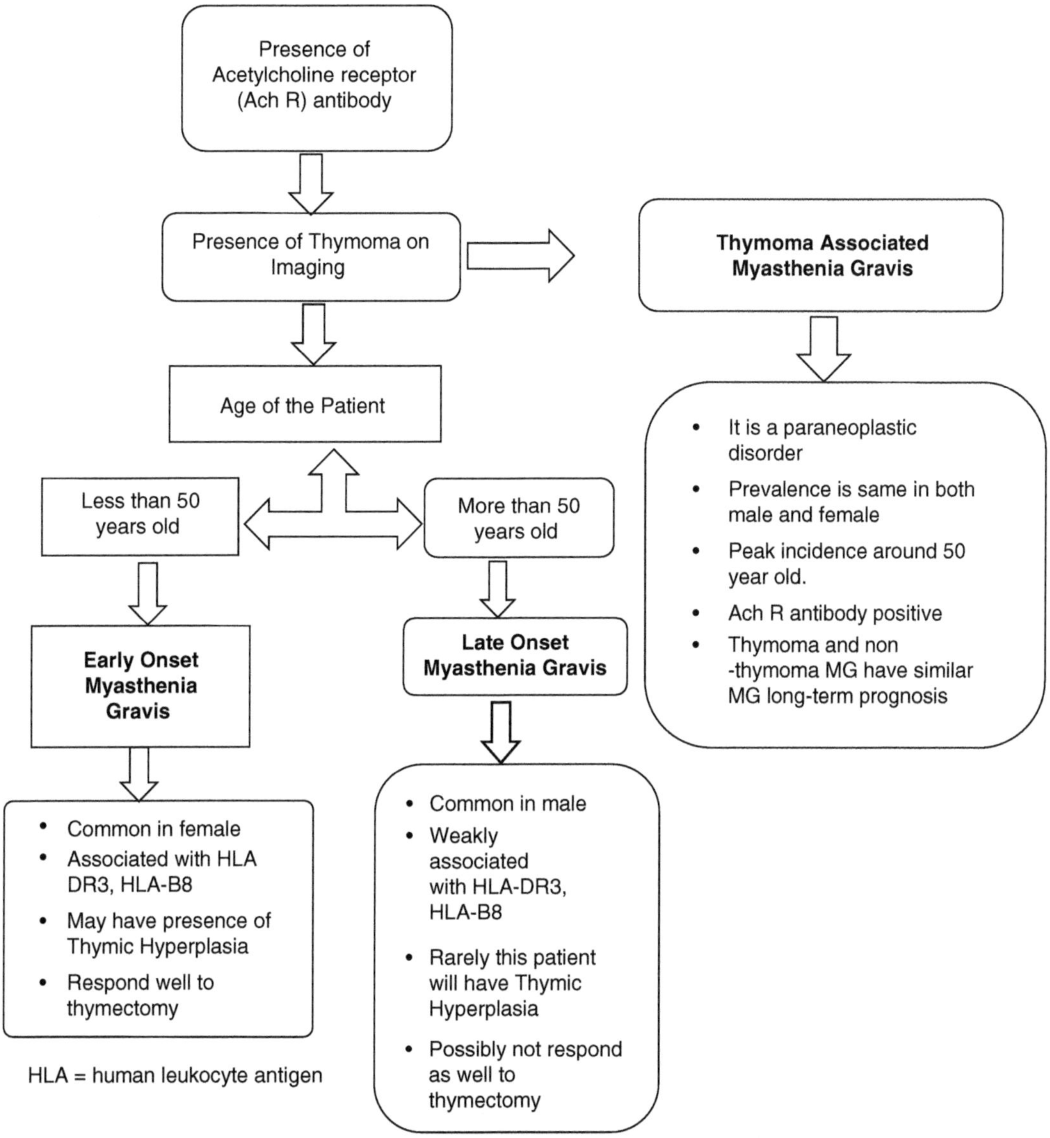

Fig. 10.2 Clinical and Pathological Features of Acetylcholine Receptor Antibody positive myasthenia gravis. *HLA* human leukocyte antigen

AChR antibodies testing was found to be unremarkable. CT chest was unremarkable for thymic abnormalities. She was started with monthly IVIG treatment along with prednisone and rituximab. Within a year, she was off of IVIG and has been maintained on low-dose prednisone and rituximab. At 2 years follow-up, swallowing and breathing difficulties, and head drop remain improved significantly.

Comment

This case highlights myasthenia gravis at a young age, female predominance with prominent bulbar, respiratory and proximal muscle weakness. MuSK antibodies are found to be positive with EDX findings consistent with a postsynaptic disorder of neuromuscular junction transmission. Typically, clinical symptoms in MuSK MG get worse with acetylcholineesterase

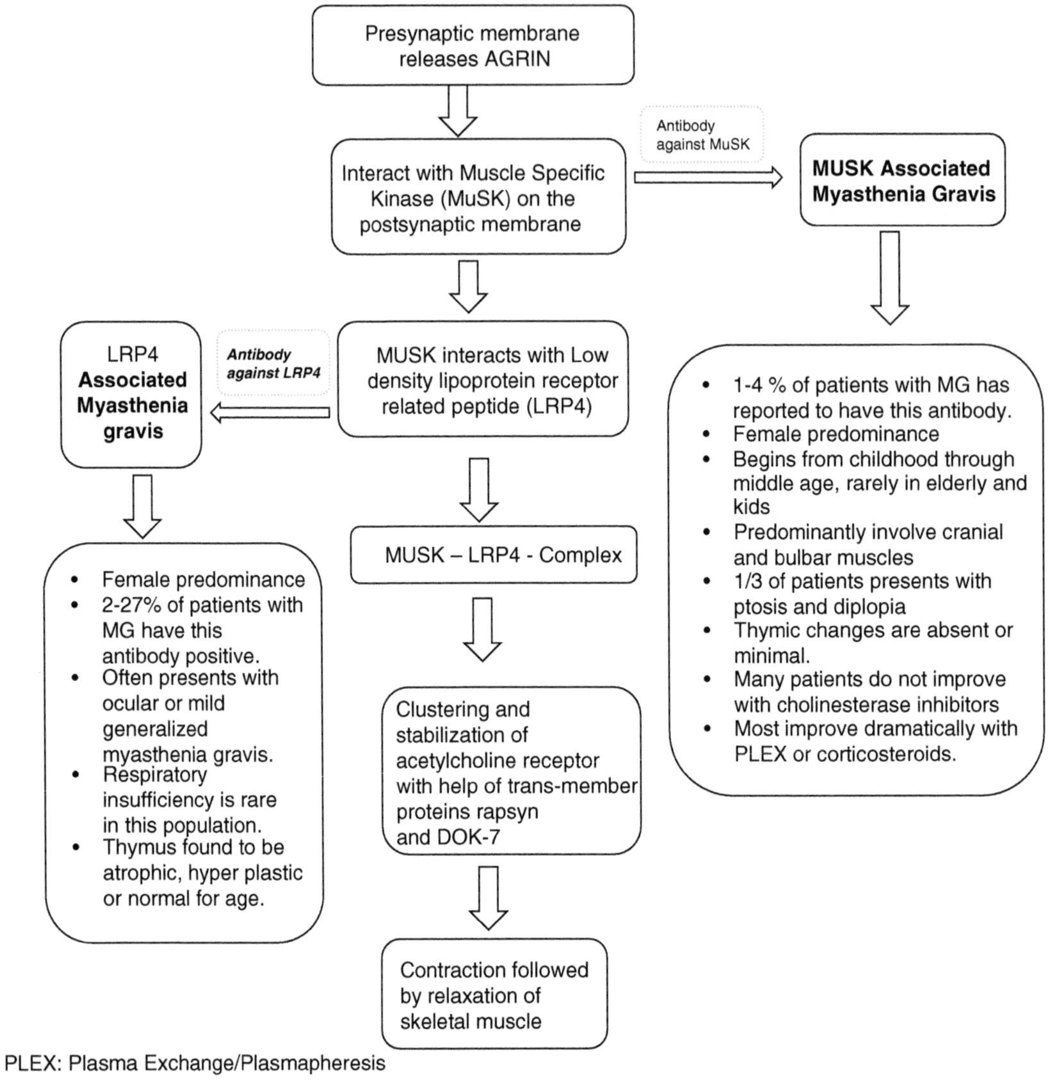

Fig. 10.3 Clinical and Pathological Features of Myasthenia Gravis with Muscle-Specific Tyrosine Kinase (MuSK) and LDL Receptor Related Protein 4 (LRP4) Receptor Antibodies. *PLEX* Plasma Exchange/Plasmapheresis

inhibitors and they respond well to immunomodulation therapy.

Diagnostic Testing

Ice Pack Test

The ice pack test is a simple and practical bedside test if the patient has ptosis on physical examination and it can also help to rule out other causes of ptosis or ophthalmoparesis. This test is performed by placing an instant cold ice pack on the affected eye for 2–5 min. If this test is positive, the patient will no longer have characteristic ptosis of MG. The sensitivity of this test has been reported as 76.9% and the specificity of 98.3%. The effect seen is attributable to inhibition of acetylcholinesterase activity at a reduced temperature which results in transient improvement of clinical symptoms [20]. However, the final diagnosis of MG needs to be confirmed by the presence of serum antibodies and electrophysiological findings.

Edrophonium Chloride Test

This is one of the classic tests for MG. It is feasible at the bedside and also in an office setting, but it is infrequently used now due to potentially serious complications such as bradycardia and syncope. The diagnostic yield is greater than 90% in patients with ptosis or diplopia, and this can also be used as ancillary testing when antibody or electrodiagnostic test is unrevealing. The response is dose-dependent and usually begins with intravenous administration of 2 mg edrophonium, with dose up to 10 mg typically accepted. The clinical response needs to be monitored for 60 seconds after administration. If there is any intermittent improvement in clinical symptoms within 60 seconds of administration, then no further dose is necessary. Some people are susceptible even to the low doses, and it is advised to have atropine available at the bedside to prevent any deleterious complications [21, 22].

Electrodiagnostic Studies

Electrophysiological studies such as RNS and Single Fiber Electromyography (SFEMG) indirectly measure the neuromuscular junction function and helps us to diagnose and characterize the specific defects i.e. presynaptic, synaptic and post synaptic disorders.

Repetitive Nerve Stimulation (RNS)

Definition

It is a neurophysiological study to assess the integrity of neuromuscular transmission.

Physiology of RNS

As we discussed earlier in this chapter, acetylcholine is stored in the presynaptic membrane inside vesicles. The amount of acetylcholine stored in vesicles is referred to as quantum. These quanta have been physiologically divided into three compartments (primary, secondary and tertiary), depending on their availability for use. The release of acetylcholine can happen either spontaneously as a single quantum or multiple quanta depending on the action potential. The spontaneous release causes a small depolarization in the postsynaptic membrane called Miniature Endplate Potential (MEPP). A large number of quanta released causes a depolarization of resting membrane at the endplate region called endplate potential (EPP). When the EPP reach a threshold which leads to a generation of action potential in the postsynaptic muscle membrane, this ultimately leads to muscle contraction. When motor nerve fibers are stimulated, the pre-synaptic region releases acetylcholine from the immediately available primary stores, and when a continuous voluntary contraction is sustained, the primary stores are depleted. To maintain the contraction, the secondary stores starts to replenish the depletion from the primary stores. Thus initiation of the secondary stores use happens with a slight lag of time. This secondary stores activation when primary stores are depleted is called the Safety Factor. At the time of secondary stores activation, the nerve releases three times the effective dose of acetylcholine.

The depletion of the primary store competes with mobilization from the secondary store. This may become apparent as impulses fail to discharge from the muscle fibers effectively (blocking), causing a decrease in the Compound muscle action potential (CMAP). CMAP is the sum of action potentials from muscle fibers, which are activated by nerve stimulation [23, 24].

Slow-Rate Stimulation

At the optimal frequency (2–5 Hz) slow rate stimulation, the primary store is maximally depleted while the secondary store mobilization is minimized. A dip in the CMAP waveform is typically visualized, with the size of the CMAP responses decreasing progressively by the fourth to sixth impulses (decline of ACh quanta from the immediately available pool), followed by a reversal. This is called as the decremental response [25].

Fast-Rate Stimulation

A high frequency (15–30, or up to 50 Hz) RNS, causes cumulative facilitation of transmitter release (due to increasing Ca^+ entry into the nerve terminal). This is the basic response to rapid nerve stimulation, leading to post activation potentiation. The CMAP responses gradually increases, this is called an incremental response [25].

Electrophysiological Findings in MG

The electrophysiological findings in MG is a classical decremental response by slow rate (2–5 Hz) RNS due to the defective postsynaptic NMJ transmission. The decremental response in slow rate occurs due to the failure of some muscle fibers to reach the threshold. This is because, even when a successive volley of acetylcholine is released from the synaptic vesicles, there is much less availability of ACh receptor in the post synaptic muscle membrane. Thus, CMAP failure occurs which corresponds to difficultly in initiating muscle contraction. This process is called *blocking*. A train of stimuli (8–10) with the supramaximal intensity is given to elicit CMAP responses from the muscle. The percentage of the amplitude decrement from first to fifth CMAP waveform should be 10% or more to be interpreted as abnormal. In some patients, the decremental response can be observed during resting and tends to worsen after activation (exercise). This is called *postexercise exhaustion* which occurs in 2–5 min after the exercise. In some patients, after activation, the decrement response tend to improve or repair, and this is called as *postexercise facilitation*. Proper technical methods, immobilization of the limb during the procedure, standard stimulus at the same point, proper voluntary activation and patient cooperation ensures a good result. RNS studies the integrity of NMJ transmission, and the decrement response is usually observed reliably in the clinically weak muscles. The decremental responses in MG are generally more prominent in the proximal muscles compared to the distal muscles [26, 27]. Electrophysiological findings are illustrated in Fig. 10.4.

Postexercise facilitation and exhaustion. 3-Hertz repetitive nerve stimulation in a patient with myasthenia gravis.

A: Decrement of compound muscle action potential (CMAP) amplitude at rest.

B: Postexercise facilitation, Decrement of CMAP immediately following 10 seconds of maximal voluntary exercise has repaired toward normal.

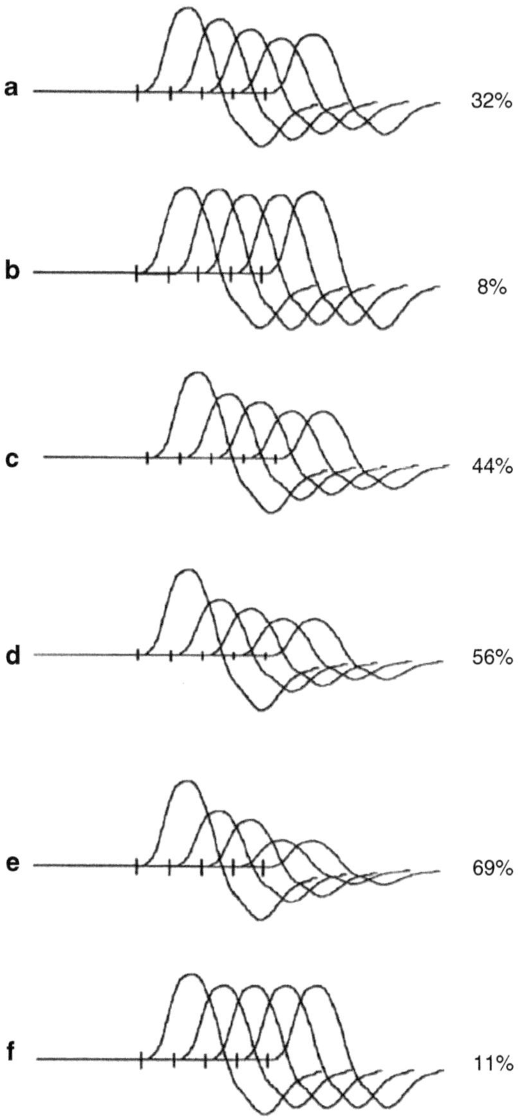

Fig. 10.4 The RNS findings in patients with myasthenia gravis (*used with permission- from Electromyography and Neuromuscular Disorders: Clinical-Electrophysiologic Correlations, second Edition by Preston, David C.; Shapiro, Barbara published by Butterworth-Heinemann*)

C–E: Postexercise exhaustion. Decrements of CMAP 1, 2, and 3 min after 1 min of maximal voluntary exercise. Decrement becomes progressively more marked over the baseline decrement.

F: Postexercise facilitation after a decrement. Immediately following another 10 seconds of maximal voluntary exercise, the decrement, which has worsened as a result of postexercise exhaustion, repairs toward normal.

Technical Aspect of RNS

The selection of a particular muscle depends on several factors which include clinical symptoms, the simplicity of performing the test, reliability of the test, and the amount of potential discomfort for the patient. It is recommended to start testing with small distal muscles that can be easily immobilized and reliably tested, followed by proximal muscles if they are needed [27, 28].

The skin should be cleaned with alcohol wipes prior to the procedure, and temperature should be maintained as close to 35 °C as possible over the recording site. The active electrode is placed over the motor endplate area (muscle belly) and the reference electrode over the distal tendon. The muscle should be at rest and immobilized [27]. The technical aspects of commonly tested muscles, their nerve supply, their stimulation site, electrode placement and activation procedures are summarized in Table 10.1.

A pathological decremental response is typical and shows a successive decrease in CMAP amplitude from the first to the fourth stimulation, then a slight recovery (facilitation) towards the tenth stimuli ("saddle shaped" response). If the amplitudes fluctuate up and down during the recording, this indicates a technical problem secondary to movements or electrode artifacts [25–29].

During activation, the examiner should inform the patient that he/she should exert full effort in activating the muscle against his/her resistance (when applied). When the contraction noise tends to drop or reduce, the examiner should advise the patient to continue with the activation exercise. If the noise reduces or drops, the patient's muscle contraction should be improved to maintain contraction for at least 1 minute.

RNS should be performed at rest and also with regular intervals after activation as above. Greater ≥10% decrement in at least one muscle is required to confirm the diagnosis.

Examination of another muscle group can be considered depending upon the patient clinical presentation.

Pretest Instructions

- Patients should be off anticholinesterase treatment for at least 12–24 h if the condition allows.
- Let the patient rest for 15 min before the recording (important for follow up studies). In LEMS 20 min rest is required.
- The patient's tested limb must be warm, if not—warm them up appropriately. (cooling increases the safety factor at NMJ)
- Stimulus-related pain must be pre-discussed to help with anticipation and tolerance,, which should reduce the liklihood of suboptimal recordings/waveforms.

Recording Protocol

The standard recoding protocol is as follows (adopted from the textbook of Electromyography and Neuromuscular Disorders: Clinical-Electrophysiologic Correlations, second Edition by Preston, David C.; Shapiro, Barbara published by Butterworth-Heinemann, utilized with permission).

1. Keep the body temperature close to 35 degrees.
2. Immobilize the muscle as best as possible.
3. Recommended to do routine nerve conduction studies before to make sure nerves are sufficiently normal;

Table 10.1 Technical Aspects of Nerve Conduction Study with Repetitive Nerve Stimulation (RNS) For Myasthenia Gravis

Muscle	Nerve supply	Stimulation site	Ground placement	Electrode placement		Activation procedure
				Active	Reference	
Abductor Pollicis Brevis	Median nerve	At the wrist, between the tendons of palmaris longus and flexor carpi radialis at the level of second crease.	At forearm, nearerthe site of stimulation	At the belly of abductor pollicis brevis.	Tendon of abductor pollicis brevis.	Ask the subject to abduct the thumb and sustain abduction for 1 min and immediately give 8–10 stimuli at 3 Hz.
Deltoid muscle	Axillary nerve	Supramaximal stimulus over the upper plexus, Erb's point, proximal to the clavicular bone.	Shoulder	Deltoid muscle belly	Shoulder bone	Ask the subject to move his elbow in a lateral direction and the examiner resists against this movement for 1 min and immediately give 8–10 stimuli at 3 Hz.
Biceps	Musculocutaneous nerve	Supramaximal stimulus over the upper plexus, Erb's point, proximal to the clavicular bone.	Shoulder	Belly of biceps muscle	Biceps tendon	Ask the patient to flex the arm against resistance for 1 min and immediately give 8–10 stimuli at 3 Hz.
Abductor digiti minimi	Ulnar nerve	At the wrist, medial or lateral to the flexor carpi ulnaris tendon at the second crease with the hand resting and with the dorsal side facing upwards.	Extensor surface of the hand	Belly of abductor digiti minimi muscle	Distal phalanx of fifth digit	Ask the patient to spread his/her fingers maximally for 1 min and immediately give 8–10 stimuli at 3 Hz.
Orbicularis oculus	Facial nerve	Beneath the ear lobe at the grove of stylomastoid foramen	Forehead	Over the orbicularis oculus muscle.	Over the canthus	Ask the subject to do continuous closure of the eyes tightly for 1 min and immediately give 8–10 stimuli at 3 Hz.
Nasalis	Facial nerve	Beneath the ear lobe at the grove of stylomastoid foramen	Forehead	Over the nasalis muscle	Over the nasal bone or nasal bridge.	Ask the subject to shrink his nose for 1 min and immediately give 8–10 stimuli at 3 Hz
Trapezius	Accessory nerve	Behind the sternocleidomastoid muscle, at the midpoint of a line connecting the mastoid and the clavicle	Placed between the recording and stimulating electrode	Placed over the belly of trapezius muscle.	Placed over the clavicle or acromion process.	Ask the subject to lift the shoulder up for 1 min and immediately give 8–10 stimuli at 3 Hz

4. Perform RNS at rest. After making sure that the stimulus is supramaximal, perform 3 Hz RNS at rest for 5–10 impulses, repeated three times, 1 min apart. Normally, there is <10% decrement between the first and fourth responses.
5. If >10% decrement occurs and is consistently reproducible:
   - Have the patient perform maximal voluntary exercise for 10 seconds.
   - Immediately repeat 3 Hz RNS post exercise to demonstrate post exercise facilitation and repair of the decrement.
6. If <10% Decrement or no Decrement Occurs
   - Have the patient perform maximal voluntary exercise for 1 min, then perform 3 Hz RNS immediately and 1,2,3 and 4 min after exercise to demonstrate post exercise exhaustion.
   - If a significant decrement occurs, have the patient perform maximal voluntary exercise again for 10 seconds and immediately repeat 3 Hz RNS to demonstrate repair of the decrement.

Pitfalls and Limitations

Technical factors play a major role in the measuring accuracy of RNS, and they are broadly classified into false positive and false negative results.

The false negative results occur when there is no decrement observed when, in fact, under the appropriate conditions, it would be seen. Two major factors that can cause false negative report include low temperature and presence of acetylcholinesterase inhibitors.

Studies show that cold temperate slows down the activity of acetylcholinesterase in the synaptic cleft and results in an increase in the availability of acetylcholine and this would account for the difference (masking of the pathological NMJ transmission deficit). The presence of acetylcholinesterase inhibitors during the procedure may similarly obscure the underlying NMJ pathophysiology, but may be suspected as the confounding factor present when there is repetitive generation of motor potentials ("afterpotentials") after single stimulation shocks [27, 29].

False-positive result happens when an obvious decrement is found when there is none.

The factors that would cause false positive test include poor electrode placement, inadequate mobilization of the limb, and inappropriate stimulus delivery. Patient cooperation and discomfort tolerance are important technical parameters that affect the RNS outcome. Patients with severe disease may have difficulty in performing the activation procedure. Intubated patients (who often have mental status effects from critical illness comorbidity and/or medications) may also have poor cooperation, and artifacts from the ventilator and other intensive care unit electronics which can affect the RNS tests results [25, 27, 29].

Single Fiber Electromyography (SFEMG)

SFEMG is a selective recording of a small number of single muscle fiber action potentials belonging to the same motor unit [27, 30]. SFEMG technique is a confirmatory test for screening the NMJ disorders even when the RNS results are negative [31].

Further details regarding SFEMG are found in the dedicated chapter (Chap. 11) covering this topic.

Treatment of MG

Patients with mild symptoms due to MG often do well with symptomatic treatment alone [6]. Drugs, which causes the reduction of acetylcholine breakdown through the inhibition of enzyme acetylcholinesterase results in an increase of acetylcholine concentration in the synaptic cleft. Pyridostigmine is the most commonly used drug,.

Immunosuppressive Therapy

Immunosuppressive therapy is warranted in patients who do not achieve complete remission with symptomatic therapy alone. The commonly used immunosuppressive drugs include azathioprine, and mycophenolate mofetil (among other similar medications). These drugs often are combined with corticosteroids such as prednisone It is recommended to start with steroids to curb the initial clinical deterioration. Once the symptoms are stable along with the addition of immunosuppressive agents over the duration of time for their onset of action (typically over several months), the steroid needs to be reduced slowly to the lowest effective level [6, 8, 32, 33].

Myasthenic crises are considered a neuromuscular emergency and should be managed in the critical care unit setting (details beyond the scope of this textbook).

Lambert-Eaton Myasthenic Syndrome (LEMS)

Lambert-Eaton myasthenic syndrome (LEMS) is a neuromuscular disorder with core clinical features consistent with proximal muscle weakness, areflexia, and autonomic dysfunction [8, 34]. It may present either as a primary autoimmune disorder or could be due to a paraneoplastic etiology. This is most commonly seen in patients with small cell lung cancer. The weakness is putatively due to the generation of auto-antibody against the voltage-gated calcium channels in the presynaptic membrane which causes selective destruction and reduction of acetylcholine which in turn leads to subsequent weakness [8]. The diagnosis is based on clinical examination and is confirmed by serologic testing and electrodiagnostic studies.

Etiology

LEMS is classified based upon the presence or absence of malignancy. Patients without any evidence of malignancy are classified as Non-Tumor Lambert-Eaton Myasthenic Syndrome (NT-LEMS) [8, 35]. Approximately 60% of the patients with the LEMS have an association with malignancy. This is most commonly seen in patients with small cell lung carcinoma (SCLC) but may occur with other malignancies including non-small cell lung cancer, prostate cancer, thymoma and lymphoproliferative disorder [36–38]. History of smoking, male gender, and weight loss are found to have a strong association in patients with LEMS [39]. The clinical symptoms of LEMS precede approximately 5 years before the evidence of malignancy. Sixty-five percent of patient with NT-LEMS were found to have an association with HLA -B8-DR 3 genetic polymorphism [39].

Epidemiology

LEMS is a rare disorder with a predicted incidence of 0.5 out of 1,00,000 and a prevalence of 2.3 out of 1,00,000 patients. The prevalence of LEMS is 46 times less than that of myasthenia gravis which is suggestive of an overall poor outcome, especially when it is associated with malignancy [40, 41]. The median age at the onset of diagnosis in patients with malignancy was 60 years, and up to 75% of them are men. Interestingly in NT-LEMS patients, age and sex distribution are similar to patients with MG with a peak age of onset of 35 years and a second larger peak at 60 years [40, 42]. NT -LEMS is most commonly seen in young females with a genetic association of HLA-B8-DR3 polymorphism which is suggestive of autoimmune etiology [39].

Pathophysiology

The voltage-gated calcium channel (VGCC) is a transmembrane protein in the presynaptic membrane, and it has approximately 4–5 subunits with a central pore. As the cell membrane depolarizes, it causes an influx of calcium through the central pore resulting in the release of acetylcholine into the synapse [8]. The tumor cells express VGCC, an antigen which induces autoantibody production. The antibody-mediated immune response in patients with LEMS is thought to be due to the crosslinking and selective destruction of VGCC which is often associated with the antibodies against the P/Q subtype of VGCC and rarely in association with N-type antibody as well [41, 43].

Clinical Features

The clinical symptoms are usually gradual in onset, but it can also progress rapidly in patients with SCLC. The classic triad consists of proximal weakness, areflexia, and autonomic dysfunction. The weakness is generally symmetrical and usually begins in the proximal lower extremities, causing gait disturbances [8, 34–36]. Patients often present with complaints of difficulty in raising from a seated position, dull aching, and stiffness in the affected limbs. The symptoms usually progress from proximal to distal, caudal to cranial distribution and then it finally reaches the oculobulbar region [44]. Deep tendon reflexes are either diminished or absent with no significant muscle atrophy. Up to 95% of patient with LEMS are reported to have autonomic dysfunction. Most commonly reported symptoms includes dry mouth, constipation, erectile dysfunction in male, orthostatic hypotension, pupillary abnormalities and loss of sweating [44, 45]. Involvement of respiratory muscles, and cranial nerves is uncommon during initial stages but it can happen as the disease progresses. In those cases, ptosis and diplopia comprise the most common presentation, followed by dysarthria and dysphagia. [8, 34]

CASE

A 62-year-old Caucasian male with a history of hypertension and smoking presented with 3 months history of bilateral lower extremity weakness and fatigue. The weakness was associated with 5-pound weight loss. The patient denied any numbness, paresthesia, and/or change in bowel and bladder habits. There has been some excessive mouth dryness and reduction in sweating. Neurological examination was significant for 3 out 5 power (Medical Research Council scale) in bilateral lower extremities at rest and increased to 4+ out of 5 after 30 seconds contraction. Deep tendon reflexes were diminished (though somewhat improved after sustained contraction as well), and rest of the neurological examination was found to be unremarkable. Routine chest X ray showed 4.3 cm left upper lobe lung mass. CT chest confirmed the mass along with the presence of central necrosis. These findings were concerning for possible LEMS. On nerve conduction studies of his right ulnar nerve, a reduced compound muscle action potential (CMAP) of 2.5 mV (normal >5) was noted recording the abductor digiti minimi muscle. The response improved to 5 mV after sustained contraction of the muscle for 10 seconds. There was no conduction block across the elbow on other ulnar motor studies. Sensory nerve conduction responses were found to be normal as well. Slow repetitive nerve stimulation (at 2 Hz) of right ulnar nerve showed more than 20% decrement in the amplitude. Paraneoplastic antibodies testing revealed the presence of P/Q voltage-gated calcium channel antibodies. The diagnosis of paraneoplastic LEMS was confirmed. She underwent surgical resection of the lung lesion and is undergoing chemotherapy along with 3,4 DAP for symptomatic therapy (seeing improvement in muscle weakness on this).

Diagnostic Evaluation

The diagnosis of LEMS is confirmed by the presence of antibodies against the P/Q type voltage gated calcium channels (VGCC). Up to 90% of patients with LEMS are found to have high titers of these antibodies. Almost all the patients with SCLC are positive for this antibody and up to 90% of patients with NT-LEMS also have detectable levels of P/Q type VGCC antibodies. Patients with undetectable levels of antibodies probably have lower concentration of antibodies or could possess antibodies to different epitopes or other structural proteins. However, the presence of these antibodies is not only reported in LEMS but are also seen in other neurological/autoimmune conditions as well [43, 46].

The N-type VGCCs antibody is more commonly seen in patients with primary lung cancer, and the presence of this antibody may increase the possibility of having an underlying malignancy as well [46]. SCLC also express an immunogenic tumor antigen called SOX1and 64% of patients with LEMS are found to have antibodies against this antigen. Reports suggest that SOX1 may play a role in predicting future predisposition to LEMS/SCLC. Accordingly, the presence of SOX1 antibodies with no underlying evidence of malignancy should be followed up very closely [47, 48].

Electrophysiological Findings in LEMS

The classical electrophysiological finding in LEMS is a low amplitude CMAP at rest. This is due to the decreased acetylcholine in the presynaptic terminal and blocking in many of the neuromuscular junctions. A decremental response is observed at supramaximal slow rate stimulus and is due to the depletion of the available acetylcholine. After brief, sustained isometric contraction (of at least 10 seconds), the amplitude of CMAP tends to increase by 100% or more. The facilitation (CMAP amplitude increment) is due to the presynaptic calcium influx which ultimately increases the available acetylcholine. Apart from demonstrating the increment with this methodology, fast-rate RNS (15–50 Hz) may be employed. In LEMS patients undergoing fast-rate RNS, there are successive CMAP amplitude increases, with the first and fifth waveforms typically demonstrating an increase by 100% or more. The limitation with fast-rate RNS is that it is painful and the associated limb movement may interfere with a technically adequate CMAP capture. The RNS and short exercise testing findings in LEMS are shown in Fig. 10.5.

For RNS in LEMS cases, 2 Proximal muscles (e.g. orbicularis oculus, nasalis, trapezius) and 1 distal muscle (e.g. abductor pollicis brevis and abductor digiti minimi) are usually selected. The details of the procedure, limitations, and pitfalls have been discussed under the MG section of this chapter.

SFEMG in LEMS

- Increased Jitter and Blocking occurs
- Contrary to what is typically seen in MG, blocking tends to improve with the surface stimulation rates.

Treatment and Management

Treatment of patients with LEMS includes resecting the underlying tumor (to the extent possible) and symptomatic management. The aim of the symptomatic treatment is to improve the acetylcholine concentration in the synaptic cleft with drugs like pyridostigmine, neostigmine, guanidine and 4-aminopyridine, and 3,4-diaminopyridine (3,4-DAP) [49, 50]. Only 3,4-DAP is studied extensively in clinical trials, and all other drugs are reported from case series.

3,4-DAP blocks potassium channels, which in turn keeps calcium channels open for longer periods, ultimately allowing more acetylcholine to be released into the synaptic cleft.

In patients with rapidly progressive symptoms, intravenous immunoglobulin (IVIG) or plasmapheresis are found to be effective in both paraneoplastic LEMS and NT LEMS [51].

Long term oral immunosuppressive medications such as prednisone, azathioprine, and rituximab have also been tried with a variable degree of success in patients when the symptoms are not adequately controlled with symptomatic treatment alone [34].

Congenital Myasthenic Syndrome (CMS) (CMS)

Congenital myasthenic syndrome is a rare group of genetic conditions that are due to functionally abnormal proteins that affect NM transmission. This results in fluctuating or fatigable weakness. The onset of symptoms varies and are commonly seen at birth but may go unrecognized until adolescence or adulthood [52–54]. Congenital myasthenia gravis is classified based upon the location of the defect. Presynaptic defects accounts for approximately 7–8%, synaptic defect are

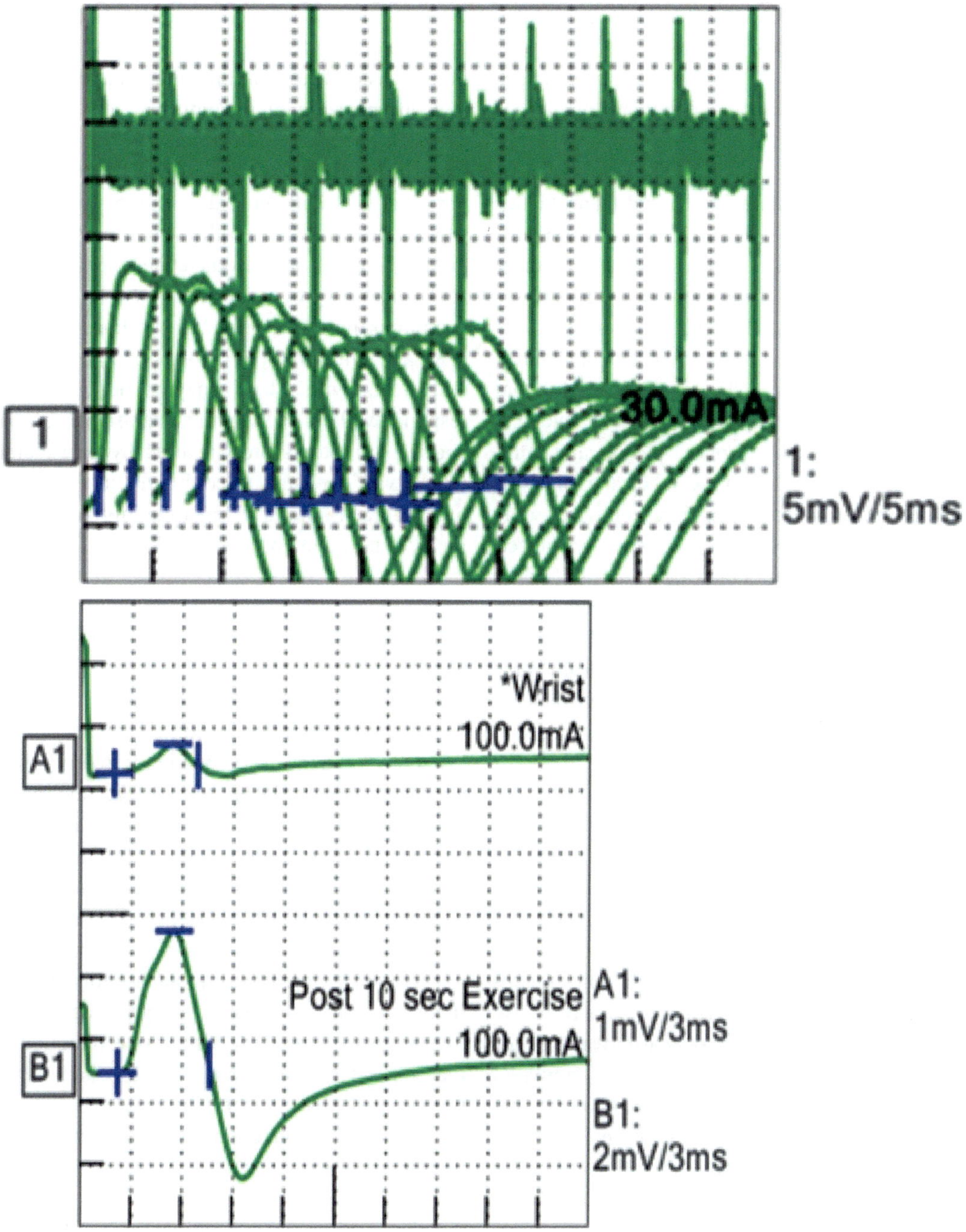

Fig. 10.5 Electrophysiological findings of RNS in a patient with LEMS

estimated at 14–15% and the remaining 75–80% are due to postsynaptic defects [52–56].

Clinical Features

Males are more commonly affected than females with an estimated ratio of 2:1. Almost all CMS subtypes follow an autosomal recessive pattern except for the slow channel syndrome which is an autosomal dominant disease. The classification and diagnosis of this syndrome is based on clinical features, response to acetyl cholinesterase inhibitors (AChEi) and electrophysiological study findings. Incomplete ophthalmoparesis, ptosis, and mild facial paresis are often seen during infancy. Ophthalmoparesis and facial paresis progress during childhood and infancy along with generalized weakness and fatigue. Often these are associated with other features such as high arched palate, facial dysmorphism, arthrogryposis, and scoliosis. Episodic respiratory crises can occur with any form of CMS but is most commonly seen in patients with acetylcholinesterase deficiency [54, 57, 58].

Diagnosis and Testing

The diagnosis is based on the presence of clinical symptoms suggestive of myasthenia gravis like fluctuating or fatigable weakness, absence of pertinent antibodies (against the acetylcholine receptor, MuSK, or LRP4), and a decremental response on RNS. [57] Genetic testing is also available for the diagnosis of the specific subtype.. Interestingly, roughly around 30–50% of patients with CMS do not carry the mutations that have been already described in the literature [52–54].

Specific Genetic Syndromes

Pre-Synaptic

Choline Acetyltransferase (ChAT) Deficiency

Choline acetyltransferase is an enzyme present in the presynaptic region which is responsible for the formation of acetylcholine. Mutations within the gene coding for this enzyme results in depletion of acetylcholine-containing vesicles. The clinical spectrum of patients with this enzyme deficiency varies significantly [59, 60]. Patients with severe disease often have severe apnea, bulbar weakness and may also require ventilation support at birth. While others may present with mild weakness and episodic apneic spells. There is also another group of patients who have milder symptoms but with proximal weakness and no respiratory involvement [59–62].

Patients with ChAT enzyme deficiency do respond well to acetylcholinesterase inhibitors, and the symptoms are triggered by or become worse with exposure to cold temperature which has not been similarly reported in other myasthenic syndromes [61].

Synaptic

Acetylcholinesterase Deficiency

Acetylcholinesterase is an enzyme present in the synaptic cleft and is responsible for hydrolysis of acetylcholine after its action. The enzyme serves as a rate limiting factor which controls the number of collisions between acetylcholine and its receptor, thereby determining the duration of the synaptic transmission [54]. This enzyme comprises catalytic subunits that bind to collagenic tails (COQL) which helps to anchor this enzyme in the synaptic cleft. The deficiency of acetylcholinesterase is caused by a recessive mutation in the gene COLQ resulting in the blockade of its binding in the basal layer. This leads to prolonged exposure of acetylcholine to the postsynaptic membrane [63, 64].

The clinical manifestations of this enzyme deficiency often present during early childhood and are rare during infancy. It is characterized by severe axial weakness, muscle atrophy and slow pupillary response to light stimulation. As the disease progresses skeletal deformities (e.g., lordosis or scoliosis), ptosis, ophthalmoplegia, dysphagia, and difficulty breathing are noted [52, 53]. NCS usually discloses repetitive CMAPs ("afterdischarges") in these patients.

Cholinesterase inhibitors such as pyridostigmine is contraindicated with COLQ deficiency. Ephedrine or albuterol seem to show improvement of symptoms via an unknown mechanism in some patients [62, 65].

Congenital Myasthenic Syndrome with Postsynaptic Defects

Anatomy of the Acetylcholine Receptor

The nicotinic acetylcholine (AChR) is a pentamer that exists in two different forms—fetal and adult form. The fetal form ($\alpha 2$ β δ γ) consists of two alpha subunits ($\alpha 2$), one beta subunit (β), one delta subunit (δ) and one gamma submit (γ) whereas in adult form ($\alpha 2$ β δ €) gamma (γ) is replaced with an epsilon (€) subunit [66].

Acetylcholine Receptor Deficiency

Patients with this deficiency are noted to have a relative reduction in the expression of acetylcholine receptors in the postsynaptic membrane. Often this follows an autosomal recessive inheritance pattern due to a mutation in the CHRNE gene. The mutation most commonly is seen is in € subunit, however, patients continue to have an expression of fetal form of the receptor which compensates for the deficiency [59].Patients with mutation of other subunits generally have more severe clinical manifestations. The clinical symptoms usually begin in childhood, adolescence or adulthood. The common clinical presentations include hypotonia, ptosis, ophthalmoplegia, weakness, skeletal deformities (e.g., arthrogryposis, lordosis, or scoliosis), muscular atrophy, dysphagia, and respiratory difficulty [67]. The diagnosis is confirmed by 2–3 Hz RNS, which shows decremental response and molecular analysis of acetylcholine receptor [57]. They often respond to treatments that increase acetylcholine receptor activation including AChE inhibitors (e.g., pyridostigmine) and 3,4-Diaminopyridine (3,4-DAP) [68].

Primary Kinetic Abnormalities of the Acetylcholine Receptor

The clinical characteristics, physiology, and pathophysiology in patients with a kinetic abnormality is summarized in the flowchart (Fig. 10.6) below.

Electrophysiologically, patients with slow channel syndrome have a decremental response to slow-rate RNS(2–3 Hz). They tend to exhibit a smaller amplitude and substantial decrement on the second peak compared to previous compound muscle action potential. NCS also often discloses repetitive CMAPs ("afterdischarges") in these patients. Needle electromyography often shows a myopathic pattern which is most likely secondary to an increase in the intracellular calcium due to prolonged opening time which eventually leads to "endplate myopathy" as the disease progresses [57]. Similarly, patients with fast channel syndrome often have a decremental response with 2–3 Hz stimulation [57]. Acetlycholinesterase inhibitors need to be avoided in the patients with slow channel syndrome because they cause a prolonged exposure of acetylcholine in the postsynaptic muscle membrane which can lead to accelerated endplate myopathy. Quinidine and fluoxetine are among agents found to be effective in patients with slow channel syndrome as they appear to block the opening of the acetylcholine receptor [69]. Medications that increase opening time of the acetylcholine receptor such as AChE inhibitors (e.g. pyridostigmine) and 3,4-DAP are found to be effective in patients with fast channel syndrome [54, 57, 70].

Defects of the Acetylcholine Receptor Complex

The acetylcholine receptor in the postsynaptic membrane is organized and clustered with the help of other structural proteins such as rapsyn, Dok-7, and MuSK. The pathophysiology of some CMS subtypes is related to reduced expression or functionality in the acetylcholine receptor secondary to an alternation in these related structural proteins.

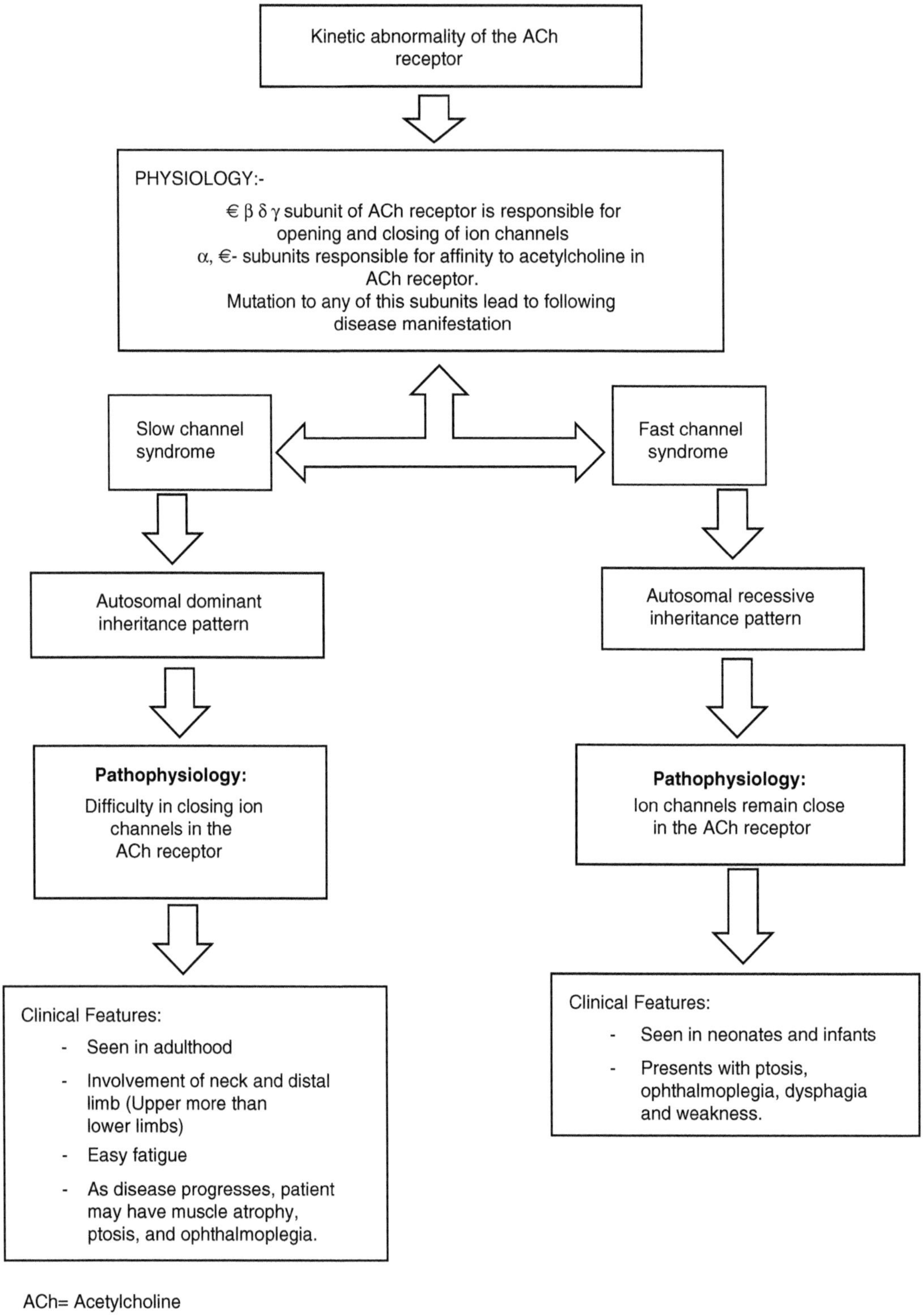

Fig. 10.6 Pathophysiology and clinical features in patients with kinetic abnormality of the Acetylcholine receptor

DOK-7 Deficiency

Patients with DOK-7 deficiency are noted to have weakness that predominately affects the proximal muscles compared to distal muscle groups. They are also regarded as limb-girdle myasthenic syndromes for this reason [71]. Slow-rate (2–3 Hz) RNS results in a decremental response [57]. This subgroup often does not respond to drugs that would increase acetylcholine concentration in the synaptic cleft, but they tend to respond to alpha adrenergic agonists such as ephedrine or albuterol [71, 72].

Rapsyn Deficiency

The mutation of Rapsyn protein leads to a deficiency in the acetylcholine receptor channels. Most often the clinical symptoms are associated with arthrogryposis and are typically neonatal in onset [73]. RNS typically shows a decremental response pattern at slow-ratestimulation (2–3 Hz) [57]. This subgroup of patients benefits from a combination of acetylcholinesterase inhibitors (e.g. pyridostigmine), 3,4-Diaminopyridine and alpha adrenergic agonists such as ephedrine or albuterol [71–73].

Voltage-Gated Sodium Channel-SCN4A Deficiency

This is a rare form of congenital myasthenic syndrome associated with mutation of the SCN4A gene. This gene encodes for voltage gated sodium channel in the muscle membrane. Patients with this mutation present with episodic weakness which involves axial, limb and respiratory muscles [74]. Treatment involves the combination of acetylcholinesterase inhibitors and acetazolamide [54, 55].

Other Rare Congenital Myasthenic Syndrome

Agrin Deficiency

Agrin is secreted from the presynaptic membrane and is responsible for the clustering and organization of acetylcholine receptors in the postsynaptic membrane. Mutation of this gene results in the production of abnormal agrin which causes a failure of neuromuscular transmission. The clinical features include ophthalmoplegia, ptosis, and proximal muscle weakness [75]. Slow-rate RNS recordings typically demonstrate a decremental response and post-exercise increment is commonly observed in the distal limb muscles. Confirmation is based on muscle biopsy and AGRN gene mutation [57]. Albuterol is usually beneficial in patients with this mutation [54].

Other Gene Defects Associated with Congenital Myasthenic Syndrome

The centronuclear myopathies are a rare group of muscle disorders due to mutations including those in the BIN1, MTM1, and DNM2 genes [76–78]. These are reported to be associated with congenital myasthenic syndrome as well. Electrophysiological features are also usually consistent with impaired neuromuscular transmission manifested by decrement as in the other subtypes aforementioned, and some of these patients are reported to have some response to pyridostigmine [78].

References

1. Lang B, Vincent A. Autoimmune disorders of the neuromuscular junction. Curr Opin Pharmacol. 2009 Jun;9(3):336–40.
2. Nishimune H, Shigemoto K. Practical Anatomy of the Neuromuscular Junction in Health and Disease. Neurol Clin. 2018 May;36(2):231–40.
3. Ganong WF. Review of medical physiology. 23rd ed. New York: McGraw-Hill Medical; 2010.
4. Guyton AC. Textbook of medical physiology. 11th ed. Philadelphia: Elsevier Saunders; 2006.
5. Khurana I Textbook of medical physiology. Elsevier, India; 2015.
6. Gilhus NE, Verschuuren JJ. Myasthenia gravis: subgroup classification andtherapeutic strategies. Lancet Neurol. 2015 Oct;14(10):1023–36.
7. Pakzad Z, Aziz T, Oger J. Increasing incidence of myasthenia gravis amongelderly in British Columbia. Canada Neurol. 2011 Apr 26;76(17):1526–8.
8. Nicolle MW. Myasthenia gravis and lambert-eaton myasthenic syndrome. Continuum (Minneap Minn). 2016 Dec;22 (6, Muscle and Neuromuscular Junction Disorders):1978–2005. Review.
9. Renton AE, Pliner HA, Provenzano C, Evoli A, Ricciardi R, Nalls MA, et al. A genome-

wideassociation study of myasthenia gravis. JAMA Neurol. 2015 Apr;72(4):396–404.
10. Meriggioli MN, Sanders DB. Autoimmune myasthenia gravis: emerging clinical and biological heterogeneity. Lancet Neurol. 2009;8:475–99.
11. Querol L, Illa I. Myasthenia and the neuromuscular junction. Curr Opin Neurol. 2013;26:459–65.
12. Skeie GO, Apostolski S, Evoli A, et al. Guidelines for treatment of autoimmune neuromuscular transmission disorders. Eur J Neurol. 2010;17:893–902.
13. Rodolico C, Toscano A, Autunno M, et al. Limb-girdle myasthenia; clinical, electrophysiological and morphological features in familial and autoimmune cases. Neuromuscul Disord. 2002;12:964–9.
14. Zhang B, Tzartos JS, Viegas S, et al. Autoantibodies to lipoprotein-related protein 4 in patients with double-negative myasthenia gravis. Arch Neurol. 2012;69:445–51.
15. Leite MI, Jacob S, Viegas S, et al. IgG1 antibodies to acetylcholine receptors in "seronegative" myasthenia gravis. Brain. 2008;131:1940–52.
16. Jacob S, Viega S, Leite MI. Presence and pathogenic relevance of antibodies to clustered acetylcholine receptor in ocular and generalized myasthenia gravis. Arch Neurol. 2012;69:994–1001.
17. Gasperi C, Melms A, Schoser B, et al. Anti-agrin autoantibodies in myasthenia gravis. Neurology. 2014;82:1976–83.
18. Gallardo E, Martinez-Hernandez E, Titulaer MJ, et al. Cortactin autoantibodies in myasthenia gravis. Autoimmun Rev. 2014;13:1003–7.
19. Kerty E, Elsais A, Argov Z, Evoli A, Gilhus NE. EFNS/ENS guidelines for the treatment of ocular myasthenia gravis. Eur J Neurol. 2014;21:687–93.
20. Chatzistefanou KI, Kouris T, Iliakis E, Piaditis G, Tagaris G, Katsikeris N, Kaltsas G, Apostolopoulos M. The ice pack test in the differential diagnosis ofmyasthenic diplopia. Ophthalmology. 2009 Nov;116(11):2236–43.
21. Oh SJ, Cho HK. Edrophonium responsiveness not necessarily diagnostic of myasthenia gravis. Muscle Nerve. 1990 Mar;13(3):187–91.
22. Pasnoor M, Dimachkie M, Farmakidis's C, Barohn R. Diagnosis of myasthenia gravis. Neurol Clin. 2018;36(2):261–74.
23. Albuquerque EX, Rash JE, Mayer RF, Satterfield JR. An electrophysiological andmorphological study of the neuromuscular junction in patients with myastheniagravis. Exp Neurol. 1976 Jun;51(3):536–63.
24. Albuquerque EX, Warnick JE, Mayer RF, Eldefrawi AT, Eldefrawi ME. Recentadvances in the molecular mechanisms of human and animal models of myastheniagravis. Ann N Y Acad Sci. 1981;377:496–518.
25. Preston DC, Shapiro BE. Electromyography and neuromuscular disorders e-book: clinical-electrophysiologic correlations (expert consult-online). Elsevier Health Sciences; 2012 Nov 1.
26. AAEM Quality Assurance Committee. American Association of Electrodiagnostic Medicine. Practice parameter for repetitive nerve stimulation and single fiber EMG evaluation of adults with suspected myasthenia gravis or Lambert-Eaton myasthenic syndrome: summary statement. Muscle Nerve. 2001 Sep;24(9):1236–8.
27. Litchy WJ, Albers JW Repetitive stimulation an AANEM workshop. https://www.aanem.org/mxonline/resources/downloads/products/REPS.pdf Used on 07/25/2018
28. Costa J, Evangelista T, Conceição I, de Carvalho M. Repetitive nerve stimulation in myasthenia gravis--relative sensitivity of different muscles. ClinNeurophysiol. 2004 Dec;115(12):2776–82.
29. Chiou-Tan FY. Electromyographic approach to neuromuscular junction disordersrepetitive nerve stimulation and single-fiber electromyography. Phys Med Rehabil Clin N Am. 2003 May;14(2):387–401. Review
30. Sarrigiannis PG, Kennett RP, Read S, Farrugia ME. Single-fiber EMG with aconcentric needle electrode: validation in myasthenia gravis. Muscle Nerve. 2006 Jan;33(1):61–5.
31. Srivastava A, Kalita J, Misra UK. A comparative study of single fiberelectromyography and repetitive nerve stimulation in consecutive patients withmyasthenia gravis. Electromyogr Clin Neurophysiol. 2007 Mar-Apr;47(2):93–6.
32. Gilhus NE. Myasthenia gravis. N Engl J Med. 2016 Dec 29;375(26):2570–81.
33. Kim JY, Park KD, Richman DP. Treatment of myasthenia gravis based on its immunopathogenesis. J Clin Neurol. 2011 Dec 1;7(4):173–83.
34. Kesner VG, Oh SJ, Dimachkie MM, Barohn RJ. Lambert-eaton myasthenic syndrome. Neurol Clin. 2018 May 31;36(2):379–94.
35. Tarr TB, Wipf P, Meriney SD. Synaptic pathophysiology and treatment of Lambert-Eaton myasthenic syndrome. Mol Neurobiol. 2015 Aug 1;52(1):456–63.
36. Nicole S, Azuma Y, Bauché S, Eymard B, Lochmüller H, Slater C. Congenital Myasthenic syndromes or inherited disorders of neuromuscular transmission: recent discoveries and open questions. J Neuromuscul Dis. 2017;(Preprint):1–6.
37. Titulaer MJ, Verschuuren JJ. Lambert–Eaton myasthenic syndrome. Ann N Y Acad Sci. 2008 Jun 1;1132(1):129–34.
38. O'Neill JH, Murray NM, Newsom-Davis J. The Lambert-Eaton myasthenic syndrome. A review of 50 cases. Brain. 1988 Jun;111(Pt 3):577–96.
39. Wirtz PW, Willcox N, van der Slik AR, Lang B, Maddison P, Koeleman BP, Giphart MJ, Wintzen AR, Roep BO, Verschuuren JJ. HLA and smoking in prediction and prognosis of small cell lung cancer in autoimmune Lambert-Eaton myasthenic syndrome. J Neuroimmunol. 2005 Feb;159(1–2):230–7.
40. Wirtz PW, Smallegange TM, Wintzen AR, Verschuuren JJ. Differences in clinical features between the Lambert-Eaton myasthenic syndrome with and without cancer: an analysis of 227 published cases. Clin Neurol Neurosurg. 2002 Sep;104(4):359–63.

41. Payne M, Bradbury P, Lang B, Vincent A, Han C, Newsom-Davis J, Talbot D. Prospective study into the incidence of Lambert Eaton myasthenic syndrome in small cell lung cancer. J Thorac Oncol. 2010 Jan 1;5(1):34–8.
42. Titulaer MJ, Maddison P, Sont JK, et al. Clinical dutch-english lambert-eaton myasthenic syndrome (LEMS) tumor association prediction score accurately predicts small-cell lung cancer in the LEMS. J Clin Oncol. 2011 Mar 1;29(7):902–8.
43. Lennon VA, Kryzer TJ, Griesmann GE, O'Suilleabhain PE, Windebank AJ, Woppmann A, Miljanich GP, Lambert EH. Calcium-channel antibodies in the Lambert-Eatonsyndrome and other paraneoplastic syndromes. N Engl J Med. 1995;332(22):1467–74.
44. Titulaer MJ, Lang B, Verschuuren JJ. Lambert-Eaton myasthenic syndrome: fromclinical characteristics to therapeutic strategies. Lancet Neurol. 2011 Dec;10(12):1098–107.
45. Titulaer MJ, Lang B, Verschuuren JJ. Lambert-Eaton myasthenic syndrome: fromclinical characteristics to therapeutic strategies. Lancet Neurol. 2011 Dec;10(12):1098–107.
46. Oh SJ, Kurokawa K, Claussen GC, Ryan HF Jr. Electrophysiological diagnosticcriteria of Lambert-Eaton myasthenic syndrome. Muscle Nerve. 2005 Oct;32(4):515–20.
47. Motomura M, Lang B, Johnston I, Palace J, Vincent A, Newsom-Davis J. Incidence of serum anti-P/O--type and anti-N-type calcium channel autoantibodies in theLambert-Eaton myasthenic syndrome. J Neurol Sci. 1997 Mar 20;147(1):35–42.
48. Sabater L, Titulaer M, Saiz A, Verschuuren J, Güre AO, Graus F. SOX1 antibodies are markers of paraneoplastic Lambert-Eaton myasthenic syndrome. Neurology. 2008 Mar 18;70(12):924–8.
49. Tim RW, Massey JM, Sanders DB. Lambert-Eaton myasthenic syndrome: electrodiagnostic findings and response to treatment. Neurology. 2000 Jun 13;54(11):2176–8.
50. Oh SJ, Kim DS, Head TC, Claussen GC. Low-dose guanidine and pyridostigmine: relatively safe and effective long-term symptomatic therapy in Lambert-Eaton myasthenic syndrome. Muscle Nerve. 1997 Sep;20(9):1146–52.
51. Bain PG, Motomura M, Newsom-Davis J, Misbah SA, et al. Effects of intravenous immunoglobulin on muscle weakness andcalcium-channel autoantibodies in the Lambert-Eaton myasthenic syndrome. Neurology. 1996 Sep;47(3):678–83.
52. Beeson D, Hantai D, Lochmuller H, Engel AG. 126th international workshop: congenital myasthenic syndromes, 24–26 September 2004, Naarden, The Netherlands. Neuromuscul Disord. 2005;15:498–512.
53. Kinali M, Beeson D, Pitt MC, et al. Congenitalmyasthenic syndromesin childhood: Diagnostic and management challenges. J Neuroimmunol. 2008;201:6e12.
54. Beeson D, Webster R, Cossins J, et al. Congenital myasthenic syndromes and the formation of the neuromuscular junction. Ann N Y Acad Sci. 2008;1132:99e103.
55. Engel AG. The therapy of congenital myasthenic syndromes. Neurotherapeutics. 2007 Apr 1;4(2):252–7.
56. Barišić N, Chaouch A, Müller JS, Lochmüller H. Genetic heterogeneity and pathophysiological mechanisms in congenital myasthenic syndromes. Eur J Paediatr Neurol. 2011 May 1;15(3):189–96.
57. Shieh PB, Oh SJ. Congenital Myasthenic Syndromes. Neurol Clin. 2018 May 31;36(2):367–78.
58. Lorenzoni PJ, Scola RH, Kay CS, Werneck LC. Congenital myasthenic syndrome: a brief review. Pediatr Neurol. 2012 Mar 1;46(3):141–8.
59. Ohno K, Tsujino A, Brengman JM, Harper CM, Bajzer Z, Udd B, Beyring R, Robb S, Kirkham FJ, Engel AG. Choline acetyltransferase mutations cause myasthenic syndrome associated with episodic apnea in humans. Proc Natl Acad Sci. 2001 Feb 13;98(4):2017–22.
60. Byring RF, Pihko H, Tsujino A, Shen XM, Gustafsson B, Hackman P, Ohno K, Engel AG, Udd B. Congenital myasthenic syndrome associated with episodic apnea and sudden infant death. Neuromuscul Disord. 2002 Aug 1;12(6):548–53.
61. Maselli RA, Chen D, Mo D, Bowe C, Fenton G, Wollmann RL. Choline acetyltransferase mutations in myasthenic syndrome due to deficient acetylcholine resynthesis. Muscle Nerve: Official Journal of the American Association of Electrodiagnostic Medicine. 2003 Feb;27(2):180–7.
62. Schara U, Christen HJ, Durmus H, Hietala M, Krabetz K, Rodolico C, Schreiber G, Topaloglu H, Talim B, Voss W, Pihko H. Long-term follow-up in patients with congenital myasthenic syndrome due to CHAT mutations. Eur J Paediatr Neurol. 2010 Jul 1;14(4):326–33.
63. Donger C, Krejci E, Serradell AP, Eymard B, et al. Mutation in the humanacetylcholinesterase-associated collagen gene, COLQ, is responsible forcongenital myasthenic syndrome with end-plate acetylcholinesterase deficiency(Type Ic). Am J Hum Genet. 1998 Oct;63(4):967–75.
64. Aldunate R, Casar JC, Brandan E, Inestrosa NC. Structural and functional organization of synaptic acetylcholinesterase. Brain Res Rev. 2004 Dec 1;47(1–3):96–104.
65. Bestue-Cardiel M, de Cabezón-Alvarez AS, Capablo-Liesa JL, López-Pisón J, Peña-Segura JL, Martin-Martinez J, Engel AG. Congenital endplate acetylcholinesterase deficiency responsive to ephedrine. Neurology. 2005 Jul 12;65(1):144–6.
66. Unwin N. Structure and action of the nicotinic acetylcholine receptor explored by electron microscopy. FEBS Lett. 2003 Nov 27;555(1):91–5.
67. Palace J, Beeson D. The congenital myasthenic syndromes. J Neuroimmunol. 2008 Sep 15;201–202:2–5.
68. Liewluck T, Selcen D, Engel AG. Beneficial effects of albuterol in congenital endplate acetylcholinesterase deficiency and Dok-7 myasthenia. Muscle Nerve. 2011 Nov;44(5):789–94.

69. Harper CM, Engel AG. Quinidine sulfate therapy for the slow-channel congenitalmyasthenic syndrome. Ann Neurol. 1998 Apr;43(4):480–4.
70. Engel AG, Shen XM, Selcen D, Sine SM. What have we learned from the congenital myasthenic syndromes. J Mol Neurosci. 2010 Jan;40(1–2): 143–53.
71. Selcen D, Milone M, Shen XM, Harper CM, Stans AA, Wieben ED, Engel AG. Dok-7 myasthenia: phenotypic and molecular genetic studies in 16 patients. Ann Neurol: Official Journal of the American Neurological Association and the Child Neurology Society. 2008 Jul;64(1):71–87.
72. Schara U, Barisic N, Deschauer M, Lindberg C, Straub V, Strigl-Pill N, Wendt M, Abicht A, Müller JS, Lochmüller H. Ephedrine therapy in eight patients with congenital myasthenic syndrome due to DOK7 mutations. Neuromuscul Disord. 2009 Dec 1;19(12):828–32.
73. Ohno K, Engel AG, Shen XM, Selcen D, Brengman J, Harper CM, Tsujino A, Milone M. Rapsyn mutations in humans cause endplate acetylcholine-receptor deficiency and myasthenic syndrome. Am J Hum Genet. 2002 Apr 1;70(4):875–85.
74. Habbout K, Poulin H, Rivier F, Giuliano S, Sternberg D, Fontaine B, Eymard B, Morales RJ, Echenne B, King L, Hanna MG. A recessive Nav1. 4 mutation underlies congenital myasthenic syndrome with periodic paralysis. Neurology. 2016 Jan 12;86(2):161–9.
75. Huzé C, Bauché S, Richard P, Chevessier F, Goillot E, Gaudon K, Ammar AB, Chaboud A, Grosjean I, Lecuyer HA, Bernard V. Identification of an agrin mutation that causes congenital myasthenia and affects synapse function. Am J Hum Genet. 2009 Aug 14;85(2):155–67.
76. Gibbs EM, Clarke NF, Rose K, Oates EC, Webster R, Feldman EL, Dowling JJ. Neuromuscular junction abnormalities in DNM2-related centronuclear myopathy. J Mol Med. 2013 Jun 1;91(6):727–37.
77. Claeys KG, Maisonobe T, Böhm J, Laporte J, Hezode M, Romero NB, Brochier G, Bitoun M, Carlier RY, Stojkovic T. Phenotype of a patient with recessive centronuclear myopathy and a novel BIN1 mutation. Neurology. 2010 Feb 9;74(6):519–21.
78. Robb SA, Sewry CA, Dowling JJ, Feng L, Cullup T, Lillis S, Abbs S, Lees MM, Laporte J, Manzur AY, Knight RK. Impaired neuromuscular transmission and response to acetylcholinesterase inhibitors in centronuclear myopathies. Neuromuscul Disord. 2011 Jun 1;21(6):379–86.

Suggested Reading

Selvan VA. Single-fiber EMG: a review. Ann Indian Acad Neurol. 2011 Jan;14(1):64.
Liveson JA, Ma DM. Laboratory reference for clinical neurophysiology. Oxford: Oxford University Press; 1992.
Jabre JF, Chirico-Post J, Weiner M. Stimulation SFEMG in myasthenia gravis. Muscle Nerve: Official Journal of the American Association of Electrodiagnostic Medicine. 1989 Jan;12(1):38–42.
Sanders DB. Clinical impact of single-fiber electromyography. Muscle Nerve. 2002;Suppl 11:S15–20.
Bromberg MB, Scott DM. Single fiber EMG reference values: reformatted in tabular form. AD HOC Committee of the AAEM Single Fiber Special Interest Group. Muscle Nerve. 1994;17(7):820–1.
Howard JF Jr. Electrodiagnosis of disorders of neuromuscular transmission. Phys Med Rehabil Clin N Am. 2013 Feb;24(1):169–92.
Titulaer MJ, Klooster R, Potman M, et al. SOX antibodies in small-cell lung cancer and Lambert-Eaton myasthenic syndrome: frequency and relation with survival. J Clin Oncol. 2009 Sep 10;27(26):4260–7.
Molgó J, Lundh H, Thesleff S. Potency of 3,4-diaminopyridine and4-aminopyridine on mammalian neuromuscular transmission and the effect of pHchanges. Eur J Pharmacol. 1980 Jan 11;61(1):25–34.

Single Fiber EMG

11

Alexandra Soriano

Single Fiber Electromyography

The technique of single fiber EMG (SFEMG) is mainly used to help with the diagnosis of myasthenia gravis when there is high clinical suspicion and other tests, including acetylcholine receptor, muscle specific tyrosine kinase (MuSK) antibodies and EMG with repetitive nerve stimulation have been negative.

This electrodiagnostic technique was developed in the 1960s by Erik Stalbërg and Jan Ekstedt with the purpose of obtaining action potentials from a single muscle fiber [1]. For optimal results with the single fiber EMG technique, a special concentric needle electrode with a small recording surface of 25 microns in diameter located 3 mm from the tip is used, so that it can selectively capture these action potentials from individual muscle fibers (see Figs. 11.1 and 11.2). The use of a high pass filter of 500 Hz when recording the action potentials further helps with the selectivity [3].

Acceptable action potentials are those with an amplitude of 200 microvolts or more.

More recently, monopolar and concentric needles have also been used to perform SFEMG, and reliable results can be obtained if the technique is done correctly by an experienced electromyographer. These needles have a lower cost and are disposable, eliminating the need to sterilize the needle electrode or to maintain the needle. It is recommended to increase the high pass filter to ~1000 Hz for better results. To the extent possible, a needle electrode with the smallest electrode surface should be used (e.g. 0.019 mm^2).

The single fiber EMG results can be obtained by using one of two techniques:

1. *Stimulation* SFEMG, in where individual motor fibers or motor axons can be activated using an intramuscular axonal stimulator in the form of a monopolar needle electrode positioned near the motor end-plate zone [1], which serves as the cathode, and a small surface electrode which serves as the anode.
2. *Voluntary activation* SFEMG, in which the patient voluntarily activates the muscle to be studied.

In either technique, the goal is to measure two parameters, the neuromuscular jitter and the presence of neuromuscular blocking.

A. Soriano (✉)
Braathen Neurological Center, Cleveland Clinic Florida, Weston, FL, USA

Cleveland Clinic Lerner College of Medicine of Case Western Reserve University, Cleveland, OH, USA
e-mail: soriana@ccf.org

Voluntary Activity SFEMG

As the patient does minimal contraction of the muscle to be examined, the SFEMG electrode is inserted into the muscle, preferably in the middle third of its length. The electrode is then placed in a

N. Galvez-Jimenez et al. (eds.), *Electrodiagnostic Medicine*,
https://doi.org/10.1007/978-3-030-74997-2_11

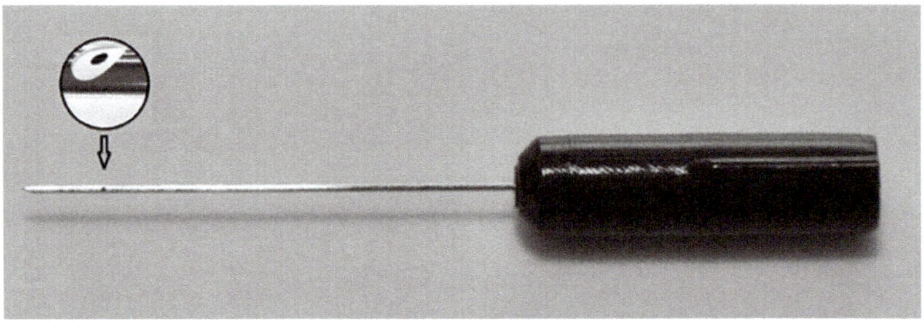

Fig. 11.1 Picture of a concentric single fiber electromyography (SFEMG) needle. Note the small recording surface (see inset) located 3 mm from the tip

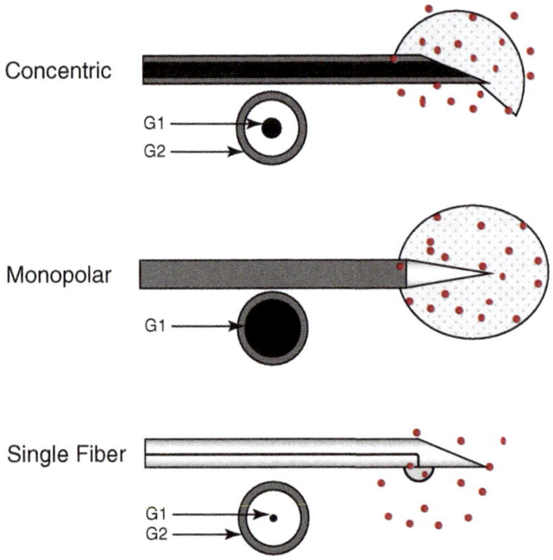

Fig. 11.2 Illustration showing the relatively small recording area (shaded) of the concentric single fiber electromyography (SFEMG) needle, compared to regular concentric and monopolar needle electrodes. G1, active recording site; G2, reference site. [Used with permission from [2]]

position where two (or at times more than two) time-locked action potentials from the same motor unit appear. Neuromuscular jitter is then recorded. The best recording is usually obtained from the superficial layer of the muscle and with minimal muscle contraction (firing frequency of the motor unit between 8 and 15 discharges per second) [4].

The most used muscles for SFEMG include the orbicularis oculi, extensor digitorum communis and frontalis muscle.

The voluntary activation SFEMG technique requires more patient cooperation but is subject to less technical errors or misinterpretations.

With the needle in position, the neuromuscular jitter is obtained, which is described as the minimal variability in latencies that exist between the appearance of one action potential and a second one from a single motor unit (Fig. 11.3). One action potential triggers the display sweep, and the second (paired) action potential appears with slightly variable position for each discharge [4]. This variability exists due to the changes in the transmission time across the synaptic gap, or the time it takes for end-plate potentials at the neuromuscular junction to reach the action potentials threshold [1]. Once the SFEMG electrode is in position where these action potentials are present, with adequate amplitude, then a minimum of 50 discharges need to be recorded. This technique is repeated several times, until a total of 20 action potential pairs, from different areas of the muscle, can be obtained. This may require a total of 3–4 skin insertions (aiming to minimize the number of these).

The jitter is then expressed as the mean value of consecutive differences (MCD) of successive interpotential intervals (IPIs), represented in Fig. 11.4 below.

Many of the modern electromyography machines have the capability of calculating the MCD directly, though it is always advisable that the operator visually analyzes the signals that are being acquired to asses for poor triggering or disturbing activity from other motor units and quality of the signal.

When obtaining jitter measurement and action potentials, errors can occur if the electrode is moved in relation to the fiber and the amplitude of the action potential decreases, affecting the calculated jitter.

Normal Jitters Findings and Values with Voluntary Activation

The measurement of jitter varies from muscle to muscle and with age. As age increases, so does

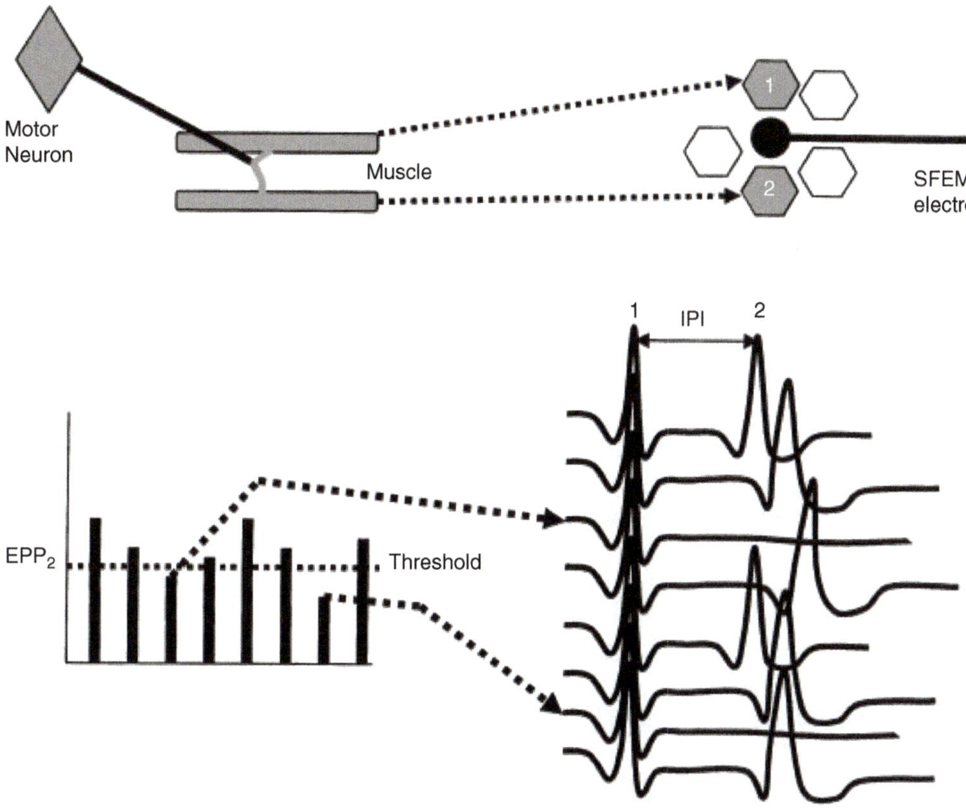

Fig. 11.3 Method of single fiber electromyography (SFEMG) with voluntary activation. The SFEMG needle is inserted into voluntarily activated muscle and is positioned so that recordings are obtained from two or more single muscle fibers belonging to the same motor unit. One single muscle fiber action potential serves as a time reference and the interpotential interval (IPI) is measured after consecutive discharges between the reference potential and subsequent time-locked potentials. In disorders of the neuromuscular junction, there may be marked variability of the IPI (abnormal jitter). If severe, neuromuscular transmission failure may occur in which the EPP amplitude fails to reach the threshold for action potential generation. This is demonstrated here by the absence of the second recorded fiber pair when the EPP in the second muscle fiber (EPP2) is subthreshold (dotted lines and arrows). [Used with permission from [5]]

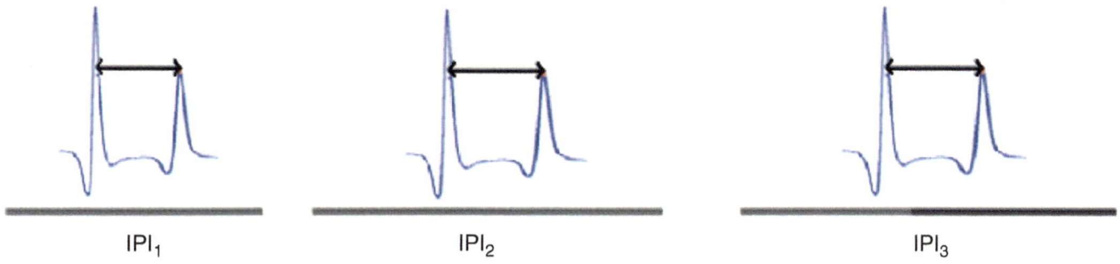

$$MCD = \frac{[IPI_1 - IP1_2] + [IPI_2 - IPI_3] + \ldots [IPI_{n-1} - IPI_n]}{n-1}$$

IPI= interpotential interval
MCD=mean value of consecutive differences

Fig. 11.4 Representation of interpotential interval (IPI) and calculation of mean value of consecutive differences (MCD) in the determination of jitter

jitter in normal subjects. Normal jitter values range from 5 to 65 microseconds, and is different to each muscle. There exist predetermined reference jitter values for the most common muscles studied with the SFEMG technique.

The value of the interpotential interval (IPI) is important and it is recommended that this stays below 4 milliseconds, as erroneous high jitter values can be obtained from recordings with long IPI [1].

The results of jitter measurements in each muscle is presented as the mean or median value of the MCD values in all the pairs or endplates measured; the percentage of paired potentials in which blocking was present (given as percentage of blocking); and the percentage of pairs in which jitter exceeds the limit of normal for that particular muscle [3].

For a study to be considered abnormal the following must be present:

1. The mean (or median) jitter exceeds the upper limit of normal for the muscle; or
2. More than 10% of pairs have increased jitter (including blocking).

In general, when blocking is present jitter values should already be abnormally increased. In MG gravis for example, blocking occurs during voluntary activation once jitter values exceed 80–100 μs.

A jitter value of 5 μS or less can be seen in some cases of myopathies and rarely with voluntary activation in normal muscle, this probably representing recording from split muscle fibers activated by a single NMJ. These values should not be counted for assessment of the neuromuscular transmission [3].

It is best to calculate mean MCD from individual muscles with data of jitter values less than 150 μs, as this can significantly increase mean jitter value, even if all other endplate potentials of this muscle show normal jitter values. Increase jitter, with or without blocking, can occasionally occur in one of 20 pairs in normal muscle [4].

Overall for reliable results, SFEMG must be performed by an electromyographer knowledgeable in the technique of data collection and analysis. Most patients cooperate well with this study and report relatively little discomfort. The SFEMG needle must be in good condition, with a sharp tip that prevents more than minimal muscle fiber damage.

Conditions that could limit SFEMG study include patients with limb tremor, in which the use of a facial muscle is generally preferred. Another challenging patient subgroup includes sedated patients, uncooperative patients or children under 8 or infants, in which the use *stimulated* SFEMG is then preferred. A decrease in intramuscular temperature below 35 °C can increase the jitter in normal muscle, so such low temperatures such be avoided.

SFEMG in Myasthenia Gravis

In patients with myasthenia gravis, the following in a tested muscle may be found:

1. Endplates with normal jitter values.
2. Endplates with jitter values above the normal range without impulse blocking.
3. Endplates with increase jitter and intermittent impulse blocking.

Jitter is found to be increased in most patients with myasthenia gravis, and this finding is more pronounced when weak muscles are tested but can also be found in muscles that do not show clinical weakness. A SFEMG tracing showing marked jitter in a clinically affected muscle is shown in Fig. 11.5 below. Jitter is abnormal in

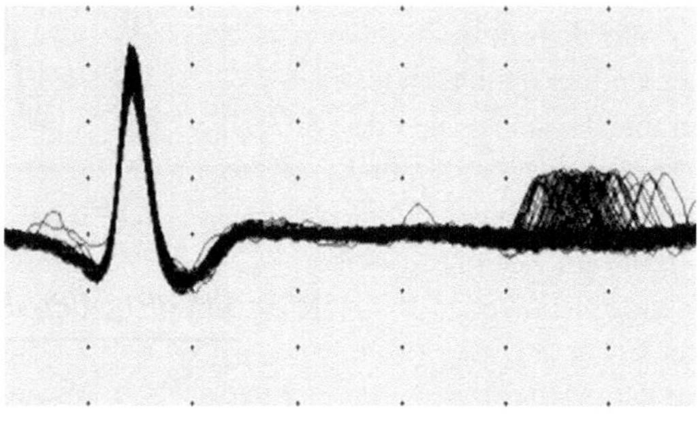

Fig. 11.5 Single fiber electromyography (SFEMG) with high jitter in the frontalis muscle, 1 kHz high-pass filtering, 200 μV/D, 0.5 ms/D. [Used with permission from [6]]

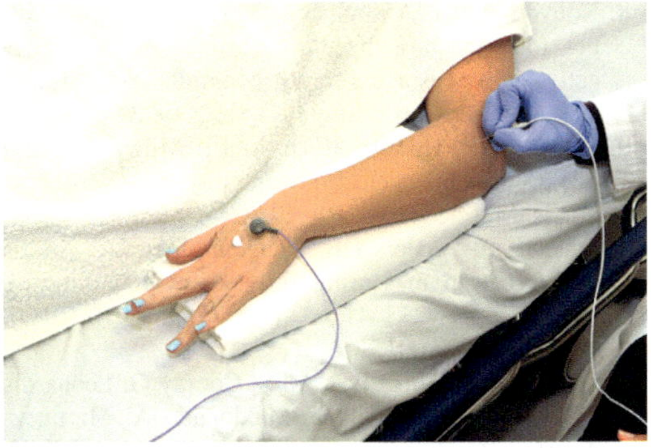

Fig. 11.6 Single fiber electromyography (SFEMG) technique recording from the extensor digitorum (communis) muscle. This is done by having the patient extend the middle finger only while the needle is inserted parallel to the muscle fibers

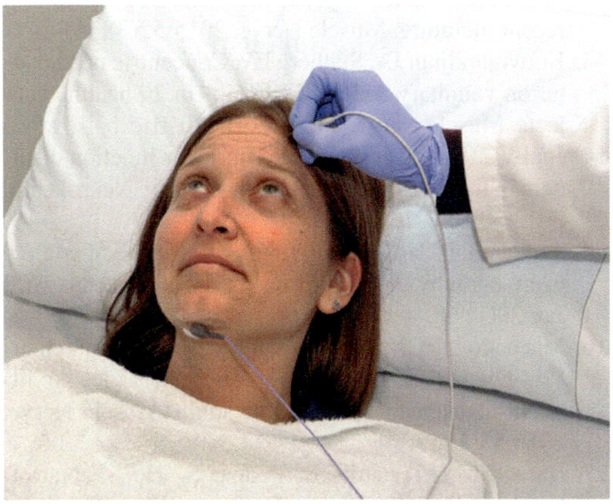

Fig. 11.7 Single fiber electromyography (SFEMG) technique recording from the frontalis muscle. This is done by having the patient gently elevate eyebrows while the needle is inserted parallel to the muscle fibers

~85% of patients with ocular MG, and in up to ~95–99% of patients with generalized MG.

The muscle to be tested should be selected depending on patients' symptoms, and it is preferable to select an unequivocally symptomatic muscle in order to increase the probability of finding abnormal jitter. We prefer the extensor digitorum (communis) (Fig. 11.6) in patients with generalized myasthenia gravis, and the frontalis (Fig. 11.7) or orbicularis oculus (Fig. 11.8) in patients with primarily ocular symptoms with or without generalized weakness.

The extensor digitorum is mostly tested first, and preferable in patients with limb or with bulbar

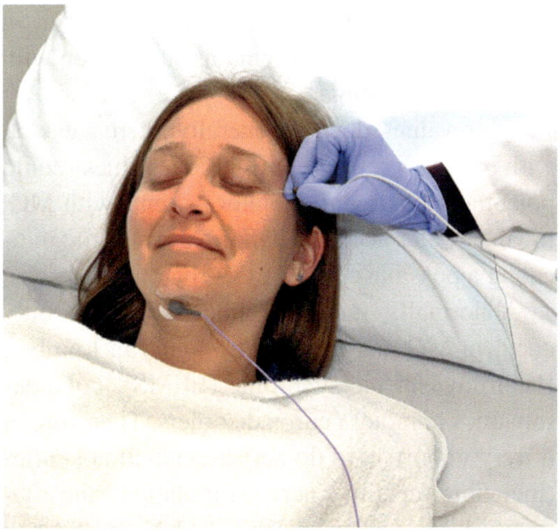

Fig. 11.8 Single fiber electromyography (SFEMG) technique recording from the orbicularis oculus muscle. This is done by having the patient close the eyes, minimally squeezing the eyelids shut. The needle is inserted parallel to the muscle fibers, directed away from the eyelid margin

muscle weakness. This muscle can be abnormal in about 85% of patients with MG during their initial electrodiagnostic assessment. This muscle is preferred due to being relatively easy to activate, with minimal patient discomfort and ease of finding pairs of action potentials. With the patient elevating the middle finger minimally, the needle is inserted parallel to the axis of the muscle fibers.

With respect to firing rate and jitter values, the jitter is most likely to be increased when the firing rate is rapid in an endplate pair, compared to when it is firing slowly.

We prefer patients discontinue the use of cholinesterase inhibitors, when clinically safe, at least 12 hours before the study. This may be more useful in patients with ocular MG or in those with minimal limb weakness as jitter can become abnormal only when these medications are discontinued. In other patients, jitter values can still be increase even when they continue to take the cholinesterase inhibitors.

If SFEMG is done in a clinically weak muscle, and jitter is normal, then the diagnosis is almost surely not MG.

In MG, jitter may not be present during initial recording of muscle activation, and measurement may need to be made for several minutes for jitter to become abnormal. This does not occur in healthy muscle, as jitter remains stable even with prolonged activation.

Jitter values do not generally correlate well with disease severity, but these values could potentially be used to monitor patients with MG, in which jitter becomes abnormal over time indicating a possible clinical exacerbation.

Abnormally increased jitter does not only occur in MG and can also be found in Lambert Eaton myasthenic syndrome (LEMS), polyneuropathies or motor neuron disorders. Therefore, it is very important to do nerve conduction studies (including repetitive nerve stimulation) and routine EMG in patients prior to SFEM, in order to exclude these diagnoses. In cases of LEMS, the jitter will be increased out of proportion to the severity of muscle weakness, and impulse blocking is commonly found. In polyneuropathies, the jitter can be increased during reinnervation, and later normalizes or reduces.

References/Suggested Reading

1. Sanders DB, Stålberg EV. AAEM minimonograph #25: single-fiber electromyography. Muscle Nerve. 1996;19:1069–83.
2. Rubin DI. Needle electromyography: basic concepts and patterns of abnormalities. Neurol Clin. 2012 May;30(2):429–56.
3. Stalberg E. Clinical electrophysiology in myasthenia gravis. J Neurol Neurosurg Psychiatry. 1980;43:622–33.
4. Selvan VA. Single-fiber EMG: a review. Ann Indian Acad Neurol. 2011;14(1):64–7.
5. Meriggioli MN, Sanders DB. Myasthenia gravis: diagnosis. Semin Neurol. 2004 Mar;24(1):31–9.
6. Sirin NG, Kocasoy Orhan E, Durmus H, Deymeer F, Baslo MB. Repetitive nerve stimulation and jitter measurement with disposable concentric needle electrode in newly diagnosed myasthenia gravis patients. Neurophysiol Clin. 2018 Oct;48(5):261–7.
7. Cherian A, Baheti NN, Iype T. Electrophysiological study in neuromuscular junction disorders. Ann Indian Acad Neurol. 2013;16:134–41.
8. Kouyoumdjian JA, Stalberg EV. Reference jitter values for concentric needle electrodes in voluntarily activated extensor digitorum communis and orbicularis oculi muscles. Muscle Nerve. 2008;37:694–9.
9. Sanders DB, Howard JF. Jr AAEE Minimonograph #25: single-fiber electromyography in myasthenia gravis. Muscle Nerve. 1986;9:809–19.
10. Stålberg E, Sanders DB, Kouyoumdjian JA. Pitfalls and errors in measuring jitter. Clin Neurophysiol. 2017;128(11):2233–41. https://doi.org/10.1016/j.clinph.2017.09.001.
11. Stålberg E, Sanders DB, Ali S, Cooray G, Leonardis L, Löseth S, Machado F, Maldonado A, Martinez-Aparicio C, Sandberg A, Smith B, Widenfalk J, Kouyoumdjian JA. Reference values for jitter recorded by concentric needle electrodes in healthy controls: a multicenter study. Muscle Nerve. 2015;53(3):351–62.
12. Chiou-Tan FY, Gilchrist JM. Repetitive nerve stimulation and single-fiber electromyography in the evaluation of patients with suspected myasthenia gravis or Lambert–Eaton myasthenic syndrome: review of recent literature. Muscle Nerve. 2015;52(3):455–62.
13. Kouyoumdjian JA, Stålberg EV. Concentric needle jitter on voluntary activated frontalis in 20 healthy subjects. Muscle Nerve. 2013;47(3):440–2.
14. Juel VC. Evaluation of neuromuscular junction disorders in the electromyography laboratory. Neurol Clin. 2012;30(2):621.
15. Sanders DB, Howard JF, Johns TR. Single-fiber electromyography in myasthenia gravis. Neurology. 1979 Jan;29(1):68.
16. Machado FCN, Kouyoumdjian JA, Marchiori PE. Diagnostic accuracy of concentric needle jitter in myasthenia: prospective study. Muscle Nerve. 2016;55(2):190–4.
17. Baruca M, Leonardis L, Podnar S, Hojs-Fabjan T, Grad A, Jerin A, Blagus R, Šega-Jazbec S. Single fiber EMG as a prognostic tool in myasthenia gravis. Muscle Nerve. 2016;54(6):1034–40.
18. Kouyoumdjian JA, Stålberg EV. Concentric needle jitter on voluntary activated frontalis in 20 healthy subjects. Muscle Nerve. 2013;47(3):440–2.
19. Stålberg E. Jitter analysis with concentric needle electrodes. Ann N Y Acad Sci. 2012;1274(1):77–85.
20. Chenevier F, Gervais-Bernard H, Bouhour F, Vial C. Myasthénies et syndromes myasthéniques. EMC Neurol. 2011;8(2):1.
21. Tidswell T, Pitt MC. A new analytical method to diagnose congenital myasthenia with stimulated single-fiber electromyography. Muscle Nerve. 2006;35(1):107–10.

Myopathies

12

Payam Soltanzadeh

Etiology and Clinical Features

Myopathies or muscle diseases are classified into acquired or genetic disease processes, which primarily affect the function and/or structure of the muscle tissue ultimately leading to various manifestations such as muscle weakness, neuromuscular hyperexcitability (including myotonia, cramps and myalgia), and physical fatigability. Due to recent advances in molecular genetics and immunology and significant clinical and pathological overlap among various muscle diseases, classification of myopathies is evolving and genetic and immunologic biomarkers are being used to further refine previous classifications that were purely based on clinical and pathologic criteria (Table 12.1). Most myopathies primarily cause symmetrical proximal muscle weakness but there are muscle diseases, like sporadic inclusion body myositis (sIBM) or myotonic dystrophy type 1, that can primarily or initially affect distal muscle groups and, later, involve the proximal muscles. Symmetry is also not a universal characteristic of myopathies as some myopathies like facioscapulohumeral muscular dystrophy (FSHD) or sIBM can have a very asymmetric presentation. Very high serum levels of creatine kinase (CK) can be a good clue to the diagnosis of a muscle disease; however, depending on the type and the stage of myopathy, CK can be either normal or only slightly elevated. Neurogenic processes like motor neuron disease, motor radiculopathies and some neuropathies can also be associated with slightly elevated CK levels. There are a few myopathies that can cause very high CK, which can help with the diagnosis (Table 12.2).

Differential Diagnosis

Subacute or chronic development of symmetric weakness in proximal muscles should raise concern for a myopathic process; however, in the neuromuscular category of neurologic diseases, some forms of motor neuron disease like late-onset spinal muscular atrophy (SMA) or atypical amyotrophic lateral sclerosis (ALS), bilateral polyradiculopathies or polyradiculoneuropathies like Chronic inflammatory demyelinating polyradiculoneuropathy (CIDP), motor predominant neuropathies, disorders of the neuromuscular junction like myasthenic syndromes, botulism or Lambert-Eaton myasthenic syndrome (LEMS) may also present with prominent proximal weakness in a relatively symmetrical fashion. If a neuromuscular process presents asymmetrically, differential

P. Soltanzadeh (✉)
Neuromuscular Program, Department of Neurology, UCLA, Los Angeles, CA, USA
e-mail: psoltanzadeh@mednet.ucla.edu

N. Galvez-Jimenez et al. (eds.), *Electrodiagnostic Medicine*,
https://doi.org/10.1007/978-3-030-74997-2_12

Table 12.1 General classification of myopathies

Acquired myopathies:

– Inflammatory or non-inflammatory necrotizing autoimmune myopathies: myositis associated with a specific antibody (anti-SRP, anti-HMGCR, anti-Jo, etc.), dermatomyositis, polymyositis
– Sporadic inclusion body myositis (sIBM)
– Granulomatous (sarcoid) myopathy
– Amyloid myopathy
– Drug-induced or toxic myopathies: self-limited statin myopathy, myopathy caused by steroids, colchicine, or alcohol
– Endocrine myopathies: thyroid or parathyroid disorders, Cushing's syndrome, vitamin D deficiency/osteomalacia, hypokalemia
– Infectious myopathies: trichinosis, cysticercosis, toxoplasmosis, HIV, coxsackie, influenza, SARS-CoV-2, Lyme disease, *staphylococcus aureus* (pyomyositis)
– Critical illness (myosin loss) myopathy

Genetic myopathies:

– Muscular Dystrophies:
  – Dystrophinopathies (X-linked): *DMD*
  – Emery-Dreifuss muscular dystrophy: *EMD, FHL1, LMNA*
  – Facioscapulohumeral muscular dystrophy (FSHD) types 1 and 2: DUX4, *SMCHD1*
  – Limb-girdle muscular dystrophies (LGMDs): many genes
– Congenital muscular dystrophies:
  – Congenital muscular dystrophy with merosin (*LAMA2)* deficiency
  – Collagen VI diseases (Bethlem and Ullrich)
  – Rigid spine syndrome: *SEPN1, FHL1, LMNA, DNM2* (dynamin 2)
  – Congenital muscular dystrophies due to defective glycosylation (Fukuyama, Walker-Warburg, muscle-eye-brain disease)
– Congenital myopathies:
  – Nemaline myopathies: *TPM3, TPM2, NEB, ACTA1* (actin alpha 1)
  – Congenital myopathy with fiber-type disproportion (CFTD): *ACTA1, SEPN1, TPM3, RYR1, MYH7*
  – Myotubular myopathy: *MTM1* (myotubularin 1)
  – Centronuclear myopathies: *DNM2* (dynamin 2), *BIN1* (amphiphysin), *RYR1, TTN*
  – Central core disease: *RYR1*
  – Multiminicore disease (classic form): *SEPN1*
  – Cap myopathy: *TPM2, TPM3, ACTA1*
– Distal Myopathies
  – Miyoshi: *DYSF*
  – Tibial muscular dystrophy (Udd): *TTN*
  – Hereditary IBM and Nonaka (now called GNE myopathy): GNE (glucosamine (UDP-N-acetyl)-2-epimerase/N-acetylmannosamine kinase)
  – Distal myopathy with VCP defect (IBMPFD): *VCP*
  – Laing Distal myopathy: *MYH7*
  – Welander distal myopathy: *TIA1* (cytotoxic granule-associated RNA binding protein)
– Myopathies due to mutant Z-disk associated proteins or Myofibrillar myopathies**:** *CRYAB* (alpha B crystallin), *DES* (desmin), LDB3 (ZASP), *MYOT* (myotilin)
– Oculopharyngeal muscular dystrophy (OPMD)
– Myotonic dystrophies
  – Myotonic dystrophy type 1 (DM-1) or Steinert's disease: *DMPK*
  – Myotonic dystrophy type 2 (DM-2) or PROMM: *ZNF9*
  – Other Myotonic syndromes (Schwartz-Jampel syndrome, etc)
– Channelopathies (include nondystrophic myotonic syndromes/periodic paralyses)
  – Chloride channel: autosomal dominant myotonia congenita (Thomsen); autosomal recessive (Becker): *CLCN1*
  – Sodium channel: hyperKPP, hypoKPP, paramyotonia congenita: *SCN4A*
  – Calcium channel: hypoKPP1: *CACNA1S*
  – Potassium channel: hypoKPP3: *KCNE3*; thyrotoxic hypokalemic: *KCNJ18*
– Metabolic myopathies
  – glycogen storage diseases: type II (Pompe disease): *GAA* (acid alpha glucosidase/acid maltase), type V (McArdle): *PYGM* (myophosphorylase)
  – glycolytic pathway
  – disorders of lipid metabolism: carnitine palmitoyltransferase deficiency: *CPT2*
  – Mitochondrial myopathies

Table 12.2 Myopathies with very high CK levels (typically, in the thousands U/L)

– Some inflammatory or necrotizing autoimmune myopathies
– Dystrophinopathies (Duchenne and Becker muscular dystrophies)
– LGMD 2A (calpainopathy)
– LGMD 2B (dysferlinopathy)
– LGMD 2C-2F (sarcoglycanopathies)
– LGMD 2I (Fukutin-related proteinopathy)
– LGMD 2L (anoctaminopathy)

diagnosis extends to multifocal motor neuropathy with conduction block (MMN), unilateral motor radiculopathies, plexopathies, and mononeuropathies. Other clinical and laboratory features especially the electrodiagnostic (EDX) findings can usually identify the cause of weakness. In addition to the data from needle EMG examination, nerve conduction study is an important component of EDX work up in a patient presenting with weakness. Although patients with myopathies may have a pre-existing length-dependent neuropathy, presence of demyelinating features like slow motor conduction, conduction block, or temporal dispersion can indicate diseases like CIDP or MMN. Significant loss of sensory amplitudes indicate pathology in the peripheral nerve or plexus. Presence of decrement or increment in compound muscle action potential amplitudes favors a disease process involving the neuromuscular junction. In patients with a neuromuscular junction transmission defect, fluctuation of muscle strength and involvement of the cranio-bulbar segments help with the diagnosis; however, diseases like LEMS or limb-girdle congenital myasthenic syndromes (including DOK7) may not show prominent ocular or bulbar deficits and fluctuations may not be as notable as in typical myasthenia gravis. Some disease processes can damage both nerves and muscles (neuromyopathies), hence creating a mixed neurogenic and myopathic picture (Table 12.3). In a pure myopathic process, nerve conduction studies are expected to be normal; however, myopathies that involve distal muscles can cause reduction of distal motor amplitudes, with preserved latencies and conduction velocities.

Table 12.3 Causes of neuromyopathy (presenting with both myopathy and neuropathy)

– HIV
– Sarcoidosis
– Amyloidosis
– Paraneoplastic neuromyopathy
– Mitochondrial neuromyopathy
– Toxic neuromyopathies (alcohol abuse, colchicine, hydroxychloroquine etc)
– Critical illness neuromyopathy
– Graft-versus-host disease (GVHD)

Electrodiagnostic Evaluation of Myopathies

EDX work up is an important component of the assessment of a patient with suspected myopathy. Despite recent advances in molecular biology and genetics, EDX data can be helpful to differentiate myopathic processes from the mimickers discussed above as well as to better characterize the myopathic process. In some genetic myopathies like Duchenne muscular dystrophy or myotonic dystrophy type 1, if clinical presentation is classic or there is known family history, one could skip EDX data and muscle biopsy and directly move on to genetic testing. If genetic test results are not consistent with the initial clinical hypothesis, a classic approach then needs to be pursued.

Needle EMG findings can help diagnose and characterize a myopathy; however, it should be emphasized that a normal needle EMG study does not exclude a myopathic process. It is worth reminding that the EDX data may be considered an extension to the clinical data and should be interpreted within the patient's clinical context. Needle EMG examination should follow the nerve conduction studies component of the EDX assessment and guided by the clinical presentation, adequate nerve conduction studies should be performed. To differentiate myopathy from a polyradiculoneuropathy like CIDP or from MMN, adequate sensory and motor responses from both upper and lower extremities should be assessed. These include one or two motor with corresponding F response(s) plus one sensory conduction study from the lower extremity; and one or two motor with corresponding F response(s) plus one sensory conduction study from the upper extremity. In the lower extremity, peroneal (fibular) and tibial motor and sural sensory responses are routinely checked and in the upper extremity, median and ulnar motor and sensory responses are usually assessed. Radial nerve studies can be useful in MMN affecting upper extremities.

If a neuromuscular junction disorder is suspected, repetitive nerve stimulation studies should be planned. Electrodiagnosis of LEMS can be difficult in the co-existence of a polyneuropathy. In the presence of low motor amplitudes, post-exercise measurements should be included in both upper and lower extremities.

Patients with myotonic dystrophies type 1 or 2, which are both systemic diseases, may have diabetes with a co-existing diabetic polyneuropathy. The presence of polyneuropathy in these cases may complicate the EDX findings but the electromyographer should note myotonic discharges and the myopathic EMG changes (discussed below).

Short and long exercise tests have been described in myotonic myopathies/periodic paralyses. Availability of genetic testing for myotonic dystrophies, non-dystrophic myotonic myopathies and other skeletal muscle channelopathies, as well as the uncomfortable technique and questionable diagnostic accuracy have made these tests of limited practical utility. Accordingly, we will defer discussing these tests in this chapter.

Needle EMG Findings in Myopathies

Needle EMG findings in patients with myopathy fall into two major categories: the ones that are associated with abnormal insertional and spontaneous activities, and those that are related to changes in motor unit potentials (MUPs).

"Insertional activity" is referred to the activity that immediately follows the mechanical stimulus by the needle and may continue after cessation of needle movement. "Spontaneous activity" does not require any mechanical trigger. Distinction between these two types of activities is often considered arbitrary and clinically irrelevant and one could use either term or the more comprehensive one "insertional/spontaneous activity". In this chapter, we will refer to both as "spontaneous activity". Increased spontaneous activity can develop in denervation or terminal motor axon injury, muscle membrane hyperexcitability or muscle membrane injury, abnormal signal transmission between the nerve endings and the motor end plate, myofiber necrosis or splitting, inflammatory changes in the muscle tissue, and vacuolar myopathologies. Based on the presence or absence of increased spontaneous activity in needle EMG examinations, myopathies are electrodiagnostically categorized into two broad categories of "irritable myopathies" (Table 12.4) and "non-irritable myopathies" (Table 12.5). Irritable myopathies show positive sharp wave or fibrillation potentials on needle examination. Positive sharp wave or fibrillation potentials are not specific to myopathies and can be seen in various neurogenic diseases as well as in botulism or following botulinum toxin injections. In non-irritable myopathies, spontaneous activity is normal. As noted in Tables 12.4 and 12.5, many myopathies can cause both irritable and non-irri-

Table 12.4 Irritable myopathies (myopathic-type MUPs with abnormal spontaneous activity, including positive sharp waves and fibrillation potentials)

Acquired muscle diseases
– Inflammatory or non-inflammatory necrotizing autoimmune myopathies
– Sporadic inclusion body myositis (sIBM)
– Sarcoid myopathy
– Amyloid myopathy
– Toxic myopathies
– Infectious myopathies
– Hypothyroid myopathy
– Critical illness (myosin loss) myopathy
Genetic muscle diseases
– Dystrophinopathies
– Other muscular dystrophies (MD): Emery-Dreifuss MD, Facioscapulohumeral muscular dystrophy (FSHD), some Limb-girdle muscular dystrophies (LGMDs), Oculopharyngeal muscular dystrophy (OPMD)
– Collagen VI diseases (Bethlem and Ullrich congenital muscular dystrophies/myopathies)
– Centronuclear, myotubular, and nemaline rod congenital myopathies
– Distal myopathies
– Myofibrillar myopathies
– Metabolic myopathies: acid maltase deficiency (Pompe disease), debrancher enzyme deficiency, carnitine deficiency, mitochondrial myopathies.

Table 12.5 Non-irritable myopathies (myopathic-type MUPs with often normal spontaneous activity)

Acquired muscle diseases
– Treated Inflammatory or non-inflammatory necrotizing autoimmune myopathies
– Steroid myopathy and myopathy from Cushing syndrome
– Myopathy due to hyper- or hypothyroidism
– Critical illness myopathy
Genetic muscle diseases
– Facioscapulohumeral muscular dystrophy (FSHD)
– Oculopharyngeal muscular dystrophy (OPMD)
– Limb-girdle muscular dystrophies (LGMDs)
– Collagen VI diseases (Bethlem and Ullrich congenital muscular dystrophies/myopathies)
– Congenital myopathies
– Distal myopathies
– Myofibrillar myopathies
– Metabolic myopathies: some glycogen storage diseases, lipid storage myopathies, carnitine deficiency, carnitine palmitoyltransferase II (CPT II) deficiency, some mitochondrial myopathies

Table 12.6 Myopathies with potentially normal EMG

Acquired muscle diseases
– Steroid myopathy
Genetic muscle diseases
– Congenital myopathies
– Metabolic myopathies: some mitochondrial myopathies, glycogen storage diseases between acute attacks, carnitine palmitoyltransferase II (CPT II) deficiency

table patterns depending on the stage of the disease, muscles involved and individual variability. In these myopathies, myopathic motor unit potentials (discussed below) can be associated with or without abnormal spontaneous activity.

Sometimes spontaneous activity and motor unit potentials are both normal and needle EMG examination does not show any abnormality (Table 12.6).

Complex repetitive discharges (CRDs) are created by a group of adjacent hyperexcitable myofibers with one serving as a pacemaker fiber and the others becoming activated via ephaptic transmission. A loop of activation is created and the spikes remain uniform from one to another. CRDs start suddenly and stop suddenly and they mimic the sound of a machine gun. CRDs tend to have higher amplitude spikes compared to fibrillation potentials. CRDs can be seen in both neurogenic and myopathic conditions and may or may not suggest chronicity of the underlying pathology.

Table 12.7 Myopathies with prominent myotonic discharges

Myotonic syndromes
– Myotonic dystrophy type 1 (Steinert's disease)
– Myotonic dystrophy type 2 (proximal myotonic myopathy or PROMM)
– Myotonia congenita (chloride channelopathy)
– Hyperkalemic periodic paralysis (sodium channelopathy)
– Paramyotonia congenita (sodium channelopathy)
Non-myotonic syndromes
– Acid maltase deficiency (Pompe disease)
– Some inflammatory myopathies
– Statin-induced myopathies
– Toxic myopathies

Myotonia is the spontaneous firing of a muscle fiber in which both amplitude and frequency wax and wane. In contrast to myotonia, fibrillation potentials fire at a regular rate. A myotonic discharge is comprised of positive sharp wave or brief spike potentials and its sound resembles that of an accelerating and decelerating motorcycle or chain saw. Although myotonia is a form of increased/abnormal spontaneous activity, muscle disorders showing prominent myotonia are electrodiagnostically categorized under a separate group, called "myotonic syndromes" (Table 12.7). Myotonic syndromes are divided into myotonic dystrophies and non-dystrophic myotonic syndromes. Myotonic dystrophies are either type 1 or type 2. Myotonic discharges are typically more prominent in type 1 than in type 2. Electrodiagnosis of myotonic dystrophy type 2 can be very difficult, as many muscles might not reveal myotonic discharges. Non-dystrophic myotonic syndromes include paramyotonia congenita (sodium channelopathy), myotonia congenita (chloride channelopathy), and hyperkalemic periodic paralysis (sodium channelopathy). Myotonia is more severe and consistent in chloride channelopathies than in patients with sodium channel mutations. Hypokalemic periodic paralysis and Andersen-Tawil syndrome are two skeletal muscle channelopathies that are not typically associated with

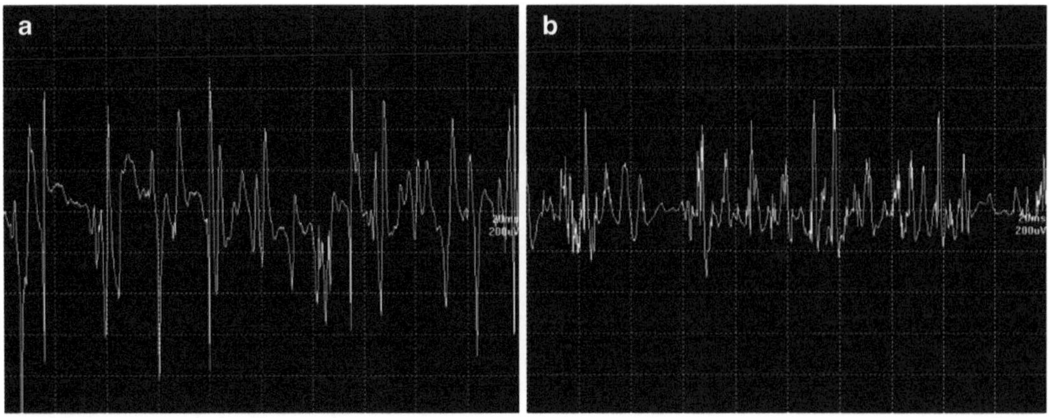

Fig. 12.1 Myopathic motor unit potentials (MUPs) compared to normal MUPs. Panel A shows normal MUPs in biceps brachii; Panel B demonstrates myopathic MUPs with early recruitment in biceps brachii (scale: 200 μV, 20 ms)

myotonia and therefore are not considered nondystrophic myotonic syndromes. Prominent myotonic discharges are also seen in some other myopathies that are not known to primarily affect the skeletal muscle ion channels and are not considered myotonic syndromes per se; these include acid maltase deficiency (Pompe disease), some inflammatory myopathies, statin-induced myopathies, and toxic myopathies.

Absent EMG activity (electrical silence) while the muscle is in the contraction phase is known as "contracture" and can be seen in McArdle disease. "Cramps" are clinically similar to contractures but during a muscle cramp, which is usually neurogenic, there is involuntary firing of normal motor unit potentials (MUPs) at a high frequency in the range of 200–300 Hz. Diminished spontaneous activity can also be seen during a periodic paralysis attack. In muscular dystrophies and progressive acquired myopathies, as the disease progresses, muscle tissue is replaced by fatty or fibrous tissue leading to end stage muscle. Spontaneous activity noted on insertion of the needle is typically decreased in such muscles.

Examination of the MUPs may provide the most specific data in support of a myopathic process. Typical myopathic MUPs demonstrate short duration, low amplitude, and polyphasia (Fig. 12.1). Short duration and low amplitude MUPs are due to destruction or dysfunction of the muscle fibers. Polyphasia results from loss of synchrony (asynchrony) in depolarization of the injured myofibers. These MUP changes may also be seen in diseases of the neuromuscular junction and during the early reinnervation phase after a severe nerve injury, when "nascent" units result.

Another EDX feature of myopathies is "early" (or "increased") recruitment of MUPs. This is caused by activation of more motor units in order to generate the required muscle force. Examination of early recruitment requires attention to the degree of patient's effort during muscle contraction. In order to assess recruitment, the patient is asked to slightly activate the muscle. In typical early recruitment, many MUPs appear almost simultaneously as the patient starts to contract. Only the electromyographer can assess early recruitment as he or she is aware of how much force is being generated. If MUP assessment starts with a rather forceful contraction, early recruitment and smaller myopathic MUPs may miss detection.

Rarely, in very chronic or advanced myopathies, entire motor units are lost and needle examination shows either mixed myopathic and neurogenic features or sometimes predominantly neurogenic changes with reduced recruitment of large MUPs. This pattern makes EDX difficult and is characteristically seen in sIBM, but also described in other chronic myopathies like muscular dystrophies (Fig. 12.2).

Disease processes involving both nerves and muscles can also cause a mixed neurogenic and myopathic pattern (Table 12.3).

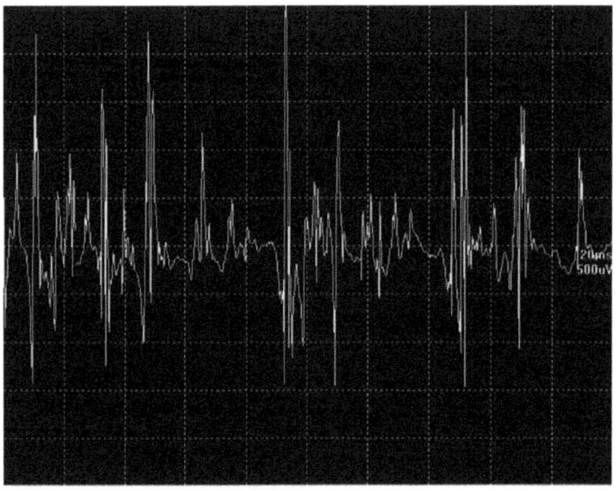

Fig. 12.2 Mixed myopathic and neurogenic motor unit potentials (MUPs) in the rectus femoris muscle of a patient with sporadic inclusion body myositis (sIBM) (scale: 500 μV, 20 ms)

EMG can help clinicians differentiate steroid myopathy from a recurrent or undertreated inflammatory or autoimmune myopathy. In such patients, an irritable myopathic pattern with abundant fibrillation or positive sharp wave potentials suggests recurrence or inadequately-treated inflammatory/autoimmune myopathy, whereas steroid myopathy typically shows normal or decreased spontaneous activity.

It is important to be mindful that in a patient with myopathy, needle examination may be normal (Table 12.6) or only a limited number of these myopathic features may be observed.

Needle EMG Protocol in Myopathies

As discussed above, nerve conduction studies are performed after a brief history and manual muscle testing. The data obtained from these studies lead to a higher yield needle EMG examination. Muscles that are weak on clinical exam are expected to show more myopathic motor units with or without increased spontaneous activity (fibrillation or positive sharp wave potentials), depending on whether the myopathy is irritable or non-irritable. It is necessary to keep in mind that if the muscle involvement is advanced or end-stage and there is significant fatty or fibrous tissue replacement, spontaneous activity is reduced. Needle EMG data can help increase the yield of the muscle biopsy. Usually, muscles with more abnormal spontaneous activity and myopathic motor units show more pathologic findings than muscles with normal EMG findings. Muscles that feel gritty or like passing a knife through butter during needle examination should be avoided because they are likely to be end-stage. Decreased insertional activity and reduced recruitment of mixed neurogenic and myopathic MUPs also suggest end-stage muscle tissue and such muscles are less preferred for biopsy. It is important to select muscles only on one side of the body and reserve the contralateral side for tissue diagnosis to avoid needle EMG (inflammatory-like) artifacts created during needle examinations. In the appendicular segments, both proximal and distal muscles should be sampled. Sampling distal muscles is more important in myopathies that sometimes start from distal segments; such myopathies include sIBM and myotonic dystrophy type 1. A comprehensive needle examination typically includes sampling at least three proximal and two distal appendicular muscles in each upper and lower extremity (total of 10 muscles) plus one or two paraspinal muscles.

Deltoid, biceps and triceps muscles in the upper extremity, and iliacus, rectus femoris, and vastus lateralis in the lower extremity are usually included in the EMG examination of a patient with proximal myopathy. To check the distal upper extremity segment, one should consider one of the finger flexors like flexor pollicis longus muscle as well as the first dorsal interosseous muscle. Brachioradialis, extensor digitorum or pronator teres muscles may also be sampled depending on the phenotype. Irritable myopathic changes in the forearm flexor muscles are commonly seen in patients with sIBM and may precede clinical weakness or atrophy. Distal lower extremity muscles that help the most include the tibialis anterior and gastrocnemius. EMG changes can be seen in distal myopathies that affect anterior or posterior compartments of the lower extremities. If posterior thigh compartment is involved, sampling the hamstring muscles or the gluteus maximus may also be added.

Involvement of the posterior leg compartments is seen in limb-girdle muscular dystrophies 2A (calpainopathy) and 2B (dysferlinopathy).

Sampling paraspinal muscles (the most proximal muscles) can be helpful in axial myopathies (including isolated neck extensor myopathy), adult-onset Pompe disease, and some inflammatory myopathies. Selection of paraspinal muscles depends on the clinical phenotype. The thoracic paraspinal muscles are more protected from degenerative changes that lead to radiculopathies, and can generally be more helpful; however, in a patient with dropped head syndrome, cervical paraspinal muscles (and possibly splenius capitis) need to be assessed.

Case Studies

Patient 1 A 23 year-old man presented with 6-month history of lower extremity weakness and muscle cramps leading to imbalance and near-falls. His examination showed severe bilateral calf atrophy and mild weakness in plantar flexors. Upper extremity strength examination was normal. Nerve conduction studies were normal. Needle EMG examination of the lower extremity showed increased spontaneous activity (fibrillation and positive sharp wave potentials) with neurogenic motor units (long duration, high amplitude, polyphasic MUPs). The EMG abnormalities were more severe in the posterior compartment muscles both below and above the knee (gastrocnemius, short head of the biceps femoris, and semitendinosus). MRI of the lumbar spine was normal. CK level was also checked showing a very high level of 11,322 (normal range: 30–220 U/L). Because of the very high CK level, a limb-girdle muscular dystrophy (LGMD) genetic panel was requested showing two mutations in *ANO5* (c.191dupA and c.2272C > T(p.R758C)). Based on the genetic results, the final diagnosis was LGMD 2L (anoctaminopathy).

Patient 2 A 33 year-old woman presented with 7 years of severe myalgia, chronic fatigue and exertion intolerance. She was originally diagnosed with "fibromyalgia". Her manual muscle testing was normal despite prominent "give-way" weakness. CK was in the 1700–5000 U/L range but her nerve conduction studies and needle EMG examination of proximal and distal muscles in both upper and lower extremities were normal. She also underwent a muscle biopsy of her vastus lateralis, which was unrevealing. An LGMD genetic panel revealed two mutations in *ANO5* (c.191dupA and c.692G > T(p.G231V)).

Discussion These two unrelated sporadic patients with LGMD 2L (anoctaminopathy) show very different clinical and EDX presentations. In patient 1, needle EMG shows neurogenic MUPs with increased spontaneous activity. Symmetrical involvement and very high CK are clues to a myopathic process. As discussed above, neurogenic MUPs can be seen in advanced or chronic myopathies. Although the patient's symptoms started about 6 months prior to the neuromuscular visit, the muscle tissue injury probably started earlier in his life. The second patient demonstrates that genetic muscle diseases can sometimes present with nonspecific neuromuscular complaints, normal EMG, and normal muscle biopsy. Very high CK is a good diagnostic clue.

Suggested Reading

1. Bonne G, Bonne G, Rivier F, Hamroun D. The 2018 version of the gene table of monogenic neuromuscular disorders (nuclear genome). Neuromuscul Disord. 2017;27(12):1152–83.
2. Fournier E, Arzel M, Sternberg D, Vicart S, Laforet P, Eymard B, Willer JC, Tabti N, Fontaine B. Electromyography guides toward subgroups of mutations in muscle channelopathies. Ann Neurol. 2004;56(5):650–61.
3. Jackson CE, Barohn RJ. A pattern recognition approach to myopathy. Continuum (Minneap Minn). 2013;19(6 Muscle Disease):1674–97.
4. Joy JL, Oh SJ, Baysal AI. Electrophysiological spectrum of inclusion body myositis. Muscle Nerve. 1990;13(10):949–51.

5. Kimura J. Electrodiagnosis in diseases of nerve and muscle: principles and practice. 4th ed. Oxford: Oxford University Press; 2013.
6. Lacomis D. Electrodiagnostic approach to the patient with suspected myopathy. Neurol Clin. 2012;30(2):641–60.
7. Logigian EL, Ciafaloni E, Quinn LC, Dilek N, Pandya S, Moxley RT 3rd, Thornton CA. Severity, type, and distribution of myotonic discharges are different in type 1 and type 2 myotonic dystrophy. Muscle Nerve. 2007;35(4):479–85.
8. Meriggioli MN, Barboi AC, Rowin J, Cochran EJ. HMG-CoA reductase inhibitor myopathy: clinical, electrophysiological, and pathologic data in five patients. J Clin Neuromuscul Dis. 2001;2(3):129–34.
9. Paganoni S, Amato A. Electrodiagnostic evaluation of myopathies. Phys Med Rehabil Clin N Am. 2013;24(1):193–207.
10. Petajan JH. AAEM minimonograph #3: motor unit recruitment. Muscle Nerve. 1991;14(6):489–502.
11. Preston D, Shapiro B. Electromyography and neuromuscular disorders: clinical-electrophysiologic correlations. 3rd ed. London: Elsevier Saunders; 2013.
12. Robinson LR. AAEM case report #22: polymyositis. Muscle Nerve. 1991;14(4):310–5.
13. Shouman K, Morren J, Soltanzadeh P. Phenotypic heterogeneity in limb-girdle muscular dystrophy type 2 L (Anoctaminopathy) (P5.446). Neurology. 2018 Apr;90(15 Supplement):P5.446.
14. Young NP, Daube JR, Sorenson EJ, Milone M. Absent, unrecognized, and minimal myotonic discharges in myotonic dystrophy type 2. Muscle Nerve. 2010;41(6):758–62.
15. Zhou C, Wu L, Ni F, Ji W, Wu J, Zhang H. Critical illness polyneuropathy and myopathy: a systematic review. Neural Regen Res. 2014;9(1):101–10.

13 Recommendations for Writing an Electrodiagnostic Study Report

Alexandra Soriano and John A. Morren

After performance of nerve conduction and electromyography studies, a written report with thorough description of the findings should be produced, with the goal of interpreting the results in a clear way that can be understood by the referring physician, and that explains the diagnosis, correlated with the findings- including the nature/character (e.g. axon loss or demyelinating), distribution, and severity of nerve, muscle or neuromuscular junction transmission disorder.

1. The performing physician must have not only the appropriate training and education to do this task, but also needs to know the patient's history and exam findings (repeating as necessary) that lead to ordering the study in the first place. With this information, the performing physician can tailor the study to answer the specific questions posed and create a report that helps correlate the final findings on the EDX study to the clinical features.

A. Soriano (✉)
Braathen Neurological Center, Cleveland Clinic Florida, Weston, FL, USA

Cleveland Clinic Lerner College of Medicine of Case Western Reserve University, Cleveland, OH, USA
e-mail: soriana@ccf.org

J. A. Morren
Neuromuscular Center, Neurological Institute, Cleveland Clinic, and Cleveland Clinic Lerner College of Medicine of Case Western Reserve University, Cleveland, OH, USA
e-mail: morrenj@ccf.org

N. Galvez-Jimenez et al. (eds.), *Electrodiagnostic Medicine*,
https://doi.org/10.1007/978-3-030-74997-2_13

2. An EDX report should include the date of the study, patient demographic data (name, medical record number, and age or birth date, also more optionally- height, weight, gender, handedness and relevant medical diagnoses), a brief description of the indication for study, including clinical findings (pertinent history and exam components), the type of EDX test that was performed (especially if a particular protocol was followed e.g. for myopathy), all nerve conduction study and needle electrode examination data collected during the study (preferably tabulated, in conjunction with normal values) and a narrative interpretation of these data with final electrodiagnosis. It is important to include these components on the report in order to allow the ordering physician, or others reviewing the results, to corroborate the conclusion to the specific findings, and/or to compare to any prior studies. Most of the data from the nerve conduction study can be given in tables that specify the side (right or left) tested, which limbs were tested, limb temperature at the time of testing, specific nerve +/– muscle tested, site of stimulation and recording, distance measured, and results of latency, amplitude and conduction velocity. It is best if the results that are outside normal range values are highlighted.
3. Findings of needle EMG are best described in addition to tabulated data, as these results can only be fully interpreted right at the time of

the study i.e. in "real time". In this part of the report, one should include muscle and side tested. The insertional activity, presence of any abnormal spontaneous activity, and the description of the motor unit action potential configuration/morphology (including amplitude, duration, and number of phases) and recruitment pattern appreciated when the muscle is activated should be described.

4. If the study featured any limitations that could have affected the results, this must be described (e.g. limb edema, suboptimal patient tolerance or inability to adequately relax during evaluation of spontaneous activity).
5. The study interpretation should specify if results are normal or abnormal, and if abnormal, which abnormalities exist. An electrophysiological diagnosis should be given, with specific location of the pathology, nature/character (e.g. axon loss versus demyelinating for polyneuropathies; with or without necrotizing/inflammatory features for myopathies), chronicity, severity, and if possible, comparison with any available prior studies. It may be optional to provide a clinical diagnosis that correlates with the electrodiagnostic test findings (e.g. median neuropathy at or distal to the wrist, consistent with a clinical diagnosis of carpal tunnel syndrome), possible differential diagnosis, and if any further testing could be of value. The further testing recommended may include other modalities within the scope of neuromuscular diagnostics, including neuromuscular ultrasound.

The name of the physician performing the EDX study should be clearly identified on the report with an appropriate signature (which may be electronic) and date/time stamp. In cases for which appropriately trained NCS technologists perform NCSs under the direction and supervision of the EDX physician, the name of the technologist and the physician should both be included on the report, along with the signature of the physician. In cases involving a resident or fellow, the name of the trainee should also be included on the report.

Sample Report

Institution/Office Address: Solveit Clinic, 1000 Madeup Ave, Fictionville, XY. 77077. USA.

Telephone: (111) 222-3333.

[**Accreditation status:** E.g. AANEM Electrodiagnostic Laboratory Accreditation status (optional but recommended)]

Patient Name: Random, John **DOB:** 06/20/1991 **Age:** 28 **Height/Weight:** 5′7″, 160 lbs

Medical Record Number: 99887766 **Gender:** Male **Handedness:** Right

Pertinent medications-Anticoagulant medication: No **Acetylcholinesterase inhibitor:** N/A

Implanted electrical devices: None.

Referring provider: John Livingston, M.D.

EMG staff: Peter Needleman, M.D. **Technician (credentials):** Susie Elektra (CNCT)

Study date: 06/05/2020 **EMG Room#:** 5

Symptoms and signs: Patient with a history of well-controlled asthma, noting right more than left hand pain/paresthesia and numbness primarily affecting digits 1–3 on both sides, with some proximal spread to the mid forearm at times. There is intermittent neck ache, sometimes spreading into the shoulders bilaterally. Hand symptoms started about 3 months ago, worse at night, causing sleep disturbance. Symptoms onset noted after about 1 month into a new job working at an assembly line for automotive parts. No significant motor symptoms apart from some loss of dexterity on the right.

Exam most notable for marked reduction of pinprick and temperature perception mostly over the palmar aspect of the thumb, index and middle finger, right more than left. There appears to be mild weakness of the right abductor pollicis brevis muscle. Tinel's sign is positive over the median nerve at the right wrist, equivocal on the left.

NCS/EMG exam type or protocol ordered (optional/depends on lab): General upper extremity screen.

Sensory nerve conduction

			B-P Amp (μV)		LatNPk (ms)		CV (m/s)		Dist (mm)					Temp (°C)	
Nerve	Stimulus	Recording	L	R	L	R	L	R	L	R	Norm B-P Amp	Norm LatNPk	Norm CV	L	R
Median	Wrist	Index	31.74	**No Response**	**3.94**	**No Response**	n/a	n/a	130	130	>20 uV	<3.3 ms	>51 m/s	32.8	33.4
Ulnar	Wrist	5th Digit		35.77		2.18		n/a		110	>18 uV	<3 ms	>51 m/s		33.9
Radial	Thumb	Forearm		45.33		1.74		n/a		100	>18 uV	<2.7 ms			33.6

Motor nerve conduction

Nerve	Recording	Stimulus	B-P Amp (mV)		LatOn (ms)		CV (m/s)		Dist (mm)		Norm B-P Amp	Norm Distal LatON	Norm CV	Temp (°C)	
			L	R	L	R	L	R	L	R				L	R
Median	Abductor pollicis brevis	Wrist	6.99	**4.91**	**4.25**	**5.60**	n/a	n/a	50	50	>6 mV	<3.9 ms	>51 m/s	32.5	34.0
		Elbow		**4.81**		9.60		56.3		225					33.8
		Post exercise		**4.96**		**5.50**		n/a							34.1
Ulnar	Abductor digiti minimi	Wrist		11.93		1.45		n/a		50	>8 mV	<3 ms	>51 m/s		33.4
		Below elbow		11.36		4.90		62.3		215					33.4
		Above elbow		11.12		6.55		61.8		315					33.4

F-wave side-to-side comparison table

Nerve	Stimulus	Recording	F-waves Lat (ms)	
			L	R
Ulnar	Wrist	Abductor digiti minimi		23.15

Needle EMG summary

Side	Muscle	Ins Act.	Fib	PW	Fasc	Other	Number	Recruit	Dur	Dur	Amp	Amp	Poly	Poly.	Descript
L	Abductor Pollicis Brevis	Norm	0	0	0		Norm	Full		Norm		Norm		Norm	NC
R	1st Dorsal Interosseous	Norm	0	0	0		Norm	Full		Norm		Norm		Norm	NC
	Abductor Pollicis Brevis	Norm	0	0	0		1–	Mod-R	Few	1+	Few	1+		Norm	NC
	Flexor Pollicis Longus	Norm	0	0	0		Norm	Full		Norm		Norm		Norm	NC
	Extensor Indicis Proprius	Norm	0	0	0		Norm	Full		Norm		Norm		Norm	NC
	Pronator Teres	Norm	0	0	0		Norm	Full		Norm		Norm		Norm	NC
	Biceps Brachii	Norm	0	0	0		Norm	Full		Norm		Norm		Norm	NC
	Triceps—lateral head	Norm	0	0	0		Norm	Full		Norm		Norm		Norm	NC
	Deltoid—middle head	Norm	0	0	0		Norm	Full		Norm		Norm		Norm	NC

Technician's comments: Patient somewhat anxious, with slightly sweaty palms.

Study Interpretation:

Extensive electrodiagnostic examination of the right upper limb and additional studies of the left upper limb reveal the following:

1. Evidence of bilateral median neuropathies at or distal to the wrist (consistent with a clinical diagnosis of carpal tunnel syndrome) which is severe in degree electrically on the right and mild in degree electrically on the left.

   Pertinent features include absence of the median nerve sensory response on the right (that on the left is normal in amplitude, with mild prolongation of its peak latency), in addition to significant prolongation of median motor distal latencies (right> left), with reduction of the median motor amplitude recording the abductor pollicis brevis (APB) on the right. There are also mild chronic (no active/ongoing) motor axon loss changes in the right APB.
2. There is no definite evidence of a superimposed right cervical (C5–C8) motor radiculopathy.
3. There is also no definite evidence of a right ulnar or radial mononeuropathy, based on screening electrodiagnostic studies in those respective nerve distributions.

EMG Staff's Signature (may be electronic, if allowed):

This examination was performed, interpreted and electronically signed by: Peter Needleman, M.D. on June 05, 2020 at 9:31 AM.

---.

Suggested Reading

1. Jablecki CK, Busis NA, Brandstater MA, Krivickas LS, Miller RG, Robinton JE, American Association of Neuromuscular & Electrodiagnostic Medicine (AANEM). Reporting the results of needle EMG and nerve conduction studies: an educational report. Muscle Nerve. 2005;32(5):682–5.

Correction to: Radiculopathies

Karen A. Karwa and John A. Morren

Corrections to: Chapter 8 in N. Galvez-Jimenez et al. (eds.), *Electrodiagnostic Medicine,* https://doi.org/10.1007/978-3-030-74997-2_8

This book was inadvertently published with a spelling error in the author's name of chapter 8. The correct name is Karen A. Karwa, this has been updated with this erratum.

The updated version of the book can be found at https://doi.org/10.1007/978-3-030-74997-2_8

N. Galvez-Jimenez et al. (eds.), *Electrodiagnostic Medicine*,
https://doi.org/10.1007/978-3-030-74997-2_14

Index

A
Abductor digiti minimi (ADM), 7, 47–48
Abductor Digiti Quinti Pedis (ADQP), 39–40
Abductor hallucis (AH), 8
Abductor pollicis brevis (APB), 7, 43, 85
Acetylcholine receptor deficiency, 243
Acetylcholinesterase, 242
Acetylcholinesterase enzyme (AChE), 227
Acute inflammatory demyelinating polyradiculoneuropathy (AIDP), 122, 134–136
Acute motor sensory axonal neuropathy (AMSAN), 136
Agrin, 245
Alcohol, 129
Amyotrophic Lateral Sclerosis (ALS), 142, 213
Anterior interosseous nerve (AIN) syndrome, 86
Anterior primary ramus (APR), 160
Axillary neuropathy, 96, 104, 107–109
Axon (A) reflex, 145
Axonal polyneuropathy, 129–131, 137, 146, 147
Axonotmesis, 6

B
B12 deficiency, 129
Behcet's disease, 19
Bell's palsy, 94
Brachial plexus
  clinical assessment, 164
  EDX assessment
    distal upper extremity sensory and motor abnormalities, 178–180
    left hand weakness and atrophy, 190, 191
    left upper extremity numbness, 180–183, 186–188, 192–194
    weakness, 175–178, 186–188, 192–194
    left upper extremity pain, 175–178, 180–183
    motor NCS, 171
    needle NCS, 171
    postoperative left ulnar neuropathy, 183–186
    progressive left upper extremity weakness, 188–190
    sensory NCS, 170
    SNAP domains, 170
  EDX exercises, 173–175
  electrodiagnostic assessment, 164, 165, 167–170
  elemental anatomy
    cords, 162
    divisions, 161
    roots, 159–161
    terminal nerves, 162
    trunks, 161
  general anatomy, 158–160
  incidence, 157
  NCS assessment, 157, 165–166
    lateral cord, 172, 173
    lower plexus, 172
    medial cord, 173
    middle plexus, 172
    posterior cord, 173
    preterminal and terminal nerves, 173
    upper plexus, 171, 172
  regional anatomy, 162–164
  site-specific disorders, 157, 158
Brachioradialis, 50

C
Carpal tunnel syndrome (CTS), 17, 43, 85
Cervical radiculopathy, 198–200
Choline acetyltransferase (ChAT) deficiency, 242
Chronic inflammatory demyelinating polyradiculoneuropathy (CIDP), 123–128, 132–135, 137–144, 146–148, 151
CMT-IA, 143
CMT-X, 143
Complex MUAP, 73
Complex repetitive discharges (CRDs), 10, 71, 259
Compound muscle action potential (CMAP) amplitude, 7, 80, 129
Concentric and monopolar needle electrodes, 75
Concentric EMG needle, 76
Conduction block, 140, 142
Conduction velocity (CV), 129
Congenital myasthenia gravis (CMS), 240, 242
Congenital myasthenic syndrome, postsynaptic defects, 243, 245
Cramp-fasciculation syndrome, 67
Cramps, 260

N. Galvez-Jimenez et al. (eds.), *Electrodiagnostic Medicine*,
https://doi.org/10.1007/978-3-030-74997-2

D
Deltoid, biceps and triceps muscles, 261
Demyelinating polyneuropathies, 133, 134
Diabetes mellitus (DM), 121, 123, 124, 128, 131–132, 135
Diabetic lumbosacral radiculoplexus neuropathy (DLRPN), 21, 132
Distal acquired demyelinating sensory neuropathy (DADS), 127
Distal acquired demyelinating symmetric neuropathy (DADS), 125
Distal symmetric polyneuropathy (DSP), 124, 130–133
DOK-7 deficiency, 245
Dorsal root ganglion (DRG), 159

E
Edaravone, 216
Edrophonium chloride test, 233
Electrodiagnostic (EDX) studies
  A-wave/axon reflex, 13–14
  biases, advantages and disadvantages, 2–5
  blink reflexes, 14–15
  concentric needle electromyography, 16
  facial nerve motor studies, 15–17
  foot drop/weakness, 22–23
  foot pain/numbness, 18–19
  F-wave response, 11–13
  hand pain/numbness/sensory disturbance, 17–18
  needle electrode examination, 9–10, 16
  nerve conduction studies, 7–9
  peripheral nerve fibers, 2
  proximal lower limb/anterior thigh weakness, 21
  radiculopathies, 19–21
  report, 265, 266, 268
  routine NCS, 11
  tibial H-reflex assesses, 13
Electromyography (EMG), 1
El Escorial criteria, 214, 216, 218
Endoneurium, 6
Endplate myopathy, 243
Endplate potential (EPP), 233
Epineurium, 6
Extensor carpi ulnaris (ECU), 49
Extensor digitorum, 253
Extensor digitorum brevis (EDB) muscle, 8
Extensor digitorum communis (EDC) muscle, 8

F
Femoral neuropathy, 93, 117, 118
Fibrillation potentials, 69
First dorsal interosseous (FDI), 8, 47
Flexor carpi radialis (FCR), 46–47
Flexor carpi ulnaris (FCU), 48
Flexor digitorum profundus (FDP), 48
Frontotemporal dementia (FTD), 213

G
Glycogen metabolism, 65
Guillain-Barré syndrome, 94, 126
Guyon's canal, 88

H
Hematoxylin, 215
Henneman size principle, 68
Hereditary neuropathy with liability to pressure palsies (HNPP), 144
Hereditary spastic paraparesis, 219
H-reflex, 200

I
Ice pack test, 232
Immune-mediated processes, 219
Inclusion body myositis (IBM), 218
Inherited polyneuropathies, 124, 125, 133, 143, 144
Innervation ratio, 159
Interpotential interval (IPI), 252
Intraspinal canal, 196
Irritable myopathies, 258

K
Kennedy's disease, 219

L
Lambert-Eaton myasthenic syndrome (LEMS), 7
  clinical features, 239
  definition, 238
  diagnostic evaluation, 239, 240
  electrophysiological finding, 240, 241
  epidemiology, 238
  etiology, 238
  pathophysiology, 238
  SFEMG, 240
  treatment and management, 240
Lateral antebrachial cutaneous (LABC) nerve, 167
Lead toxicity, 133
Lower motor neurons (LMN), 213
Lumbosacral radiculopathy, 199, 200

M
McArdle disease, 260
Microtubules, 121
Miller Fisher syndrome, 136
Miniature Endplate Potential (MEPP), 233
Moment-to-moment amplitude variation (MMAV), 78
Monoclonal gammopathy with undetermined significance (MGUS), 127, 143

Mononeuritis multiplex, 143
Mononeuropathies
  anterior interosseous neuropathy, 109, 110
  axillary neuropathy, 96, 107–109, 1104
  facial nerve, 94, 95
  femoral nerve, 93, 94
  femoral neuropathy, 93, 117, 118
  focal demyelination, 83
  long thoracic neuropathy, 96–97
  median nerve, 83–86
  median neuropathy, 83, 97–98
  musculocutaneous neuropathy, 96
  peroneal (fibular) nerve, 90–92
  peroneal (fibular) neuropathy, 111–113
  radial nerve, 89–90
  radial neuropathy, 101
  sciatic nerve, 93
  sciatic neuropathy, 111
  spinal accessory neuropathy, 97
  superficial radial sensory neuropath, 83
  suprascapular neuropathy, 95, 101–104
  tibial nerve, 92
  tibial neuropathy, 113–117
  ulnar nerve, 86–89
  ulnar neuropathy, 83, 87–89, 98–101
Monopolar EMG needle, 76
Motor F-wave, 200
Motor neuron diseases (MND), 2
  anatomy, 215, 216
  clinical features, 216–218
  differential diagnosis, 218, 219
  electrodiagnostic evaluation, 219–221
  electrodiagnostic limitations, 221–223
  etiology
    ALS, 213, 214
    PBP, 214, 215
    PLS, 214
    PMA, 214
    UMN symptoms, 213
  patient history, 223, 224, 226
Motor unit action potentials (MUAPs), 65, 131, 136, 221
Multifocal acquired demyelinating sensory and motor neuropathy (MADSAM), 142
Multifocal axonal motor neuropathy (MAMN), 142
Multifocal motor neuropathy (MMN), 142
Multifocal motor neuropathy with conduction block (MMNCB), 219
Muscle-specific tyrosine kinase (MuSK), 227
Muscle stretch reflexes (MSRs), 164
Musculocutaneous neuropathy, 96
Myasthenia gravis (MG), 228, 230–232, 252–254
Myelin sheath, 122
Myokymia, 10
Myokymic potentials, 70
Myopathy
  differential diagnosis, 255, 257
  electrodiagnostic evaluation, 257, 258
  etiology and clinical features, 255–257
  MUAPs, 78
  needle EMG findings, 258–261
  needle EMG protocol, 261, 262
  patient history, 262
Myotonia, 259
Myotonic potentials, 70
Myotonic syndromes, 259

N

Needle electrode examination (NEE)
  abductor hallucis, 58–59
  adductor longus, 63
  ADM, 47–48
  anconeus, 50
  APB, 43
  biceps brachii, 51
  brachioradialis, 50
  cervical paraspinal muscles, 56
  deltoid, 52
  ECU, 49
  extensor digitorum, 49–50
  extensor digitorum brevis, 56–57
  extensor hallucis longus, 57
  extensor indicis, 49
  FCR, 46–47
  FCU, 48
  FDI, 47
  FDP, 48
  flexor digitorum longus, 59
  flexor digitorum profundus, 45–46
  flexor digitorum superficialis, 46
  flexor hallucis brevis, 59
  flexor pollicis brevis, 44
  flexor pollicis longus, 45
  gluteus maximus, 62
  gluteus medius, 61–62
  iliopsoas/iliacus, 59
  infraspinatus, 54
  latissimus dorsi, 55
  long head of biceps femoris, 60
  lumbar paraspinal muscles, 64
  opponens pollicis, 44
  pectoralis major, 51–52
  peroneus longus, 58
  peroneus tertius, 57
  pronator quadratus (PQ), 44–45
  pronator teres (PT), 47
  rectus femoris, 63
  rhomboids, 54–55
  semimembranosus, 60–61
  semitendinosus, 61
  serratus anterior, 55–56
  short head of biceps femoris, 60
  sternocleidomastoid, 53
  supraspinatus, 54
  surface localization, 43
  tensor fascia lata, 61
  teres minor, 52
  tibialis anterior, 58
  triceps brachii, 50–51
  upper trapezius, 53

vastus lateralis, 62
Needle Electrode examination (NEE), 201, 203, 204
Needle electromyography (EMG)
abnormal spontaneous activity, 67
acute discontinuity lesion, 75
advantages and limitations of NCS, 66
CMAP amplitude, 81
complex fasciculation potential, 67
complex MUAP, 73
concentric needles, 72, 76
cooling of muscle, 68
cramp potentials, 71
CRDs, 71
decreased insertional activity, 65
early recruitment, 72
end-plate noise, 65, 66
end-plate spikes, 66
fasciculation potentials, 67
fibrillation potentials, 69
focal demyelination, 80
Henneman size principle, 68
"inferred" block, 81
insertional activity, 65
monopolar EMG needle, 76
MUAP abnormalities, 78
MUAP appearance and recruitment, 65
myokymic potentials, 70
myopathy, 80
"myopathic" MUAPs, 79
myotonic potentials, 70
neurogenic-appearing and myopathic-appearing, 80
neuromyotonia, 70
normal insertional activity, 66
normal recruitment pattern, 74
optimal needle EMG, 76, 77
positive sharp wave potentials, 69
reduced recruitment, 69
spontaneous activity, 65
tremor tracing- normal MUAPs, 71
Needle EMG, 77, 78
Nerve conduction studies (NCS), 2, 83, 129
filter settings, 25
lower extremity
lateral femoral cutaneous nerve recording, 36
medial and lateral plantar mixed nerve response recording, 36–37
saphenous nerve recording, 35–36
superficial peroneal (fibular) sensory recording, 35
sural (sensory) recording, 34–35
motor NCS
facial motor recording, 41–42
femoral motor recording, 40, 41
peroneal (fibular) motor recording, 37–38
spinal accessory motor recording, 41
tibial motor recording, 38–40
upper extremities
axillary recording, 34
dorsal ulnar cutaneous sensory recording, 27–28
lateral antebrachial cutaneous sensory, 29–30
medial antebrachial cutaneous sensory recording, 29
median motor recording, 30–31
median palmar mixed nerve, 28–29
median sensory recording, 26–27
musculocutaneous recording, 33–34
radial motor recording, 32–33
radial sensory recording, 28
ulnar motor recording, 31, 32
ulnar palmar mixed nerve, 29
ulnar sensory recording, 27
Neural foramina, 196
Neurapraxia, 6
Neuromuscular jitter, 250, 252
Neuromuscular junction (NMJ)
anatomy and physiology, 227, 228
clinical presentation, 229
CMS, 240, 242
congenital myasthenic syndrome, postsynaptic defects, 243, 245
diagnostic testing
edrophonium chloride test, 233
ice pack test, 232
RNS, 233–235, 237
SFEMG, 237, 239
epidemiology, 228, 229
genetic syndromes, 242, 243
immunosuppressive therapy, 237
LEMS, 238–241
myasthenia gravis, 228, 230–232
transmission, 78
Neuromyotonia, 70
Neurotmesis, 6
Nodopathies, 122
Non-irritable myopathies, 259
Normal motor unit action potential (MUAP), 73
Nutritional deficiency, 132

O

Oculopharyngeal muscular dystrophy, 218
Opponens pollicis, 85

P

Paraneoplastic processes, 219
Paraproteinemic polyneuropathy, 127
Paraspinal muscle NEE abnormalities, 20
Perineurium, 6
Plasma cell dyscrasias, 127
Polyneuropathy
definition, 121
electrodiagnosis
AIDP, 134–136
AMAN/AMSAN, 136
asymmetric, 129–132, 134
axonal polyneuropathy, 129–131
CIDP, 133, 134, 137–140, 142, 143
demyelinating polyneuropathies, 133, 134, 143
diabetes mellitus, 131, 132

distal symmetric polyneuropathy, 133
electromyography, 146, 147
examination techniques and protocol for evaluation, 144, 145
GBS, 136
inherited polyneuropathies, 143, 144
nerve conduction, 145–151
nutritional deficiency, 132
symmetric, 129, 134, 141
toxic polyneuropathies, 133
length dependent/non–length dependent, 125
pathogenesis, 121, 122
patient history, 143, 148, 151
symmetry/asymmetry
CIDP, 126, 127
DADS, 125
DSP, 124
etiology, 128, 129
GBS, 126
inherited polyneuropathies, 124, 125
length dependent polyneuropathy, 124
paraproteinemic polyneuropathy, 127
predominantly proximal weakness, 125
weakness, 128
temporal evolution, 122
type of modality, 123, 124
type of nerve fiber, 123, 124
upper limb predominant weakness, 128
Polyphasic MUAP, 10
Postexercise exhaustion, 234
Postexercise facilitation, 234
Predominantly proximal weakness, 125
Preganglionic sympathetic axons, 161
Primary lateral sclerosis (PLS), 214
Progressive bulbar palsy (PBP), 214
Progressive muscular atrophy (PMA), 214
Pronator teres syndrome, 86
Proximal median neuropathies, 47

Q
Quadrilateral space, 96

R
Radiculopathy
anatomy, 196, 197
clinical features
cervical radiculopathy, 198–200
lumbosacral radiculopathies, 199, 200
sensory loss and weakness, 197
thoracic radiculopathies, 198
diagnosis, 205, 206
electrodiagnostic evaluation
NEE, 201, 203, 204
nerve conduction studies, 200, 201
etiology, 195, 196
patient history, 206–210
Rapsyn protein, 245
Repetitive nerve stimulation (RNS), 2
definition, 233
electrophysiological findings in MG, 234, 235
fast-rate stimulation, 233
physiology, 233
slow-rate stimulation, 233
technical aspects, 235–237
Reversible conduction failure (RCF), 136
Riluzole, 216

S
Sensory nerve action potentials (SNAPs), 7, 130, 139
Single fiber electromyography (SFEMG), 237
development, 249
monopolar and concentric needles, 249, 250
myasthenia gravis, 252–254
stimulation, 249
voluntary activation, 249–252
Single MUAP (SMU), 72
Slow firing MUAPS, 72
Somatosensory evoked potentials (SEPs), 200
Spinal accessory neuropathy, 97
Spontaneous activity, 65, 68
Spurling's test, 198
S-Radial response, 188
Superficial part of flexor pollicis brevis, 85
Suprascapular neuropathy, 95

T
Terminal latency index (TLI), 143
Thoracic radiculopathy, 198
Tibial neuropathy, 113–117
Tibialis anterior (TA) muscle, 8
Toxic polyneuropathies, 133

U
Upper limb predominant weakness, 128
Upper motor neurons (UMN), 213

V
Voltage-gated calcium channel (VGCC), 238, 245

Batch number: 10732809

Printed by Printforce, the Netherlands